Contributors

GUEST EDITORS

BACHIR TAOULI, MD
Assistant Professor, Department of Radiology,
New York University Langone Medical Center,
New York, New York

VIVIAN S. LEE, MD, PhD
Professor of Radiology, Physiology and
Neuroscience, and Vice Dean of Science, and
Senior Vice President, and Chief Scientific
Officer, Department of Radiology, New York
University Langone Medical Center, New York,
New York

AUTHORS

JELLE O. BARENTSZ, MD, PhD
Department of Radiology, Radboud University,
Nijmegen Medical Centre, Nijmegen,
The Netherlands

MARC BAZOT, MD
Doctor of Medicine, Division of Radiology,
Hôpital Tenon-Assistance Publique des
Hopitaux de Paris, Paris, France

LOUISA BOKACHEVA, PhD
Assistant Research Scientist, Department
of Radiology, New York University School
of Medicine, New York, New York

CHRISTIAN COMBE, MD, PhD
Département de Néphrologie, Groupe
Hospitalier Pellegrin, Bordeaux-Cedex,
France

FRANK COUILLAUD, PhD
UMR-CNRS Imagerie Moléculaire et
Fonctionnelle, Université Victor
Segalen-Bourdeaux 2, Bordeaux-Cedex,
France

CHARLES A. CUENOD, MD, PhD
Researcher, Laboratoire de Recherche en
Imagerie, Université Paris René Descartes;
Professor of Medicine, Division of
Radiology, Hopital Européen Georges
Pompidou-Assistance Publique des
Hopitaux de Paris, Paris, France

EMILE DARAI, MD, PhD
Professor of Medicine, Division of Gynecology
and Obstetrics, Hôpital Tenon-Assistance
Publique des Hopitaux de Paris, Paris, France

OMER EKER
Radiology Student, Service d'Imagerie
Diagnostique et Thérapeutique
de l'Adulte, Groupe Hospitalier Pellegrin,
Bordeaux-Cedex, France

JURGEN J. FÜTTERER, MD, PhD
Department of Radiology; and Department
of Interventional Radiology, Radboud
University, Nijmegen Medical Centre,
Nijmegen, The Netherlands

KOJI FUJIMOTO, MD
Graduate Student, Department of Diagnostic
Radiology, Kyoto University Hospital, Kyoto,
Japan

J. DAMIEN GRATTAN-SMITH, MBBS
Department of Radiology, Children's
Healthcare of Atlanta; and Department
of Radiology, Emory University School of
Medicine, Atlanta, Georgia

NICOLAS GRENIER, MD
UMR-CNRS Imagerie Moléculaire et
Fonctionnelle, Université Victor Segalen-
Bourdeaux 2; Service d'Imagerie Diagnostique
et Thérapeutique de l'Adulte, Groupe
Hospitalier Pellegrin, Bordeaux-Cedex, France

SARAH HALTER, BA
Center for Advanced Imaging, Department of Radiology, Evanston Northwestern Healthcare, Evanston, Illinois

THOMAS HAMBROCK, MD
Department of Radiology, Radboud University, Nijmegen Medical Centre, Nijmegen, The Netherlands

OLIVIER HAUGER, MD, PhD
UMR-CNRS Imagerie Moléculaire et Fonctionnelle, Université Victor Segalen-Bourdeaux 2; Service d'Imagerie Diagnostique et Thérapeutique de l'Adulte, Groupe Hospitalier Pellegrin, Bordeaux-Cedex, France

RICHARD A. JONES, PhD
Department of Radiology, Children's Healthcare of Atlanta; and Department of Radiology, Emory University School of Medicine, Atlanta, Georgia

SOOAH KIM, MD
Assistant Professor, Department of Radiology, Abdominal Imaging, New York University Medical Center, New York, New York

TAKASHI KOYAMA, MD, PhD
Assistant Professor, Department of Diagnostic Radiology, Kyoto University Hospital, Kyoto, Japan

JOHN KURHANEWICZ, PhD
Professor of Radiology, Urology, and Pharmaceutical Chemistry, University of California, San Francisco, San Francisco, California

VIVIAN S. LEE, MD, PhD
Professor of Radiology, Physiology and Neuroscience, and Vice Dean of Science, and Senior Vice President, and Chief Scientific Officer, Department of Radiology, New York University Langone Medical Center, New York, New York

TIM LEINER, MD, PhD
Assistant Professor, Department of Radiology, Maastricht University Hospital; Cardiovascular Research Institute Maastricht, Maastricht, The Netherlands

LU-PING LI, PhD
Center for Advanced Imaging, Department of Radiology, Evanston Northwestern Healthcare, Evanston; Feinberg School of Medicine, Northwestern University, Chicago, Illinois

VIBEKE B. LOGAGER, MD
Department of Diagnostic Radiology, Copenhagen University Hospital Herlev, Herlev, Denmark

JEFFREY H. MAKI, MD, PhD
Associate Professor and Director of Body MRI, Department of Radiology, University of Washington; Department of Radiology, Puget Sound VAHCS, Seattle, Washington

PETER MARCKMANN, MD
Department of Nephrology, Copenhagen University Hospital Herlev, Herlev, Denmark

CLAUDE MARSAULT, MD, PhD
Professor of Medicine, Division of Radiology, Hôpital Tenon-Assistance Publique des Hopitaux de Paris, Paris, France

HENRIK MICHAELY, MD, PhD
Assistant Professor of Radiology, Institute of Clinical Radiology and Nuclear Medicine, University Medical Center Mannheim, Mannheim, Germany

CHRIT MOONEN, PhD
UMR-CNRS Imagerie Moléculaire et Fonctionnelle, Université Victor Segalen-Bourdeaux 2, Bordeaux-Cedex, France

ASAKO NAKAI, MD, PhD
Assistant Professor, Department of Diagnostic Radiology, Kyoto University Hospital, Kyoto, Japan

MOHIT NAIK, MD
Clinical Body MRI Fellow, Department of Radiology, Abdominal Imaging, New York University Medical Center, New York, New York

SILKE POTTHAST, MD
Department of Radiology, University of
Washington, Seattle, Washington

POTTUMARTHI V. PRASAD, PhD
Center for Advanced Imaging, Department of
Radiology, Evanston Northwestern Healthcare,
Evanston; Feinberg School of Medicine,
Northwestern University, Chicago, Illinois

HENRY RUSINEK, PhD
Associate Professor of Radiology, Department
of Radiology, New York University School of
Medicine, New York, New York

ERIC SIGMUND, PhD
Assistant Professor, Department of Radiology,
New York University Medical Center, Center for
Biomedical Imaging, New York, New York

DIEDERIK M. SOMFORD, MD
Department of Urology, Radboud University,
Nijmegen Medical Centre, Nijmegen, The
Netherlands

BACHIR TAOULI, MD
Assistant Professor, Department of Radiology,
New York University Langone Medical Center,
New York, New York

ISABELLE THOMASSIN-NAGGARA, MD
Doctor of Medicine, Division of Radiology,
Hôpital Tenon-Assistance Publique des
Hopitaux de Paris; Researcher, Laboratoire de
Recherche en Imagerie, Université Paris René
Descartes, Paris, France

HENRIK S. THOMSEN, MD
Professor, Department of Diagnostic
Radiology, Copenhagen University Hospital
Herlev; Department of Diagnostic Sciences,
Faculty of Health Sciences, University of
Copenhagen, Herlev, Denmark

KAORI TOGASHI, MD, PhD
Professor and Chairman, Department of
Diagnostic Radiology, Kyoto University
Hospital, Kyoto, Japan

DANIEL B. VIGNERON, PhD
Professor of Radiology, University of California,
San Francisco, San Francisco, California

JEFF L. ZHANG, PhD
Assistant Research Scientist, Department of
Radiology, New York University School of
Medicine, New York, New York

Contents

Update on Nephrogenic Systemic Fibrosis 551

Henrik S. Thomsen, Peter Marckmann, and Vibeke B. Logager

Gadolinium-based contrast agents were for many years considered safe, but this is no longer the case. The least stable agents may trigger the development of nephrogenic systemic fibrosis (NSF), a generalized fibrotic disorder, in renal failure patients. The use of gadodiamide and gadopentetate dimeglumine is now contraindicated in Europe and Japan in patients who have a glomerular filtration rate less than 30 mL/min/1.73 m^2, including those on dialysis. The fear of NSF, however, should not lead to an enhanced MR imaging examination being denied when there is a good clinical indication to give a gadolinium-based contrast agent.

Advances in Contrast-Enhanced MR Angiography of the Renal Arteries 561

Tim Leiner and Henrik Michaely

Renal artery stenosis (RAS) is a potentially curable cause of renovascular hypertension (RVH) and is caused by either atherosclerosis or fibromuscular dysplasia in the vast majority of patients. Although intra-arterial digital subtraction angiography is still considered the standard of reference test for the anatomic diagnosis of RAS, MR angiography and functional renal MR imaging are promising alternatives that also allow for functional characterization of RAS. This article provides an overview of these techniques and discusses their relative merits and shortcomings. Because missing RVH may have serious consequences the most important requirement for an alternative test is that it has high sensitivity. An unresolved issue is the prediction of functional recovery after therapy.

Non–Contrast-Enhanced MR Imaging of the Renal Arteries 573

Silke Potthast and Jeffrey H. Maki

In this article, we focus on non-contrast magnetic resonance angiography techniques for evaluating renal artery imaging. Time-of-flight, phase contrast, steady-state free procession, and arterial spin labeling are discussed.

Diffusion-weighted MR Imaging of the Kidneys and the Urinary Tract 585

Sooah Kim, Mohit Naik, Eric Sigmund, and Bachir Taouli

There is currently a growing interest in applications of diffusion-weighted imaging (DWI) in the abdomen and pelvis. DWI provides original functional information where the signal and contrast are determined by the microscopic mobility of water. DWI can provide additional information over conventional MR sequences, and could potentially be used as an alternative to contrast-enhanced sequences in patients with

greater insights into the pathophysiology of not only urologic disorders but also disorders of the kidney itself.

Dynamic Contrast-Enhanced MR Imaging of Ovarian Neoplasms: Current Status and Future Perspectives   661

Isabelle Thomassin-Naggara, Charles A. Cuenod, Emile Darai, Claude Marsault, and Marc Bazot

MR imaging is useful for characterizing ovarian tumors. Dynamic contrast-enhanced MR imaging is a promising new technique useful for characterizing perfusion and angiogenesis of ovarian masses. This article describes the dynamic contrast-enhanced MR imaging technique examines the current and future applications of this technique in patients with ovarian tumors.

Functional MR Imaging of the Uterus   673

Asako Nakai, Takashi Koyama, Koji Fujimoto, and Kaori Togashi

Recent developments in MR imaging techniques have enabled the functional assessment of the uterus. Cine MR imaging is a useful tool for evaluating uterine kinematic functions derived from myometrial contractility, and for investigating the alteration of uterine contractility in a variety of conditions and gynecologic disorders. Diffusion-weighted imaging can demonstrate abnormal signal in pathologic foci based on differences in molecular diffusion, and could provide useful information in evaluating malignant conditions. Dynamic contrast-enhanced MR imaging has the potential to improve tumor detection and local staging, and quantitative information may be useful for both monitoring therapeutic effects and predicting outcome. These state-of-the-art functional MR imaging techniques are beneficial for elucidating various uterine conditions when used appropriately, and the findings further provide the basis of future MR imaging investigations.

Diffusion and Perfusion MR Imaging of the Prostate   685

Diederik M. Somford, Jurgen J. Fütterer, Thomas Hambrock, and Jelle O. Barentsz

Conventional anatomic MR imaging has evolved to a superior modality in the evaluation of prostate carcinoma and is now a widely established technique in the detection and staging of this disease, aiding in clinical decision making on treatment and therapy evaluation. Recent improvements in functional MR techniques, such as diffusion-weighted MR imaging and dynamic contrast-enhanced MR imaging, have greatly increased the impact of MR imaging in prostate cancer. The combination of T2-weighted imaging, diffusion-weighted MR imaging, and dynamic contrast-enhanced MR imaging may overcome the limitations of conventional T2-weighted MR imaging of the prostate and may be able accurately to detect, localize, stage, and grade prostate carcinoma and guide biopsies.

Advances in MR Spectroscopy of the Prostate   697

John Kurhanewicz and Daniel B. Vigneron

Commercial MR imaging/magnetic resonance spectroscopic imaging (MRSI) packages for staging prostate cancer on 1.5-T MR scanners are now available. The technology is becoming mature enough to begin assessing its clinical utility in selecting, planning, and following prostate cancer therapy. Before therapy, 1.5-T MR imaging/MRSI has the potential to improve the local evaluation of prostate cancer presence and volume and has a significant incremental benefit in the prediction of pathologic stage when added to clinical nomograms. After therapy, two metabolic biomarkers of effective and ineffective therapy have been identified and are being validated with 10-year outcomes. Accuracy can be improved by performing MR imaging/MRSI at higher magnetic field strengths, using more sensitive hyperpolarized ^{13}C MRSI techniques and through the addition of other functional MR techniques.

Magnetic Resonance Imaging Clinics of North America

FORTHCOMING ISSUES

February 2009

MRA From Head to Toe
William Weadock, MD and Thomas
Chenevert, MD, *Guest Editors*

May 2009

Clinical Applications of MR
Diffusion/Perfusion/Tractography
Scott Reeder, MD and Pratik Mukerjee,
MD, PhD, *Guest Editors*

RECENT ISSUES

August 2008

Pediatric MR
Marilyn J. Siegel, MD and Diego Jaramillo,
MD, MPH, *Guest Editors*

May 2008

Chest MR
Michael Gotway, MD, *Guest Editor*

RELATED INTEREST

Radiologic Clinics of North America January 2008 (Vol. 46, No. 1)
Genitourinary Tract Imaging
Michael A. Blake and Manudeep Kalra, *Guest Editors*

THE CLINICS ARE NOW AVAILABLE ONLINE!

Access your subscription at:
www.theclinics.com

GOAL STATEMENT

The goal of *Magnetic Resonance Imaging Clinics of North America* is to keep practicing physicians up to date with current clinical practice by providing timely articles reviewing the state of the art in patient care.

ACCREDITATION

The *Magnetic Resonance Imaging Clinics of North America* is planned and implemented in accordance with the Essential Areas and Policies of the Accreditation Council for Continuing Medical Education (ACCME) through the joint sponsorship of the University of Virginia School of Medicine and Elsevier. The University of Virginia School of Medicine is accredited by the ACCME to provide continuing medical education for physicians.

The University of Virginia School of Medicine designates this educational activity for a maximum of 15 *AMA PRA Category 1 Credits*™. Physicians should only claim credit commensurate with the extent of their participation in the activity.

The American Medical Association has determined that physicians not licensed in the US who participate in this CME activity are eligible for 15 *AMA PRA Category 1 Credits*™.

Credit can be earned by reading the text material, taking the CME examination online at: http://www.theclinics.com/home/cme, and completing the evaluation. After taking the test, you will be required to review any and all incorrect answers. Following completion of the test and evaluation, your credit will be awarded and you may print your certificate.

FACULTY DISCLOSURE/CONFLICT OF INTEREST

The University of Virginia School of Medicine, as an ACCME accredited provider, endorses and strives to comply with the Accreditation Council for Continuing Medical Education (ACCME) Standards of Commercial Support, Commonwealth of Virginia statutes, University of Virginia policies and procedures, and associated federal and private regulations and guidelines on the need for disclosure and monitoring of proprietary and financial interests that may affect the scientific integrity and balance of content delivered in continuing medical education activities under our auspices.

The University of Virginia School of Medicine requires that all CME activities accredited through this institution be developed independently and be scientifically rigorous, balanced and objective in the presentation/discussion of its content, theories and practices.

All authors/editors participating in an accredited CME activity are expected to disclose to the readers relevant financial relationships with commercial entities occurring within the past 12 months (such as grants or research support, employee, consultant, stock holder, member of speakers bureau, etc.). The University of Virginia School of Medicine will employ appropriate mechanisms to resolve potential conflicts of interest to maintain the standards of fair and balanced education to the reader. Questions about specific strategies can be directed to the Office of Continuing Medical Education, University of Virginia School of Medicine, Charlottesville, Virginia.

The authors/editors listed below have identified no professional or financial affiliations for themselves or their spouse/partner:

Jelle O. Barentz, MD, PhD; Marc Bazot, MD; Louisa Bokacheva, PhD; Christian Combe, MD, PhD; Frank Couillaud, PhD; Emile Darai, MD, PhD; Eduard de Lange, MD (Test Author); Omer Eker; Koji Fujimoto, MD; Jurgen J. Fütterer, MD, PhD; John Damien Grattan-Smith, MBBS; Nicolas Grenier, MD; Sarah Halter, BA; Thomas Hambrock, MD; Olivier Hauger, MD, PhD; Richard A. Jones, PhD; Sooah Kim, MD; Takashi Koyama, MD, PhD; Vivan S. Lee, MD, PhD, MBA (Guest Editor); Lu-Ping Li, PhD; Vibeke Berg Løgager, MD; Peter Marckmann, MD; Claude Marsault, MD, PhD; Chrit Moonen, PhD; Mohit M. Naik, MD; Asako Nakai, MD, PhD; Silke Potthast, MD; Pottumarthi V. Prasad, PhD; Lisa Richman (Acquisitions Editor); Henry Rusinek, PhD; Eric Sigmund, PhD; Diederik M. Somford, MD; Bachir Taouli, MD (Guest Editor); Isabelle Thomassin-Naggara, MD; Kaori Togashi, MD, PhD; and Jeff L. Zhang, PhD.

The authors/editors listed below identified the following professional or financial affiliations for themselves or their spouse/partner:

Charles A. Cuenod, MD, PhD is an industry funded research/investigator for the Guerbet Group (Aulnay France.)
John Kurhanewicz, PhD is an industry funded research/investigator for GE Healthcare.
Tim Leiner, MD, PhD has received research support and a grant from Bayer Schering Pharma.
Jeffrey H. Maki, MD, PhD serves on the Advisory Committee/Board for Bracco Diagnostics.
Henrik Michaely, MD, PhD is a consultant for Bayer Healthcare.
Henrik S. Thomsen, MD serves on the Advisory Committee and holds a patent with CMC Contrast.
Daniel B. Vigneron, PhD is an industry funded research/investigator for GE Healthcare.

Disclosure of Discussion of non-FDA approved uses for pharmaceutical products and/or medical devices:
The University of Virginia School of Medicine, as an ACCME provider, requires that all faculty presenters identify and disclose any "off label" uses for pharmaceutical and medical device products. The University of Virginia School of Medicine recommends that each physician fully review all the available data on new products or procedures prior to instituting them with patients.

TO ENROLL

To enroll in the Magnetic Resonance Imaging Clinics of North America Continuing Medical Education program, call customer service at 1-800-654-2452 or visit us online at: www.theclinics.com/home/cme. The CME program is available to subscribers for an additional fee of $99.95.

Preface

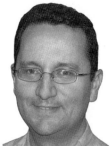 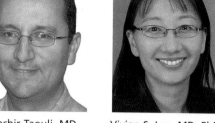

Bachir Taouli, MD   Vivian S. Lee, MD, PhD
Guest Editors

Powered by the tremendous advances in technology over the last few years, MR imaging is poised to realize its potential of going beyond morphology and providing functional information about organ physiology and tumor pathophysiology. Whether the methods relate to dynamic kinetic imaging of the uterus or diffusion-weighted imaging of the kidneys, these new tools enable us to begin asking new scientific questions and to explore new diagnostic applications with MR. Some of the interest in noncontrast-enhanced techniques (such as arterial spin labeling for vascular or perfusion imaging and diffusion or blood oxygen level dependent MR imaging for functional organ assessment) has been fueled by the risk of nephrogenic systemic fibrosis in patients who have renal disease who are exposed to gadolinium contrast agents. A review of this hot topic is included in this issue.

Many of the functional imaging methods in this issue of *Magnetic Resonance Imaging Clinics of North America* are ready for clinical implementation; some methods require further development and evaluation. In all cases, the potential to translate emerging technologies into expanded and improved diagnostic capabilities make the future of genitourinary MR brighter than ever.

Bachir Taouli, MD
Vivian S. Lee, MD, PhD
Department of Radiology
New York University Langone Medical Center
560 First Avenue
New York, NY 10016, USA

E-mail addresses:
bachir.taouli@nyumc.org (B. Taouli)
vivian.lee@nyumc.org (V.S. Lee)

Magn Reson Imaging Clin N Am 16 (2008) xiii
doi:10.1016/j.mric.2008.07.009
1064-9689/08/$ – see front matter

Update on Nephrogenic Systemic Fibrosis

Henrik S. Thomsen, MD[a,b],*, Peter Marckmann, MD[c],
Vibeke B. Logager, MD[a]

KEYWORDS
- Gadolinium-based contrast agents
- Late adverse reactions • Nephrogenic systemic fibrosis

For many years it was believed that gadolinium-based contrast agents (Gd-CAs) were safe, which led to the free use of these agents. Gd-CAs have been preferred in patients who have reduced renal function instead of iodine-based contrast agents (I-CAs).[1,2] Because of their favorable radiographic characteristics, Gd-CAs have been used in very high doses (8–440 mL) in a single examination;[3] however, time has shown that Gd-CAs are not inert.[4] Today we know that when Gd-CAs are given intravascularly, there are the following safety risks: (1) nephrotoxicity requiring dialysis, (2) NSF, (3) anaphylactoid/anaphylactic reactions requiring immediate intervention, and (4) reactions at the injection site.[4] With the exception of NSF, the reactions are similar to those seen after administration of I-CAs. Significant differences in safety have even been shown between different Gd-CAs. When the chelates are cyclic, the toxic gadolinium ion is more tightly bound than it is with linear chelates.[5] Since early 2006, evidence has accumulated that some Gd-CAs, particularly gadodiamide, may cause the potentially devastating or even fatal sclerodermalike, fibrosing condition NSF in patients who have renal failure.[6] Recently it has been shown that gadopentetate dimeglumine may also trigger NSF, but not with the same high frequency as gadodiamide. This review concentrates on gadolinium-associated NSF.

GADOLINIUM

The lanthanide metal ion gadolinium has the strongest effect of all elements on T1 relation time because it has seven unpaired electrons.[5] It has a large magnetic moment; it shortens the longitudinal (T1) and transverse (T2) relaxation times of protons in the water of tissues.[7] Gadolinium alone is highly toxic in vivo because it is distributed to the liver, where it rapidly produces liver necrosis, to bone, and to lymph nodes.[8,9] It competes with calcium ions in muscle cell calcium channels, reducing neuromuscular transmission, and interferes with intracellular enzymes and cell membranes by the process of transmetallation, a phenomenon by which Gd^{3+} replaces endogenous metals such as zinc, iron, and copper. To prevent the harmful effects of Gd^{3+} and to make it usable in humans, Gd^{3+} needs to be sequestered by nontoxic substances.[7] At the same time, its contrast enhancement must be maintained. These two goals are achieved by binding Gd^{3+} to a chelate. Chelates are large organic molecules that form a more or less stable complex around Gd^{3+}. The gadolinium ion has nine coordination sites, of which eight are used for binding with the chelate. The various gadolinium chelates have different physicochemical properties (**Table 1**), including bonds between the gadolinium atom and the chelates, which are of differing stability.[5,10,11] Bonds between

[a] Department of Diagnostic Radiology, Copenhagen University Hospital Herlev, Herlev Ringvej 75, DK-2730 Herlev, Denmark
[b] Department of Diagnostic Sciences, Faculty of Health Sciences, University of Copenhagen, Blegdamsvej 3, DK-2200 Copenhagen N, Denmark
[c] Department of Nephrology, Copenhagen University Hospital Herlev, Herlev Ringvej 75, DK-2730 Herlev, Denmark
* Corresponding author. Department of Diagnostic Radiology 54E2, Copenhagen University Hospital Herlev, Herlev Ringvej 75, DK-2730 Herlev, Denmark.
E-mail address: hentho01@heh.regionh.dk (H.S. Thomsen).

Magn Reson Imaging Clin N Am 16 (2008) 551–560
doi:10.1016/j.mric.2008.07.011

Table 1
The various gadolinium-based agents

Brand Name	Generic Name	Acronym	Chemical Structure	Charge	Elimination Pathway	Protein Binding	Cases of NSF[a]
Omniscan	Gadodiamide	Gd-DTPA-BMA	Linear	Non-ionic	Kidney	None	Yes
OptiMARK	Gadoversetamide	Gd-DTPA-BMEA	Linear	Non-ionic	Kidney	None	Yes
Magnevist	Gadopentetate dimeglumine	Gd-DTPA	Linear	Ionic	Kidney	None	Yes
MultiHance	Gadobenate dimeglumine	Gd-BOPTA	Linear	Ionic	97% kidney 3% bile	<5%	No
Primovist	Gadoxetic acid disodium salt	Gd-EOB-DTPA	Linear	Ionic	50% kidney 50% bile	<15%	No
Vasovist	Gadofosveset trisodium	Gd-DTPA	Linear	Ionic	91% kidney 9% bile	>85%	No
ProHance	Gadoteridol	Gd-HP-DO3A	Cyclic	Non-ionic	Kidney	None	No[b]
Gadovist	Gadobutrol	Gd-BT-DO3A	Cyclic	Non-ionic	Kidney	None	No
Dotarem	Gadoterate meglumine	Gd-DOTA	Cyclic	Ionic	Kidney	None	No

[a] Unconfounded cases published in the peer-reviewed literature.
[b] A single case of stage 0 NSF (a small plaque on the upper back, an unusual location for NSF) has been reported in the non-peer-reviewed literature after multiple injections (total dose 6 × 32 mL) over a short period. Sufficient data (eg, histopathology), however, have not yet been published.

carboxyl groups and amino nitrogen atoms and the gadolinium ion are the strongest, whereas bonds involving amide carbonyl groups are the weakest.[9]

Extracellular Gd-CAs are linear or macrocyclic chelates, and both types are available as ionic or nonionic preparations (**Fig. 1**). Linear chelates are flexible open chains that do not bind as strongly to Gd^{3+} as macrocyclic chelates; the macrocyclic rings are of almost optimal size to cage the gadolinium atom. Nonionic linear compounds are also less stable than ionic ones because the binding between Gd^{3+} and the negatively charged carboxyl groups in the ionic compounds is stronger than that with amides or alcohol in the nonionic compounds. Based on their stability constants and kinetic measurements, the

least stable agents are the nonionic linear chelates, such as gadodiamide and gadoversetamide. Concern about the stability of the nonionic linear chelates was expressed in the early 1990s.[12–15] The benefits of high kinetic and thermodynamic stability offered by a cagelike structure that holds the gadolinium tightly (such as DOTA for use as MR imaging contrast agents) were established in the 1980s, whereas DTPA-based chelates were considered to be kinetically labile, raising the possibility of in vivo transmetallation with endogenous metal ions.[13] The superiority of the cyclic chelate over the linear chelate was demonstrated by an 85% improvement in safety: the ratio of median lethal dose to effective dose was 53 for the cyclic chelate versus 28 for the linear chelate.[14] The cyclic chelate also showed significantly higher

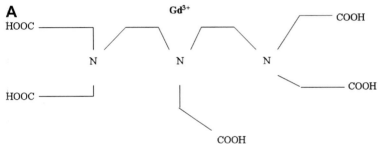

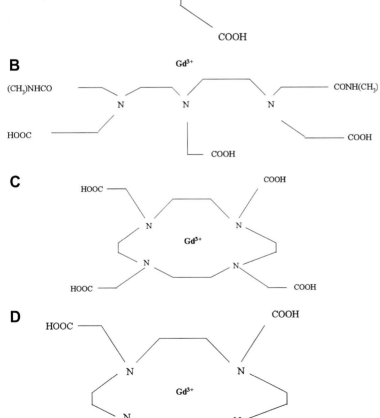

Fig. 1. Principal chemical structures of the various Gd-CAs. Linear chelates: (*A*) ionic (gadopentetate dimeglumine) and (*B*) nonionic (gadodiamide). Cyclic chelates: (*C*) ionic (gadoterate meglumine) and (*D*) nonionic (gadoteridol).

stability in serum based on metal retention: less than 2% gadolinium was released after 150 hours, with 10% to 20% gadolinium being released from the linear chelate.

Gadolinium deposition occurs in human body tissues and has been identified in tissue samples from patients who have NSF up to several years after exposure to gadodiamide. Gadolinium does not occur naturally in human beings; it is there because it has been injected. Abraham and colleagues[16] found increasing amounts of gadolinium in the skin up to 3 years after exposure to gadodiamide. The increase in gadolinium amounts in the skin over time might be explained by gadolinium having been deposited in the bone and slowly released over a period of time. No gadolinium was identified in the skin from a gdodiamide exposed patient who did not have NSF. Other metals found in the tissue of NSF patients included large deposits of iron, copper, and zinc. Gadolinium in the tissue samples is intracellular, and gadolinium may therefore be phagocytosed by macrophages. Intracellular gadolinium, such as in the skin and other organs, may increase the number of profibrotic cytokines or growth factors, leading to dermal or systemic fibrosis, and this may have a role in the development of NSF. Gadolinium deposition in patients who have NSF may occur at sites where there is also deposition of calcium phosphate, a complication associated with renal failure patients who have hyperphosphatemia.

NEPHROGENIC SYSTEMIC FIBROSIS

NSF was first described in San Diego, California, in 1997 as an idiopathic skin condition characterized by thickening and hardening of the skin of the extremities and sometimes the trunk, with an increase in the number of dermal fibroblastlike cells associated with collagen remodeling and mucin deposition. It took another 3 years, however, before the observation was reported in the peer-reviewed literature.[17]

The typical patient has end-stage renal disease.[6,18] NSF affects all ages and races. Most reported patients are on regular hemodialysis treatment, but there are centers at which patients are not on hemodialysis. The first signs of NSF may be seen within hours of exposure to Gd-CA but may also occur as late as 3 months after exposure.[19] It has been claimed that NSF may occur several years after exposure to a Gd-CA. In the meantime, gadolinium may have accumulated in tissue other than skin (eg, bone). Tweedle and colleagues[20] studied [153]Gd release from four different Gd-CAs in mice and rats and found that gadolinium was retained in liver and bone.

In most patients, the condition begins with subacute swelling of the distal extremities, followed in subsequent weeks by severe skin induration and sometimes extension to involve the thighs, forearms, and lower abdomen.[18,19] The skin induration may be aggressive and associated with constant pain, muscle restlessness, and loss of skin flexibility (Fig. 2). In some cases, NSF leads to serious physical disability including becoming wheelchair bound. For many patients, the skin thickening inhibits flexion and extension of joints, resulting in contractures (Fig. 3). Severely affected patients may be unable to walk or fully extend the upper and lower limb joints. Complaints of muscle weakness are common, and deep bone pain in the hips and ribs has been described. Radiography may show soft tissue calcification. There is great variability. NSF severity may be graded from 0 to 4 (0 = no symptoms; 1 = mild physical, cosmetic, or neuropathic symptoms not causing any kind of disability; 2 = moderate physical or neuropathic symptoms limiting physical performance to some extent; 3 = severe symptoms limiting daily physical activities such as walking, bathing, shopping, and so forth; 4 = severely disabling symptoms causing dependence on aid or devices for common, daily activities).[19]

NSF was initially observed in and thought to affect only the skin, so it was called nephrogenic fibrosing dermopathy, but it is now known that it may involve organs such as the liver, lungs, muscles, and heart. Involvement of internal organs

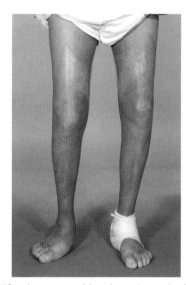

Fig. 2. Fifty-three-year-old male patient who has end-stage diabetic kidney disease and late-stage severe NSF involving both legs symmetrically, from the feet to the upper thighs. The affected skin is shiny, hairless, indurated, sclerotic, and brawny.

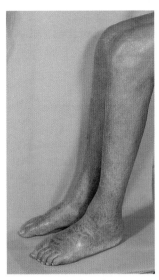

Fig. 3. Thirty-five-year-old female patient on hemodialysis for several years who has late-stage severe, disabling NSF primarily affecting the lower limbs and causing contractures, loss of walking ability, and wheelchair requirement.

may explain the suspected increased mortality of NSF patients. In up to 50% of patients, the disease is progressive and severe. NSF may contribute to death by causing scarring of organs (which impairs normal function), by restricting effective ventilation, or by restricting movement, leading to falls that may cause fractures or hemorrhage. Other patients have died as a result of renal disease or transplant surgery. In one study it was shown that 18-month mortality was increased significantly in NSF patients compared with those who did not have NSF (40% versus 16%), with an adjusted hazard ratio of 2.9 (95% confidence interval: 1.3–6.5; $P = .008$);[21] however, it is difficult in this high-risk group to differentiate deaths caused by complications of the underlying disease and its treatment from those due to NSF.

In several studies based on pathologic or nephrologic registers, the prevalence of NSF after exposure to gadodiamide has been reported to be between 3% and 7% in patients who have reduced renal function.[22] In patients who have a (glomerular filtration rate (GFR) of less than 15 mL/min/1.73 m^2), it may be closer to 20%.[23] The prevalence is higher after two or more injections than after a single injection, indicating a cumulative effect.[23] The incidence after gadopentetate dimeglumine and gadoversetamide is unknown. In the peer-reviewed literature, only one center has reported a large number (>10) of NSF cases after gadopentetate dimeglumine,[21] whereas many centers, including the authors',

have reported more than 10 cases after gadodiamide.[22] This difference is not just a reflection of the market share of the two products, because gadopentetate dimeglumine has been administered to as many as four to five times the number of patients who have had gadodiamide. For many years, it has been known that gadodiamide is not as stable as gadopentetate dimeglumine and that the cyclic agents are the most stable agents.[10,13] Thirty months after the first article indicating a link between Gd-CAs and the development of NSF, no case of NSF after exposure to a cyclic agent or to the high-relaxivity agents (eg, gadobenate dimeglumine) has been published in the peer-reviewed literature.

VALIDATION OF NEPHROGENIC SYSTEMIC FIBROSIS CASES

Because NSF may mimic other skin lesions that occur in patients who have end-stage renal failure (**Box 1**), the diagnosis of NSF should never be made without a histologic evaluation by an experienced dermatopathologist.[24] Some cases reported outside the peer-reviewed literature as NSF (eg, to the health authorities), have, after investigation, turned out not to be NSF.

Box 1
Skin lesions that may mimic nephrogenic systemic fibrosis on clinical examination

Scleromyxedema

Eosinophilic fasciitis

Eosinophilia-myalgia syndrome

Toxic oil syndrome

Sclerodermoid graft-versus-host disease

Fibrosis (induced by drugs, silica, or organic solvents)

Fibroblastic rheumatism

Borreliosis

B2-microglobulin amyloidosis

Systemic sclerosis/morphea

Scleroderma of Buschke

Amyloidosis

Carcinoid syndrome

Porphyria cutanea tarda

Calciphylaxis

Lipodermatosclerosis

Data from Cowper SE. Nephrogenic systemic fibrosis. Adv Dermatol 2007;23:139.

Correlation of the disease with exposure to drugs or contrast media requires adequate documentation of patient exposure. Not all radiology departments have adequate registration systems for the dose and name of the contrast medium used. Sometimes nicknames are used independently of the product administered, or a brand name continues to be used even though a new product has been introduced. In addition, the patient's weight is often not recorded. The lack of complete records causes problems in retrospective studies for detecting unsuspected NSF cases. In the future, it is very important that a record is kept of the type and amount of each injection of Gd-CA given and that all new cases of NSF are reported to the appropriate national regulatory authority. Of interest, no National Medicines Agency had any record of NSF before we submitted 20 cases of gadodiamide-induced NSF to them on March 30, 2006.[25] The authorities need only four simple facts: (1) the initials, birth date, and sex of the patient; (2) the adverse event; (3) the name of the drug; and (4) the name and occupation of the reporting person. The information requires validation, which is the responsibility of the vendor in most parts of the world.

Validation becomes even more difficult when several gadolinium products have been used in a short period of time. Thus, if two different Gd-CAs have been injected, for example, within 8 weeks of each other or longer, it may be impossible to determine with certainty which agent triggered the development of NSF, and the situation is described as "confounded." The agent that is most likely to be responsible, however, is the one that has triggered NSF in other unconfounded situations.

Diagnosis must be confirmed by clinical examination and by the presence of specific histopathologic features on deep skin biopsy, which is a prerequisite because of the many lesions that may mimic NSF clinically and histopathologically (**Box 2**; see **Box 1**).

COFACTORS IN THE DEVELOPMENT OF NEPHROGENIC SYSTEMIC FIBROSIS

Time has shown that two factors are important: (1) reduced renal function and (2) exposure to one of the less stable Gd-CAs. NSF, however, does not develop in all at-risk patients after exposure to the less stable Gd-CAs;[6] therefore, many investigators have been looking for cofactors that may destabilize the agent.

The following cofactors have been suggested: high doses of erythropoietin, metabolic acidosis, iron and ferritin, chronic inflammation,

---

Box 2
Histopathologic differential diagnosis for nephrogenic systemic fibrosis

Scleromyxedema

Eosinophilic fasciitis

Eosinophilia-myalgia syndrome

Toxic oil syndrome

Sclerodermoid graft-versus-host disease

Fibroblastic rheumatism

B2-microglobulin amyloidosis

Systemic sclerosis/morphea

Scleroderma of Buschke

Amyloidosis

Carcinoid syndrome

Porphyria cutanea tarda

Calciphylaxis

Lipodermatosclerosis

Dermatofibrosarcoma protuberans

Melanoma (spindle-cell variant)

Granuloma annulare

Data from Cowper SE. Nephrogenic systemic fibrosis. Adv Dermatol 2007;23:143.

---

hypercoagulability, thrombotic events, recent vascular surgery, recent renal transplant failure, recent surgery, anion gap, and increased phosphate, although no universal cofactor apart from renal failure has been identified. Marckmann and colleagues[26] could not identify any exposure/event other than gadodiamide common to more than a minority of the patients who developed NSF. The Centers for Disease Control and Prevention found that only exposure to Gd-CAs during the preceding 6 months or the preceding year remained statistically significant in their case-control study of 19 NSF cases.[27]

Our current knowledge suggests that there may be several cofactors that increase the risk of NSF after some Gd-CAs; however, some of the factors may have been listed just by chance because enhanced MR imaging was performed when the particular factors were present. For example, in some departments, enhanced MR imaging is done as part of the evaluation of thromboembolic symptoms, postsurgical complications, and so forth, whereas in other departments, MR imaging is not used in these situations. Therefore, one institution may report that NSF occurs more frequently in patients who have particular conditions, but others cannot confirm it because they use enhanced MR imaging differently.

NEPHROGENIC SYSTEMIC FIBROSIS REGISTRIES

Many different registries have collected data about NSF cases, and this has led to confusion. The International Center for Nephrogenic Fibrosing Dermopathy Research (http://www.icnfdr.org) has collected cases of NSF submitted to them since 2000. Most cases are from the United States, and a case can be registered only if the head of the registry, Dr. Shawn Cowper, has evaluated the histologic specimen and agrees with the diagnosis of NSF. Since June 8, 2007, the Food and Drug Administration has encouraged the reporting of American cases through Med-Watch. The cases are not validated, and many do not fulfill the criteria mentioned previously or the criteria for being included in the international registry. Nonetheless, the figures are quoted frequently. The same applies to the reports submitted to national regulatory authorities in the various European countries—all of which rely on the vendor to collect the validating data. The Contrast Media Committees of the American College of Radiology and the European Society of Urogenital Radiology have asked their members to report cases but, again, these are not validated. In addition, the vendors have a registry, which should be identical to that of the national regulatory authorities. Finally there is the peer-reviewed literature, which provides the most reliable information, but suffers from delays in the collection of data and the publication process. By February 1, 2008, 190 cases of NSF (confirmed by biopsy and by clinical examination) were reported in the literature. Gadodiamide was administered in 157 of these cases, gadopentetate in 8, gadoversetamide in 3, and no exposure could be verified in 5. In 18 cases, the agent could not be identified, and several agents were administered in 4 cases.[28]

PATIENTS AT RISK FOR NEPHROGENIC SYSTEMIC FIBROSIS

Patients at higher risk are those who have severe, acute, or chronic renal insufficiency (GFR <30 mL/min/1.73 m^2), those on hemo- or peritoneal dialysis, and patients who have reduced renal function and have had or are awaiting liver transplantation.[6,29] Patients at lower risk are those who have GFR between 30 and 59 mL/min/1.73 m^2 and children under age 1 year, because of their immature renal function. To date, no cases in which the patient had GFR above 60 mL/min/1.73 m^2 have been reported in the literature. Patients who have acute renal failure are at particular risk because the reduced renal function may be overlooked by a single determination of their estimate GFR. If they have the injection of a less-stable gadolinium agent when they have low renal function and then develop NSF, then NSF does not disappear when the renal function improves.[30]

Determination of Glomerular Filtration Rate

Accurate determination of the GFR is not easy. The most precise method measures inulin clearance; isotope methods give similar results. Both methods, however, are cumbersome and impractical for daily use.[31] Measurement of serum creatinine is not satisfactory because more than 25% of older patients have normal serum creatinine levels but reduced GFRs. A single determination of the GFR does not exclude acute renal insufficiency.

Renal function can also be estimated using specially derived predictive equations that use not only serum creatinine but also characteristics such as weight, height, race, and sex. The most accurate results are obtained with the Cockroft-Gault equation,[32] whereas the most precise formula is the Modification of Diet in Renal Disease (MDRD) study equation.[33–35] It is unfortunate that the predictive capabilities of these formulae are suboptimal.[36] In addition, they are not useful for patients who have a GFR above 60 mL/min/1.73 m^2.[37] Different methods also can result in very different values for GFR.[37–39] For example, a 43-year-old 70-kg male patient who has a creatinine level of 264 μmol/L would have a GFR of 32 mL/min/1.73 m^2 if it was calculated by the Cockcroft-Gault equation. When calculated by the MDRD equation, the same patient would have a GFR of 33 mL/min/1.73 m^2 if he was African American and 27 mL/min/1.73 m^2 if he was Caucasian. Thus it would have been illegal to use one of the less stable agents in the Caucasian if the GFR had been estimated by the MDRD equation but not if it had been estimated by the Cockcroft-Gault equation. The situation is further complicated in Asian patients, in whom GFRs are lower but equations have not been established.

In practice, it is easier to use one of the more stable gadolinium agents for which measurement of estimate GFR before administration may not be mandatory. If one of the less stable agents is still used, patients who have reduced renal function must be identified. Serum creatinine should be measured within 7 days of contrast medium administration in patients who have had a previously elevated serum creatinine or who have a history suggesting the possibility of elevated serum creatinine, namely, renal disease, renal surgery, proteinuria, diabetes mellitus, hypertension, gout, or recent nephrotoxic drugs.[31]

Laboratory Analyses

Gadodiamide interferes with the technique of measurement of serum calcium commonly used in hospitals. Cases of spurious hypocalcemia caused by the formation of a complex between Gd^{3+} and a reagent (o-cresol-phthalein) used in the measurement technique have been reported with gadodiamide and gadoversetamide.[40–43] As a general rule, laboratory measurements on blood and urine should not be performed within 24 hours of administration of any contrast medium.[44]

Legal Aspects

In the United States, the Food and Drug Administration last summer required that an identical black box warning be placed on package inserts for all approved Gd-CAs. The European Medicines Agency concluded that the agents have different risks. In their recent public assessment report[45] of June 26, 2007, the European Medicines Agency wrote,

Are all Gd-based CA associated with the same risk of NSF? No. Current evidence suggests that the risk of developing NSF is related to the physicochemical and pharmacokinetic properties of Gd-based CA. The physicochemical properties affect the release of toxic Gd^{3+} from the chelate complex, and the pharmacokinetic properties influence how long the agent remains in the body.

Today in Europe, gadodiamide and gadopentetate dimeglumine are contraindicated in patients who have a GFR less than 30 mL/min/1.73 m², including those on dialysis. The European recommendation is that these agents should be used only with caution in patients who have moderately reduced kidney function (GFR = 30–60 mL/min/1.73 m²). The Japanese authorities have recently taken the same position as the Europeans.

Alternative Imaging

There are several conditions in which alternative imaging is diagnostically inferior and cannot replace enhanced MR imaging. The risk of NSF is low when the nonionic linear chelates are avoided and when the stable agents are used in the smallest dose consistent with a diagnostic result in at-risk patients. Despite the American College of Radiology recommendations,[47] initiating dialysis should be considered with care because the risk associated with hemodialysis in a patient not already adjusted to hemodialysis is higher and more serious than the risk of NSF after exposure to a macrocyclic gadolinium agent. The risk of complications (procedural, allergylike reactions, contrast-induced nephropathy, radiation) following conventional or CT arteriography with iodinated contrast medium must also be weighed carefully against performing MR imaging using a stable gadolinium agent. In most cases, there is no better alternative to enhanced MR imaging.[46,48]

GADOLINIUM AND NORMAL RENAL FUNCTION—A THREAT IN THE FUTURE?

Gadolinium has been demonstrated in skin[16,49] and in bone.[50] The bone accumulation is about four times greater after a linear chelate agent is used than after a nonionic cyclic agent in patients who have normal renal function.[50] The rates of dissociation of gadolinium from macrocyclic ligands are several orders of magnitude slower than their dissociation from linear systems.[51] Bone has a slow turnover. In patients who undergo multiple enhanced MR imaging examinations (eg, in women at increased risk of breast cancer who may follow recommendations to undergo annual enhanced MR imaging), after each examination, some gadolinium accumulates in the bone and stays there for many years.[52] What will happen when the gadolinium is released from bone, for example, when osteoporosis increases bone turnover? The release of an overload of gadolinium might cause classic toxicity symptoms, not NSF. The safety of multiple injections of Gd-CAs has never been studied; the studies that led to approval by the health authorities included only a single injection in humans, and in most cases, it was 0.1 mmol/kg body weight. In the meantime, there has been a major evolution with regard to enhanced MR imaging. The likelihood of having several enhanced MR imaging examinations within a shorter period is much higher now than it was 15 years ago.

Another risk group could be patients who have diabetes mellitus; after approximately 10 years, 50% may develop diabetic nephropathy. These patients cannot be identified when they have normal renal function. When the patient has severely reduced GFR (CKD 5), if some gadolinium is left from an MR imaging examination when the patient had normal function, it cannot be excluded that the patient could develop more severe NSF after enhanced MR imaging with a less stable agent. Marckmann and colleagues[26] showed that patients who had severe NSF had had a higher lifetime (independent of renal function) dose of the gadolinium-based agent than those developing nonsevere NSF.

SUMMARY

NSF is an important delayed adverse reaction with some Gd-CAs that occurs in patients who have impaired renal function.[53] The recognition of this reaction to agents previously considered safe emphasizes the need to have a good clinical indication for all enhanced MR imaging examinations, to choose an agent that leaves the smallest amount of gadolinium in the body (stable agents and high-relaxivity agents), and to keep complete records of the type and dose of agent given.

REFERENCES

1. Hammer FD, Gofette PP, Malaise J, et al. Gadolinium dimeglumine: an alternative contrast agent for digital subtraction angiography. Eur Radiol 1999;9:128–36.
2. Spinosa DJ, Matsumoto AH, Hagspiel KD, et al. Gadolinium-based contrast agents in angiography and interventional radiology. AJR Am J Roentgenol 1999; 173:1403–9.
3. Gemmete JJ, Fortauer AR, Kazanjian S, et al. Safety of large volume gadolinium angiography. J Vasc Interv Radiol 2001;12(Part 2):S28.
4. Marzaellla L, Blank M, Gelperin K, et al. Safety risks with gadolinium-based contrast agents. J Magn Reson Imaging 2007;26:816.
5. Morcos SK. Extracellular gadolinium contrast agents (Gd-CA): differences in stability. Eur J Radiol 2008; 66:175–9.
6. Thomsen HS, Marckmann P, Logager VB. Nephrogenic systemic fibrosis (NSF): a late adverse reaction to some of the gadolinium based contrast agents. Cancer Imaging 2007;7:130–7.
7. Greenen RWF, Krestin GP. Non-tissue specific extracellular MR contrast media. In: Thomsen HS, editor. Contrast media. Safety issues and ESUR guidelines. Heidelberg (Germany): Springer; 2006. p. 107–14.
8. Dawson P. Gadolinium chelates: chemistry. In: Dawson P, Cosgrove DO, Grainger RG, editors. Textbook of contrast media. Oxford (UK): Isis Medical Media; 1999. p. 291–6.
9. Desreux JF, Gilsoul D. Chemical synthesis of paramagnetic complexes. In: Thomsen HS, Muller RN, Mattrey RF, editors. Trends in contrast media. Heidelberg (Germany): Springer Verlag; 1999. p. 161–9.
10. Idee J-M, Port M, Raynal I, et al. Clinical and biological consequences of transmetallation induced by contrast agents for magnetic resonance imaging: a review. Fundam Clin Pharmacol 2006;20:563–76.
11. Sherry AD, Cacheris WP, Kuan K-T. Stability constants for Gd3+ binding to model DTPA-conjugates and DTPA-proteins: implications for their use as magnetic resonance contrast agents. Magn Reson Med 1988;8:180–90.
12. Harpur ES, Worah D, Halz P-A, et al. Preclinical safety assessment and pharmacokinetics of gadodiamide injection. A new magnetic resonance imaging contrast agent. Invest Radiol 1993;28(Suppl 1):S28–43.
13. Varadarajan JA, Crofts SP, Carvalho JF, et al. The synthesis and evaluation of macrocyclic gadolinium-DTPA-bis(amide) complexes as magnetic resonance imaging contrast agents. Invest Radiol 1994;24(Suppl 2):S18–20.
14. Watson AD, Rocklage SM, Carvlin MJ. Contrast agents. In: Stark DD, Bradley WG Jr, editors. Magnetic resonance imaging. 2nd edition. St. Louis (MO): Mosby Year book; 1992. p. 372–437.
15. Cacheris WP, Quay SC, Rocklage SM. The relationship between thermodynamics and the toxicity of gadolinium complexes. Magn Reson Imaging 1990;8:467–81.
16. Abraham JL, Thakral C, Skov L, et al. Dermal inorganic gadolinium concentrations: evidence for in vivo transmetallation and long-term persistence in nephrogenic systemic fibrosis. Br J Dermatol 2008; 158:273–80.
17. Cowper SE, Robin HS, Steinberg SM, et al. Scleromyxoedema-like cutaneous disease in renal dialysis patients. Lancet 2000;356:1000–1.
18. Cowper SE, Rabach M, Girardi M. Clinical and histological findings in nephrogenic systemic fibrosis. Eur J Radiol 2008;66:200–7.
19. Marckmann P, Skov L, Rossen K, et al. Clinical manifestations of gadodiamide-related nephrogenic systemic fibrosis. Clin Nephrol 2008;69:161–8.
20. Tweedle MF, Wedeking P, Kumar K. Biodistribution of radiolabeled, formulated gadopentetate, gadoteridol, gadoterate, and gadodiamide in mice and rats. Invest Radiol 1995;30:372–80.
21. Todd DJ, Kagan A, Chibnik LB, et al. Cutaneous changes of nephrogenic systemic fibrosis. Predictor of early mortality and association with gadolinium exposure. Arthritis Rheum 2007;56:3433–41.
22. Thomsen HS, Marckmann P. Extracellular Gd-CA: differences in prevalences of NSF. Eur J Radiol 2008;66:180–3.
23. Rydahl C, Thomsen HS, Marckman P. High prevalence of nephrogenic systemic fibrosis in chronic renal failure patients exposed to gadodiamide, a gadolinium (Gd)-containing magnetic resonance contrast agent. Invest Radiol 2008;43:141–4.
24. Cowper SE. Nephrogenic systemic fibrosis. Adv Dermatol 2007;23:131–54.
25. Stenver DI. Pharmacovigilance: what to do if you see an adverse reaction and the consequences. Eur J Radiol 2008;66:184–6.

26. Marckmann P, Skov L, Rossen K, et al. Case-control study of gadodiamide-related nephrogenic systemic fibrosis. Nephrol Dial Transplant 2007;22:3174–8.

27. Center for Disease Control and Prevention (CDC). Nephrogenic fibrosing dermopathy associated with exposure to gadolinium-containing contrast agents—St. Louis, Missouri, 2002–2006. MMWR Morb Mortal Wkly Rep 2007;56:137–41.

28. Broome DR. Nephrogenic systemic fibrosis associated with gadolinium based contrast agents: a summary of the medical literature reporting. Eur J Radiol 2008;66:230–4.

29. Thomsen HS. ESUR guideline: gadolinium-based contrast media and nephrogenic systemic fibrosis. Eur Radiol 2007;17:2692–6.

30. Kalb RE, Helm TN, Sperry H, et al. Gadolinium-induced nephrogenic systemic fibrosis in a patient with an acute and transient kidney injury. Br J Dermatol 2008;8:607–10.

31. Thomsen HS, Morcos SK. Members of Contrast Media Safety Committee of European Society of Urogenital Radiology (ESUR). In which patients should serum-creatinine be measured before contrast medium administration? Eur Radiol 2005;15:749–54.

32. Cockroft DW, Gault MH. Prediction of creatinine clearance from serum creatinine. Nephron 1976; 16:31–41.

33. Levey AS, Bosch JP, Lewis JB, et al. A more accurate method to estimate glomerular filtration rate from serum creatinine: a new prediction equation. Ann Intern Med 1999;130:461–70.

34. Levey AS, Greene T, Kusek J, et al. A simplified equation to predict glomerular filtration rate from serum creatinine. J Am Soc Nephrol 2000;11:155A.

35. Levey AS, Coresh J, Greene T, et al. Expressing the modification of diet in renal disease study equation for estimating glomerular filtration rate with standardized serum creatinine values. Clin Chem 2007; 53:766–72.

36. Bostom AG, Kronenberg F, Ritz E. Predictive performance of renal function equations for patients with chronic kidney disease and normal serum creatinine levels. J Am Soc Nephrol 2002;13:2140–4.

37. Stevens LA, Coresh J, Greene T, et al. Assessing kidney function—measured and estimated glomerular filtration rate. N Engl J Med 2006;354:2473–83.

38. Band RA, Gaieski DF, Mills AM, et al. Discordance between serum creatinine and creatinine clearance for identification of ED patients with abdominal pain at risk for contrast induced nephropathy. Am J Emerg Med 2007;25:268–72.

39. Eken C, Kilicaslan I. Differences between various glomerular filtration rate calculation methods in predicting patients at risk for contrast-induced nephropathy. Am J Emerg Med 2007;25:487 [Correspondance].

40. Prince MR, Erel HE, Lent RW, et al. Gadodiamide administration causes spurious hypocalcemia. Radiology 2003;227:639–46.

41. Proctor KA, Rao LV, Roberts WL. Gadolinium magnetic resonance contrast agents produce analytic interference in multiple serum assays. Am J Clin Pathol 2004;121:282–92.

42. Normann PT, Frøysa A, Svaland M. Interference of gadodiamide injection (OMNISCAN®) on the colorimetric determination of serum calcium. Scand J Clin Lab Invest 1995;55:421–6.

43. Choyke PL, Knopp MV. Pseudohypocalcemia with MR imaging contrast agents: a cautionary tale. Radiology 2003;227:627–8.

44. Morcos SK, Thomsen HS, Exley CM. Members of Contrast Media Safety Committee of European Society of Urogenital Radiology (ESUR). Contrast media: interaction with other drugs and clinical tests. Eur Radiol 2005;15:1463–8.

45. European Medicines Agency. Public assessment report, June 26th 2007. Available at: www.esur.org. Accessed December 22, 2007.

46. Diego DR. Nephrogenic system fibrosis: a radiologist's practical perspective. Eur J Radiol 2008;66: 220–4.

47. Kanal E, Barkovich AJ, Bell C, et al. ACR blue ribbon panel on MR safety. ACR guidance document for safe MR practices: 2007. AJR Am J Roentgenol. 2007;188:1447–74.

48. Thomsen HS, Marckmann P, Logager VB. Enhanced computed tomography or magnetic resonance imaging: a choice between contrast medium-induced nephropathy and nephrogenic systemic fibrosis? Acta Radiol 2007;48:593–6.

49. High W, Ayers RA, Chandler J, et al. Gadolinium is detectable within the tissue of patients with nephrogenic systemic fibrosis. J Am Acad Dermatol 2007; 56:27–30.

50. White GW, Gibby WA, Tweedle MF. Comparison of Gd (DTPA-BMA) (Omniscan) versus Gd(HP-DO3A) (ProHance) relative to gadolinium retention in human bone tissue by inductively coupled plasma mass spectroscopy. Invest Radiol 2006;41:272–8.

51. Rosky NM, Sherry AD, Lenkinski RE. Nephrogenic systemic fibrosis: a chemical perspective. Radiology 2008;247:608–12.

52. Abraham JL, Thakral C. Tissue distribution and kinetics of gadolinium and nephrogenic systemic fibrosis. Eur J Radiol 2008;66:200–7.

53. Thomsen HS. Nephrogenic systemic fibrosis: a serious late adverse reaction to gadodiamide. Eur Radiol 2006;16:2619–21.

Advances in Contrast-Enhanced MR Angiography of the Renal Arteries

Tim Leiner, MD, PhD[a,b,*], Henrik Michaely, MD, PhD[c]

KEYWORDS
- Renal arteries • Hypertension • Kidney • MR imaging
- MR angiography • Contrast-enhanced MR imaging
- Functional MR imaging

Renal artery stenosis (RAS) is a relatively common and well-known condition and potentially curable cause of secondary hypertension.[1] The main clinical syndromes associated with RAS are renovascular hypertension (RVH), ischemic nephropathy, proteinuria, and flash pulmonary edema.[2] Diagnosis and management of RAS remains an important clinical problem especially considering that the prevalence of RAS is increasing, mainly because of greater awareness of the long-term deleterious consequences of untreated RVH and the increase in patients who have diabetes mellitus.[3]

In recognition of this problem it is incumbent on the medical community to noninvasively identify patients who have RAS in whom an intervention might delay the decline of or even improve renal function. Although it was formerly believed that the mere presence and subsequent endovascular treatment of RAS of more than 50% luminal narrowing would improve renal function, several randomized trials have shown this is not necessarily the case and only certain patients will benefit from intervention.[4–9]

Recent advances in magnetic resonance (MR) gradient hardware in combination with the migration to 3.0 T now enable the acquisition of isotropic submillimeter spatial resolution data sets, facilitating the detection of renal artery narrowing with high accuracy.[10,11] Although these advances are evolutionary, the real value of MR is that it is now also possible to demonstrate the functional consequences of RAS, such as a decline in renal perfusion and glomerular filtration. The unique capability of MRI to study not only the anatomy of the renal arteries and kidneys but also various physiologic phenomena has culminated in a set of tools that are of high value for this particular clinical problem.

This article discusses recent advances in contrast-enhanced MR angiography (MRA) of the renal arteries and kidneys, and how they can be applied to improve the diagnostic work-up of suspected RAS.

MR ANGIOGRAPHY OF THE RENAL ARTERIES

Renal MRA is primarily focused on the detection of RAS. Atherosclerosis accounts for 70% to 90% of cases of RAS and usually involves the ostium and proximal third of the main renal artery.[1,12] Fibromuscular dysplasia (FMD) is a collection of vascular diseases that affects the intima, media, and adventitia and is responsible for 10% to 30% of cases of RAS.[1,12,13]

[a] Department of Radiology, Maastricht University Hospital, Peter Debijelaan 25, Maastricht NL-6229 HX, The Netherlands
[b] Cardiovascular Research Institute Maastricht, Peter Debijelaan 25, Maastricht NL-6229 HX, The Netherlands
[c] Institute of Clinical Radiology and Nuclear Medicine, University Medical Center Mannheim, Theodor-Kutzer-Ufer 1-3, 68167 Mannheim, Germany
* Corresponding author. Department of Radiology, Maastricht University Hospital, Peter Debijelaan 25, Maastricht, NL-6229 HX, The Netherlands.
E-mail address: leiner@rad.unimaas.nl (T. Leiner).

Magn Reson Imaging Clin N Am 16 (2008) 561–572
doi:10.1016/j.mric.2008.07.013
1064-9689/08/$ – see front matter © 2008 Published by Elsevier Inc.

Although intra-arterial digital subtraction angiography (IA-DSA) is traditionally regarded as the definitive test to diagnose the presence of RAS, the invasive nature of IA-DSA and the difficulty in assessing the pathophysiologic significance of stenotic lesions have encouraged the search for widely available noninvasive or minimally invasive diagnostic tests. In addition, IA-DSA is by no means a perfect test for the detection of RAS because it is subject to substantial interobserver variation.[14] With the introduction of high spatial resolution contrast-enhanced MR angiography (CE-MRA) a reliable alternative for IA-DSA has emerged.

Anatomic Considerations

The renal arteries arise from the abdominal aorta and assume a dorsoinferolateral course until they enter the kidney at the renal hilum. In about one third of the general population there are variations in number, location, and branching patterns of the renal arteries, with more than 30% of subjects having one or more accessory renal arteries.[15,16] This finding is clinically important because RAS in an accessory renal artery can, albeit rarely, also be responsible for RVH.[17] In healthy adults the mean maximum diameter of the renal artery lumen is about 5 to 6 mm. The diameter of accessory renal arteries is highly variable but is generally equal to or smaller than the main renal artery.[15] There is no consensus on what constitutes a significant stenosis but most authors use a reduction in luminal diameter of 50% or greater as the cutoff point.[18]

Precise knowledge of renal arterial anatomy is important because it determines the spatial resolution of the MR imaging sequence to reliably differentiate a stenosed from a healthy vessel. At least three pixels are needed across the lumen of an artery to quantify the degree of stenosis with an error of less than 10%.[19] Taking into account the average diameter of 5 to 6 mm, the spatial resolution of any given imaging technique must ideally be on the order of $1.0 \times 1.0 \times 1.0$ mm^3. In addition to the arterial supply it is important to evaluate renal size, cortical thickness, and corticomedullary differentiation and to compare these parameters with the contralateral kidney.[1]

MR Angiography for Detection of Renal Artery Stenosis

Because of the relative ease of use and high reliability, CE-MRA is the preferred MR technique for the detection of RAS.[20] In addition, phase-contrast (PC) MR flow measurements should be obtained to supplement the anatomic information (see the section on functional renal MR imaging later in this article).

In CE-MRA the renal arteries are imaged in the coronal plane during initial arterial passage of 0.1 to 0.2 mmol/kg 0.5 M extracellular gadolinium chelate contrast medium. Because of the increase in T1 of tissue at 3.0 T the contrast dose can be reduced relative to 1.5 T.[21] For best results patients are required to hold their breath during the acquisition, which typically lasts about 10 to 20 seconds, depending on the resolution and other technical factors related to system performance. Contrast medium is injected at speeds up to 3.0 mL/s, followed by 25 mL saline flush, and spatial resolution in current reports is typically in the order of $1.5 \times 1.5 \times 2.0$ mm^3 (craniocaudal/frequency direction $\times$ left-right/phase-encoding direction $\times$ anteroposterior/slice direction) or better. Using this approach, the abdominal aorta and renal arteries, including accessory arteries, can be visualized with high accuracy (**Figs. 1** and **2**). Arteries can usually be evaluated down to the proximal part of the segmental arteries. Distal segmental and interlobar branches cannot be evaluated reliably at this time.[20,22] To obtain a study with maximum arterial and minimum venous enhancement it is important to ensure careful synchronization of peak arterial contrast concentration with sampling of central k-space profiles.[23] This synchronization is typically done by performing a timing sequence with 1 to 2 mL of contrast medium before the contrast-enhanced acquisition, or by the use of real-time bolus monitoring software. With the latter technique the entire contrast bolus is injected and simultaneously monitored by either the operator or the MR scanner, and when sufficient enhancement is present in the descending aorta the MR fluoroscopy sequence is aborted, the patient is given a breath-hold command, and the three-dimensional (3D) CE-MRA acquisition is started. A third option, available on the most advanced systems, is the use of a time-resolved technique to obtain a series of high spatial resolution 3D volumes by using view-sharing techniques.[11]

Because of the risk for motion artifacts it is important to limit breath-hold length. Motion artifacts may occur when patients are unable to sustain the breath-hold because the acquisition is too long, and because even while performing a breath-hold the kidneys are subject to linear caudocranial motion.[22] Application of parallel imaging technology leads to higher spatial resolution CE-MRA and shorter acquisition durations. On current systems, parallel imaging factors ranging from to 2 to 6 can be achieved, relative to standard nonaccelerated sequences.[24]

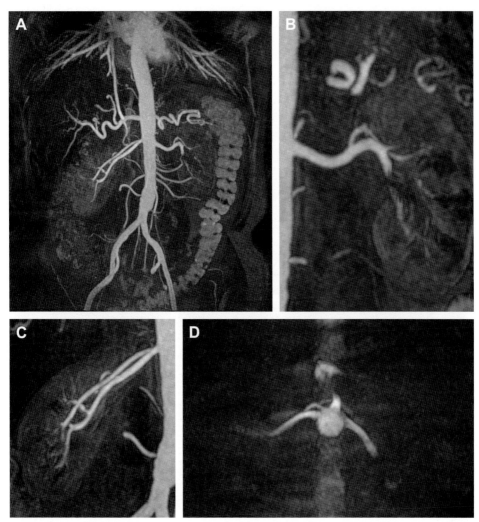

Fig. 1. A 63-year-old male patient who had refractory hypertension. Whole volume maximum intensity projection (MIP) (*A*) depicts renal arterial anatomy with exquisite detail, clearly demonstrating the early bifurcation of the right renal artery. Thin-slab sliding MIPs of the left (*B*) and right (*C*) renal arteries allow for more detailed inspection. Phase-contrast (PC) imaging (axial MIP; *D*) confirms brisk flow through to both kidneys. Both renal arteries were considered normal.

Nonenhanced (two-dimensional time-of-flight and PC) and CE-MRA techniques have been investigated for detection of RAS. The results of these studies were summarized in a meta-analysis by Vasbinder and colleagues[18] Of the 306 studies published up to mid-2000 in which the usefulness of renal MRA was investigated, 18 studies were performed because of clinical suspicion of RVH, used explicitly defined criteria for the presence of RAS, and used IA-DSA as the standard of reference test. Reported sensitivities and specificities for the detection of atherosclerotic RAS in these CE-MRA studies are uniformly high.[18]

The reported sensitivity of CE-MRA for the visualization of accessory renal arteries is greater than 90%.[25,26] At present a single study has been published that specifically investigated the usefulness of CE-MRA for the detection of FMD. Willoteaux and colleagues[27] retrospectively analyzed the accuracy of CE-MRA compared with IA-DSA in 25 subjects who had angiographically proven FMD. The authors evaluated the sensitivity, specificity, and accuracy of CE-MRA for the detection of FMD-associated stenosis, "string-of-pearls" sign, and aneurysm formation. Although the sensitivity for FMD-associated stenosis in their study was only 68%, the sensitivity for the detection of the string-of-pearls sign and aneurysm formation were 95% and 100%, respectively. The overall sensitivity and specificity for the diagnosis FMD

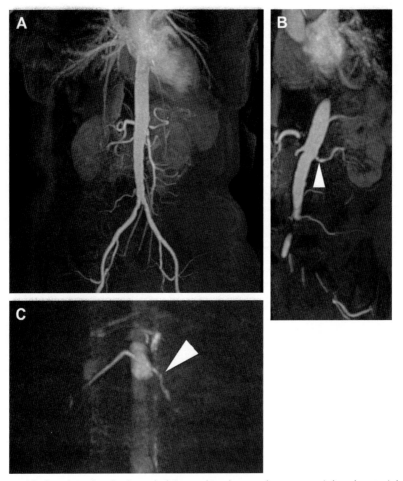

Fig. 2. A 50-year-old female who had underlying scleroderma, known peripheral arterial disease, and unexplained hypertension. (*A*) The whole volume MIP suggests a stenosis in the left renal artery of moderate to severe intensity. The subvolume MIP, however, suggests a mild stenosis (*arrowhead, B*). Supplemental PC imaging confirms relatively preserved flow in the left renal artery confirming mild instead of severe stenosis (*arrowhead, C*). In the presence of conflicting information on PC and CE-MRA, we consider the lower grade of stenosis as suggested by PC more realistic.

were 97% and 93%.[27] Although overt cases of FMD can be diagnosed with CE-MRA (**Fig. 3**A, B), the general opinion is that CE-MRA is currently not able to detect FMD with high accuracy in the presence of only subtle anatomic changes.

The favorable results of the aforementioned CE-MRA studies are, however, in contrast with the results of a large multicenter study from The Netherlands in which the validity of CE-MRA and CTA were prospectively investigated in 356 patients suspected of having RVH, using IA-DSA as the standard of reference. Two panels of three observers judged CE-MRA and CTA examinations, and were blinded for each other's results and the results of all other imaging modalities. Overall, sensitivity ranged from 61% to 69% for CTA and 57% to 67% for CE-MRA.

Specificity ranged from 89% to 97% for CTA and 77% to 90% for CE-MRA.[16] Additional analyses revealed that selecting a subgroup of patients who had high prevalence of RAS could increase the diagnostic performance of both tests, but not to levels as commonly reported in the literature. Possible explanations for these discrepant findings are suboptimal technique, low overall disease prevalence, a high proportion of patients who had FMD, and imperfect standard of reference.[16] Strikingly similar results were obtained in a more recent multicenter trial by Soulez and colleagues[28] who investigated the diagnostic performance of gadobenate dimeglumine for the detection of RAS using IA-DSA as the reference standard in 268 patients who had hypertension or suspected renal artery stenosis. Sensitivity, specificity, and

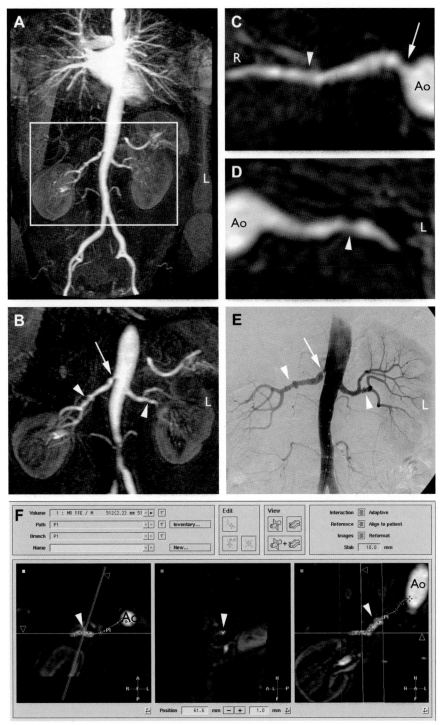

Fig. 3. A 61-year-old male patient who had therapy-resistant hypertension. (*A*) A whole volume MIP of the abdominal aorta and renal arteries show the typical "string-of-pearls" sign suggestive of FMD. (*B*) A zoomed, thin-slab MIP is shown of the area enclosed by the white box in (*A*). There is a high-grade stenosis at the origin of the right renal artery (*arrow*). In addition, both renal arteries show the string-of-pearls sign characteristic for FMD (*arrowheads*). Multiplanar reformations (viewed in transverse orientation) are helpful to confirm location and severity of high-grade stenosis in the right main renal artery (*C*, *arrow*), and the string-of-pearls sign in the distal right (*C*, *arrowhead*) and left renal arteries (*D*, *arrowhead*). (*E*) The corresponding intra-arterial digital subtraction angiogram is shown, which confirms the MRI findings. Diagnostic accuracy can be increased further by measuring reduction in cross-sectional area in a stenosis (as opposed to reduction in diameter) as shown in (*F*) (right renal artery). This functionality is available on most commercially available postprocessing workstations. Ao, aorta; L, left; R, right.

accuracy for the detection of 51% or more RAS on patient level in this study ranged from 65.2% to 79.9%, 81.3% to 91.4%, and 73.6% to 83.8%, respectively.[28]

Postprocessing and Display of Contrast-Enhanced MR Angiography and CT Angiography Data

As mentioned earlier, most authors use a stenosis grade of more than 50% as the cutoff separating significant from nonsignificant stenoses.[18] Historically, most authors have measured stenosis grade on source images in the coronal plane. Unfortunately this technique is subject to substantial interobserver variability.[16]

Because CE-MRA and multidetector-CTA data sets are truly 3D, they can be viewed from an infinite number of angles after acquisition without the need for additional injections of contrast medium. Data sets are usually displayed using ray-casting algorithms, such as (targeted) maximum intensity projection (MIP) or volume rendering. Although these techniques are useful to get an overview of renal arterial anatomy, the true degree of stenosis is best assessed by combining review of original partitions, multiplanar reformations along the vessel axis, and reformations orthogonal to the stenosis (see **Fig. 3**C–F). The latter postprocessing technique significantly increases diagnostic accuracy compared with in-plane evaluation.[29] In addition, recent developments in quantitative vessel analysis are promising with regard to reduction of intra- and interobserver variation for measuring renal artery geometry.[30]

The use of gadolinium-based contrast media in patients who have impaired renal function

Because of the extensive experience with CE-MRA and the superior results obtained with this technique compared with nonenhanced MRA it remains the preferred technique for the detection of RAS and the study of renal perfusion (see later discussion). There is an increased risk for nephrogenic systemic fibrosis (NSF) after administration of gadolinium-based contrast agents (GdBCA) in patients who have acute or chronic severely impaired renal function (stages 4 and 5).[31] NSF is a rare idiopathic systemic fibrosing disorder characterized by pain, dermopathy, and joint contractures.[32] To date, virtually all unconfounded cases of NSF have been associated with the administration of the linear group of GdBCA (gadodiamide [Omniscan, GE Healthcare, Chalfont-St. Giles, United Kingdom] and gadopentetate dimeglumine [Magnevist, Bayer Schering Pharma, Berlin, Germany]). These agents are therefore contraindicated in patients who have

severe renal impairment. The macrocyclic agents gadobutrol (Gadovist BayerSchering Pharma, Berlin, Germany), Gd-HPDO3A (ProHance; Bracco, Milan, Italy) and Gd-DOTA (Dotarem; Guerbet, Aulnay-sur-Bois, France)[33] have not been convincingly associated with NSF, and some experts deem them to be safe in patients who have severely impaired renal function.[34] Although the exact pathogenesis of NSF is a rapidly moving target, we would advise caution at present in this group of patients. In patients who have normal or mildly decreased renal function (chronic kidney disease stages 1–3) GdBCA can be used without problems.[31]

ASSESSMENT OF THE FUNCTIONAL SIGNIFICANCE OF RENAL ARTERY STENOSIS

MRI has the advantage of not only providing MR angiographic data with high spatial resolution and high image contrast but also offering the possibility of acquiring functional data. Functional data allow one to characterize the blood flow in the renal artery and vein,[35] to measure the renal parenchymal blood flow with[36–39] or without contrast agent,[40,41] and to determine the glomerular filtration rate and the split renal function.[42,43] Functional renal imaging techniques have been studied extensively in preclinical studies and volunteer studies. Their clinical application is also increasing as the combination of MRA and functional renal imaging techniques allow comprehensive assessment of renal morphology and renal function. For example, in many cases the hemodynamic relevance of RAS cannot be assessed correctly, particularly in intermediate-grade RAS. In this case the measurement of renal artery flow or of renal parenchymal perfusion fosters a correct assessment of the hemodynamic relevance of RAS. Other applications of functional renal imaging sequences include the detection of renoparenchymal damage in the absence of renovascular disease.

Technical Concepts

Renal artery flow and kidney perfusion can be measured using nonenhanced and contrast-enhanced techniques. The underlying principles and techniques are discussed in detail in the article by Dr. Lee elsewhere in this issue.

In brief, PC techniques allow measurement of renal artery flow. PC MR flow measurements can be acquired using standard gradient-echo sequences (GRE) with resulting measurement times of 3 to 5 minutes depending on the cardiac cycle.[35] Faster approaches for flow measurements include the use of interleaved echoplanar imaging sequences and spatio-temporal undersampling, such as k-t-BLAST.[44,45] Arterial spin labeling (ASL) techniques, on the other hand, can provide estimates of renal perfusion without administration of contrast agents by magnetically labeling blood outside of the imaging plane, and performing the readout after the blood enters the imaging plane where stationary tissues are selectively suppressed.[41,46]

The most widely used and promising technique, however, is dynamic contrast-enhanced (DCE)–MRI of the kidneys. In DCE MRI fast repetitious imaging of the kidney is performed during the first pass of the contrast agent. The temporal resolution has to be chosen high enough to monitor the arrival of the contrast agent in the kidneys. A recent study investigating the minimal temporal resolution found a minimum temporal resolution of 4 seconds.[47] Parallel imaging and echo sharing have significantly decreased the acquisition times of these data sets without major degradation of the image quality. The perfusion sequence and the administration of the contrast agent should be started at the same time. By this means a few images can be acquired before the arrival of the contrast agent. These images serve as baseline images for the postprocessing of the perfusion data. A fast injection rate of at least 2 mL/s followed by a saline chaser of 30 mL at the same injection rate should be chosen to allow for a compact contrast agent bolus even after the pulmonary passage. A compact contrast agent bolus yields maximal T1 shortening during the first pass and hence yields optimal enhancement of the aorta and kidneys.

Before functional renal parameters can be derived from DCE-MRI the data have to be postprocessed. For this purpose various automated and semiautomated segmentation algorithms are becoming available that will facilitate extraction of quantitative parameters of renal function.[48,49]

Evidence-based indications and applications for functional renal imaging

MR-PC flow measurements of the renal arteries have been extensively studied. Their main application is to detect and grade renal artery stenoses.[50] The flow profile derived from the renal artery shows characteristic changes with increasing degree of renal artery narrowing. If used in combination with high spatial resolution MRA of the renal arteries MR-PC flow measurements minimized the interobserver variability and led to an improved accuracy in a tricenter study of 43 renal arteries.[51] In combination with ASL perfusion measurements can be used to differentiate healthy kidneys from abnormal kidneys. In a study with 24 volunteers and 46 patients who had suspected renal artery

stenosis a specificity of 99% and sensitivity of 69% with a positive/negative predictive value of 97%/84% was achieved for the separation of healthy kidneys from kidneys with vascular, parenchymal, or combined disease.[46]

Most publications on DCE-MRI focus on the technical concepts and postprocessing. At this time there are only a limited number of clinical studies on the topic available. An initial study focused on the parenchymal blood flow changes in patients who had renal artery stenosis.[11] In this study with 73 patients who had semiquantitative postprocessing significant differences in blood flow parameters between patients who did not have renal artery stenosis and those who had significant (>75%) renal artery stenosis were found. Patients who had intermediate renal artery stenosis showed nonsignificantly decreased perfusion parameters. In this study and in another study by Michoux and colleagues,[52] significant correlations between raising serum creatinine levels and decreasing renal perfusion parameters were found also indicating that renal first pass perfusion parameters may reflect, at least to a certain degree, renal function. A smaller study by Vallee and colleagues[39] included four renal transplant patients who had renal artery stenosis and seven renal transplant patients who had renal failure and reported on significantly reduced blood flow in transplant patients who had either renal artery stenosis or renal failure, in which the latter showed a smaller residual perfusion. In a further study the same group investigated in 30 patients who had normal renal function or chronic renal failure the cortical and medullary perfusion.[52] Significant reductions of the cortical perfusion and medullary perfusion and of the accumulation of contrast media in the medulla were found in presence of renal failure. Similarly, detection of segmental perfusion deficits in renal transplant patients who had focal rejection were also reported with DCE-MRI.[53]

A further application of DCE-MRI is the evaluation of kidneys after stent placement[11,54] when the renal artery cannot be assessed with CE-MRA because of stent-induced susceptibility artifacts (Fig. 4). DCE-MRI allows demonstration of normalized perfusion parameters after successful stent placement and hence proves the patency of the stent.

FUTURE APPLICATIONS

Several clinical trials aimed at elucidating the optimal treatment strategy in patients who have RAS are currently underway or in the final phase of follow-up. The conventional wisdom (ie, to dilate or stent in the presence of 50% or greater RAS)

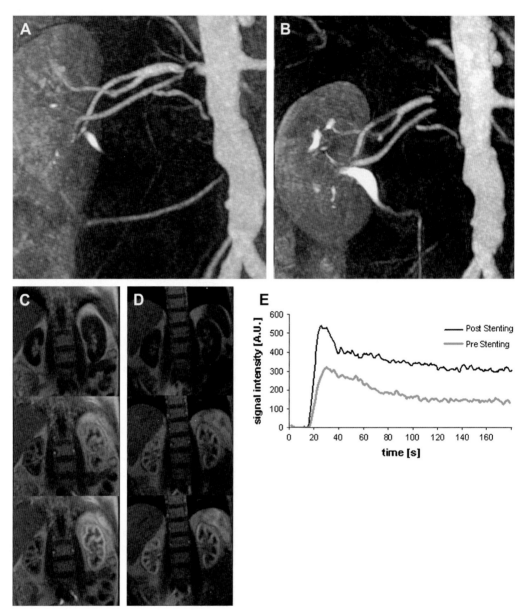

Fig. 4. Renal MRA and perfusion measurements pre and post intervention. (*A*) A coronal thin-slab MIP of the MRA (1.5 T, 1 × 0.9 × 1 mm³, parallel imaging factor 2) of a 55-year-old male patient who had hypertension who presented with a proximal high-grade stenosis of the right renal artery is shown. After stenting (*B*) the stent artifact disrupts the local magnetic field so that no vascular enhancement can be appreciated at this site. To assess the renal parenchymal blood flow and success of the intervention renal perfusion measurements were performed at the baseline visit (*C*) and after the intervention (*D*). Before the intervention delayed perfusion of the affected right side could be appreciated with hypo-enhancement compared with the left side. After the intervention there was again a bilateral regular enhancement of both kidneys. The perfusion changes of the affected right kidney can be visualized semiquantitatively by using signal-intensity versus time curves as done in this example (*E*). Comparing the pre-interventional signal (*red line*) with the post-interventional signal (*black line*) a significant change can be appreciated. The impaired perfusion of the right kidney before intervention is reflected by the slower upslope and the delayed and lowered peak signal intensity in the semiquantitative assessment. (*Reprinted from* Michaely HJ, Dietrich O, Reiser MF, et al. Neue Konzepte für die funktionelle MRT bei Nierenerkrankungen. Der Nephrologe 2006;1:40–9; with permission.)

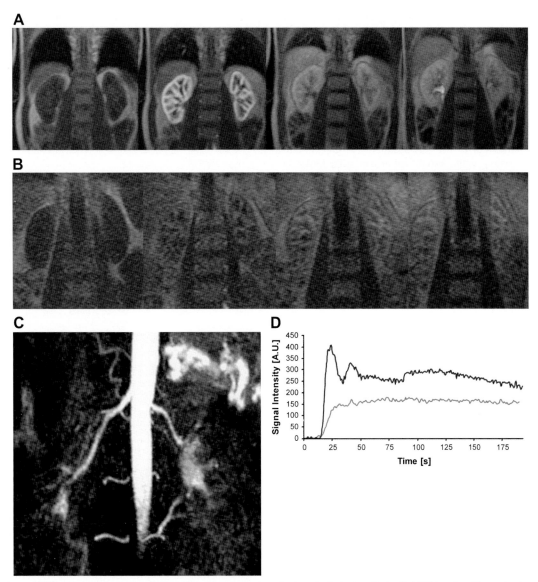

Fig. 5. Different time frames from a contrast-enhanced perfusion study (using TurboFLASH) in a healthy volunteer, which demonstrates a good corticomedullary differentiation and a normal excretory function of the kidney (*A*). In contrast, different time frames of the same sequence in a patient who had hypertension show poor cortical enhancement after contrast agent administration; also no excretion can be demonstrated (*B*). In the absence of renal artery stenosis, as can be seen on this thin MIP of the arterial phase MRA, the patient underwent biopsy, which revealed extensive nephrosclerosis (*C*). Comparison of the cortical signal intensity versus time curve of the healthy volunteer (*green upper line*) and of the patient (*red lower line*) shows normal signal intensity versus time curve for the volunteer (*D*). The patient's signal intensity versus time curve is grossly pathologic with a delayed upslope, lacking first pass peak, and a diminished overall signal. (*Reprinted from* Michaely HJ, Herrmann KA, Nael K, et al. Functional renal imaging: nonvascular renal disease. Abdom Imaging 2007;32:1–16; with permission.)

was greatly challenged in 2000 with the appearance of the results of the study by van Jaarsveld and colleagues,[8] who found no difference at 12-month follow-up in 106 patients who had RAS and hypertension randomized between medical antihypertensive therapy and angioplasty. The

Dutch benefit of stent placement and blood pressure and lipid lowering for the prevention of progression of renal dysfunction caused by atherosclerotic ostial stenosis of the renal artery (STAR) trial has just completed enrollment and results of 2-year follow-up are expected later in

2008.[55] The large-scale angioplasty and stent for renal artery lesions (ASTRAL) trial will compare renal function in 750 patients who have RAS randomized to either medical management or revascularization[56] and is specifically powered to detect a reduction in the decline of renal function of more than 20% as assessed by reciprocal serum creatinine over time. Results with 5-year follow-up are also expected in 2008. The final ongoing trial is the 1000-patient cardiovascular outcomes with renal atherosclerotic lesions (CORAL) study,[57] which aims to address a similar question to ASTRAL.

Common to all of these trials is selection of patients purely based on the presence of RAS, not taking into account the functional consequences of the stenosis or the degree of renal impairment. Future trials using combined MRA/renal MRI protocols will have to be performed to investigate whether such a protocol leads to optimized selection of patients in whom revascularization therapy is indeed beneficial. Apart from the above, the detection and differentiation of renoparenchymal disease independent from the presence of RAS may be another suitable indication for functional MRI techniques (**Fig. 5**). Larger single-center studies on this topic are currently being undertaken.

SUMMARY

Although IA-DSA is still regarded as the most accurate test for anatomic detection of RAS, MRA is an attractive noninvasive alternative in the diagnostic work-up of patients suspected of having RVH. In addition to anatomic diagnosis of RAS, CE-MRA enables precise quantification of the degree of renal impairment using MR perfusion sequences. Additional studies are needed to establish reference values, to determine the optimal postprocessing protocols, and to investigate whether such a comprehensive MRI protocol improves selection of patients in whom revascularization is beneficial.

Because the prevalence of RAS among patients who have hypertension is low, the cost effectiveness of any diagnostic strategy is sensitive to the pretest probability of RVH. Careful clinical evaluation to achieve a pretest probability of at least 20% is an essential component in the work-up of patients suspected of having RVH.[58,59] Because missing RVH may have serious consequences the most important requirement for an alternative test is that it has high sensitivity. The combination of renal artery imaging and assessment of renal perfusion will undoubtedly lead to better selection of patients who will benefit from interventional therapy.

REFERENCES

1. Safian RD, Textor SC. Renal-artery stenosis. N Engl J Med 2001;344:431–42.
2. Textor SC, Wilcox CS. Renal artery stenosis: a common, treatable cause of renal failure? Annu Rev Med 2001;52:421–42.
3. Crook ED. The role of hypertension, obesity, and diabetes in causing renal vascular disease. Am J Med Sci 1999;317:183–8.
4. Cheung CM, Hegarty J, Kalra PA. Dilemmas in the management of renal artery stenosis. Br Med Bull 2005;73–74:35–55.
5. Ives NJ, Wheatley K, Stowe RL, et al. Continuing uncertainty about the value of percutaneous revascularization in atherosclerotic renovascular disease: a meta-analysis of randomized trials. Nephrol Dial Transplant 2003;18:298–304.
6. Plouin PF, Chatellier G, Darne B, et al. Blood pressure outcome of angioplasty in atherosclerotic renal artery stenosis: a randomized trial. Essai Multicentrique Medicaments vs Angioplastie (EMMA) Study Group. Hypertension 1998;31:823–9.
7. van de Ven PJ, Kaatee R, Beutler JJ, et al. Arterial stenting and balloon angioplasty in ostial atherosclerotic renovascular disease: a randomised trial. Lancet 1999;353:282–6.
8. van Jaarsveld BC, Krijnen P, Pieterman H, et al. The effect of balloon angioplasty on hypertension in atherosclerotic renal-artery stenosis. Dutch Renal Artery Stenosis Intervention Cooperative Study Group. N Engl J Med 2000;342:1007–14.
9. Webster J, Marshall F, Abdalla M, et al. Randomised comparison of percutaneous angioplasty vs continued medical therapy for hypertensive patients with atheromatous renal artery stenosis. Scottish and Newcastle Renal Artery Stenosis Collaborative Group. J Hum Hypertens 1998;12:329–35.
10. Leiner T. Magnetic resonance angiography of abdominal and lower extremity vasculature. Top Magn Reson Imaging 2005;16:21–66.
11. Michaely HJ, Sourbron S, Dietrich O, et al. Functional renal MR imaging: an overview. Abdom Imaging 2006 [epub ahead of print].
12. Working Group on Renovascular Hypertension. Detection, evaluation, and treatment of renovascular hypertension. Final report. Arch Intern Med 1987; 147:820–9.
13. Slovut DP, Olin JW. Fibromuscular dysplasia. N Engl J Med 2004;350:1862–71.
14. Schreij G, de Haan MW, Oei TK, et al. Interpretation of renal angiography by radiologists. J Hypertens 1999;17:1737–41.

15. Kaufman JA. Renal arteries. In: Kaufman JA, Lee MJ, editors. Vascular and interventional radiology. The requisites. Philadelphia: Mosby; 2004. p. 323–49.

16. Vasbinder GB, Nelemans PJ, Kessels AG, et al. Accuracy of computed tomographic angiography and magnetic resonance angiography for diagnosing renal artery stenosis. Ann Intern Med 2004; 141:674–82 [discussion: 682].

17. Bude RO, Forauer AR, Caoili EM, et al. Is it necessary to study accessory arteries when screening the renal arteries for renovascular hypertension? Radiology 2003;226:411–6.

18. Vasbinder GB, Nelemans PJ, Kessels AG, et al. Diagnostic tests for renal artery stenosis in patients suspected of having renovascular hypertension: a meta-analysis. Ann Intern Med 2001;135:401–11.

19. Hoogeveen RM, Bakker CJ, Viergever MA. Limits to the accuracy of vessel diameter measurement in MR angiography. J Magn Reson Imaging 1998;8: 1228–35.

20. Schoenberg SO, Prince MR, Knopp MV, et al. Renal MR angiography. Magn Reson Imaging Clin N Am 1998;6:351–70.

21. Michaely HJ, Kramer H, Oesingmann N, et al. Intraindividual comparison of MR-renal perfusion imaging at 1.5 T and 3.0 T. Invest Radiol 2007;42:406–11.

22. Vasbinder GB, Maki JH, Nijenhuis RJ, et al. Motion of the distal renal artery during three-dimensional contrast-enhanced breath-hold MRA. J Magn Reson Imaging 2002;16:685–96.

23. Maki JH, Chenevert TL, Prince MR. Three-dimensional contrast-enhanced MR angiography. Top Magn Reson Imaging 1996;8:322–44.

24. Weiger M, Pruessmann KP, Kassner A, et al. Contrast-enhanced 3D MRA using SENSE. J Magn Reson Imaging 2000;12:671–7.

25. Bakker J, Beek FJ, Beutler JJ, et al. Renal artery stenosis and accessory renal arteries: accuracy of detection and visualization with gadolinium-enhanced breath-hold MR angiography. Radiology 1998;207:497–504.

26. Shetty AN, Bis KG, Kirsch M, et al. Contrast-enhanced breath-hold three-dimensional magnetic resonance angiography in the evaluation of renal arteries: optimization of technique and pitfalls. J Magn Reson Imaging 2000;12:912–23.

27. Willoteaux S, Faivre-Pierret M, Moranne O, et al. Fibromuscular dysplasia of the main renal arteries: comparison of contrast-enhanced MR angiography with digital subtraction angiography. Radiology 2006;241:922–9.

28. Soulez G, Pasowicz M, Benea G, et al. Renal artery stenosis evaluation: diagnostic performance of gadobenate dimeglumine-enhanced MR angiography—comparison with DSA. Radiology 2008;247: 273–85.

29. Schoenberg SO, Rieger J, Weber CH, et al. High-spatial-resolution MR angiography of renal arteries with integrated parallel acquisitions: comparison with digital subtraction angiography and US. Radiology 2005.

30. van Assen HC, Vasbinder GB, Stoel BC, et al. Quantitative assessment of the morphology of renal arteries from X-ray images: quantitative vascular analysis. Invest Radiol 2004;39:365–73.

31. Marckmann P. Nephrogenic systemic fibrosis: epidemiology update. Curr Opin Nephrol Hypertens 2008;17:315–9.

32. Cowper SE, Rabach M, Girardi M. Clinical and histological findings in nephrogenic systemic fibrosis. Eur J Radiol 2008;66:191–9.

33. Idee JM, Port M, Medina C, et al. Possible involvement of gadolinium chelates in the pathophysiology of nephrogenic systemic fibrosis: a critical review. Toxicology 2008;248:77–88.

34. Thomsen HS, Marckmann P. MRI contrast media re used to improve visualization of abnormal structures or lesions in various parts of the body. Eur J Radiol 2008;66:153–9.

35. Schoenberg SO, Just A, Bock M, et al. Noninvasive analysis of renal artery blood flow dynamics with MR cine phase-contrast flow measurements. Am J Physiol 1997;272:H2477–84.

36. Montet X, Ivancevic MK, Belenger J, et al. Noninvasive measurement of absolute renal perfusion by contrast medium-enhanced magnetic resonance imaging. Invest Radiol 2003;38:584–92.

37. Schoenberg SO, Aumann S, Just A, et al. Quantification of renal perfusion abnormalities using an intravascular contrast agent (part 2): results in animals and humans with renal artery stenosis. Magn Reson Med 2003;49:288–98.

38. Sourbron SP, Michaely HJ, Reiser MF, et al. MRI-measurement of perfusion and glomerular filtration in the human kidney with a separable compartment model. Invest Radiol 2008;43:40–8.

39. Vallee JP, Lazeyras F, Khan HG, et al. Absolute renal blood flow quantification by dynamic MRI and Gd-DTPA. Eur Radiol 2000;10:1245–52.

40. Boss A, Martirosian P, Graf H, et al. High resolution MR perfusion imaging of the kidneys at 3 Tesla without administration of contrast media. Rofo 2005;177: 1625–30.

41. Martirosian P, Klose U, Mader I, et al. FAIR true-FISP perfusion imaging of the kidneys. Magn Reson Med 2004;51:353–61.

42. Lee VS, Rusinek H, Noz ME, et al. Dynamic three-dimensional MR renography for the measurement of single kidney function: initial experience. Radiology 2003;227:289–94.

43. Teh HS, Ang ES, Wong WC, et al. MR renography using a dynamic gradient-echo sequence and low-dose gadopentetate dimeglumine as an alternative

to radionuclide renography. AJR Am J Roentgenol 2003;181:441–50.

44. Baltes C, Kozerke S, Hansen MS, et al. Accelerating cine phase-contrast flow measurements using k-t BLAST and k-t SENSE. Magn Reson Med 2005;54: 1430–8.

45. Bock M, Schoenberg SO, Schad LR, et al. Interleaved gradient echo planar (IGEPI) and phase contrast CINE-PC flow measurements in the renal artery. J Magn Reson Imaging 1998;8:889–95.

46. Michaely HJ, Schoenberg SO, Ittrich C, et al. Renal disease: value of functional magnetic resonance imaging with flow and perfusion measurements. Invest Radiol 2004;39:698–705.

47. Michaely HJ, Sourbron SP, Buettner C, et al. Temporal constraints in renal perfusion imaging with a 2-compartment model. Invest Radiol 2008;43:120–8.

48. Attenberger UI, Sourbron SP, Notohamiprodjo M, et al. MR-based semi-automated quantification of renal functional parameters with a two-compartment model—an interobserver analysis. Eur J Radiol 2008;65:59–65.

49. Rusinek H, Boykov Y, Kaur M, et al. Performance of an automated segmentation algorithm for 3D MR renography. Magn Reson Med 2007;57:1159–67.

50. Schoenberg SO, Knopp MV, Bock M, et al. Renal artery stenosis: grading of hemodynamic changes with cine phase-contrast MR blood flow measurements. Radiology 1997;203:45–53.

51. Schoenberg SO, Knopp MV, Londy F, et al. Morphologic and functional magnetic resonance imaging of renal artery stenosis: a multireader tricenter study. J Am Soc Nephrol 2002;13:158–69.

52. Michoux N, Montet X, Pechere A, et al. Parametric and quantitative analysis of MR renographic curves for assessing the functional behaviour of the kidney. Eur J Radiol 2005;54:124–35.

53. Michaely HJ, Herrmann KA, Nael K, et al. Functional renal imaging: nonvascular renal disease. Abdom Imaging 2007;32:1–16.

54. Michaely HJ, Schoenberg SO, Oesingmann N, et al. Renal artery stenosis: functional assessment with dynamic MR perfusion measurements—feasibility study. Radiology 2006;238:586–96.

55. Bax L, Mali WP, Buskens E, et al. The benefit of STent placement and blood pressure and lipid-lowering for the prevention of progression of renal dysfunction caused by Atherosclerotic ostial stenosis of the Renal artery. The STAR-study: rationale and study design. J Nephrol 2003;16:807–12.

56. Mistry S, Ives N, Harding J, et al. Angioplasty and STent for Renal Artery Lesions (ASTRAL trial): rationale, methods and results so far. J Hum Hypertens 2007;21:511–5.

57. Murphy TP, Cooper CJ, Dworkin LD, et al. The Cardiovascular Outcomes with Renal Atherosclerotic Lesions (CORAL) study: rationale and methods. J Vasc Interv Radiol 2005;16:1295–300.

58. Mounier-Vehier C, Haulon S, Devos P, et al. Renal atrophy outcome after revascularization in fibromuscular dysplasia disease. J Endovasc Ther 2002;9: 605–13.

59. Mounier-Vehier C, Haulon S, Lions C, et al. Renal atrophy in atherosclerotic renovascular disease: gradual changes 6 months after successful angioplasty. J Endovasc Ther 2002;9:863–72.

Non–Contrast-Enhanced MR Imaging of the Renal Arteries

Silke Potthast, MD[a], Jeffrey H. Maki, MD, PhD[a,b],*

KEYWORDS
- Magnetic resonance angiography
- Non-contrast enhanced • Renal arteries

Renal artery stenosis (RAS) is the most common cause of secondary hypertension and renal impairment,[1] affecting between 1% and 6% of the general population[2] and up to 45% of patients with atherosclerotic disease.[3,4] As many as 60% to 97% of the cases of RAS are due to arteriosclerosis, with the second most common cause of RAS being fibromuscular dysplasia, representing 30% to 40% of cases.[5] Other less common etiologies include aortic dissection, congenital stenosis, transplant arteriopathy, arteritis, status post embolization, and trauma.[6] RAS is a progressive disease, and more than 50% of all high-grade stenoses progress to occlusion within 2 years.[7,8]

It is known that atherosclerotic lesions are not symmetric, but instead cause eccentric and irregular stenoses. Hemodynamically significant stenosis has been defined in different ways, with a diameter cutoff of 50% often used in studies.[9,10] But recent experimental studies have demonstrated that a significant drop in mean arterial blood flow does not occur until a stenosis reaches 75%.[11] Physiologically, RAS is perhaps better defined as inadequate renal blood flow leading to reduction in glomerular filtration rate and loss of renal parenchyma.[5]

Most patients with mild to moderate RAS and hypertension respond to drug therapy. But renovascular and renal parenchymal disease often coexist in the kidney, and this may be one reason why only about one third of patients improve with regard to hypertension or renal function after undergoing renal artery dilatation or revascularization.[12–14] Thus, a critical goal in the workup of RAS is to identify those patients who have true hemodynamically significant RAS and accordingly might benefit from interventional or surgical revascularization. This has been shown by several studies.[15–18]

IMAGING MODALITIES FOR ASSESSMENT OF RENAL ARTERY STENOSIS

Intra-arterial digital subtraction angiography (DSA) is the accepted gold standard for the anatomic depiction and grading of RAS. This test, however, is invasive and uses nephrotoxic contrast agents and ionizing radiation, making it a poor choice for first-line diagnosis of RAS.

Doppler ultrasound is a widely used noninvasive modality to perform clinical nephrologic imaging; useful for determining renal size, evaluating parenchymal thickness, and visualizing flow in the renal arteries.[19] But this technique is highly operator dependent, with lengthy examination times and a substantial percentage of failed exams. Up to 22% failed exams were reported in one recent study,[20] usually a result of an inadequate acoustic window

In this article, we focus on non-contrast magnetic resonance angiography techniques for evaluating renal artery imaging. Time-of-flight (TOF), phase contrast (PC), steady-state free procession (SSFP), and arterial spin labeling (ASL) are discussed.

[a] Department of Radiology, University of Washington, Box 357115, 1959 NE Pacific Street, Seattle, WA 98195, USA

[b] Department of Radiology (114), Puget Sound VAHCS, 1660 S. Columbian Way, Seattle, WA 98108, USA

* Corresponding author.

E-mail address: jmaki@u.washington.edu (J.H. Maki).

Magn Reson Imaging Clin N Am 16 (2008) 573–584
doi:10.1016/j.mric.2008.07.007
1064-9689/08/$ – see front matter. Published by Elsevier Inc.

or patient habitus. Radionuclide renal scintigraphy has also been shown to have a high accuracy in patients with unilateral RAS, but its accuracy decreases in patients suffering from bilateral RAS or azotemia and in patients with a single functioning kidney.[21] For these reasons, scintigraphy is considered a second-line imaging modality.

Intravascular ultrasound (IVUS) is the first modality that can accurately assess stenosis and directly visualize plaque morphology, but because of its cost and highly invasive nature it is not now or likely ever an appropriate method for primary grading of RAS.[22]

Less invasive alternatives such as computed tomography angiography (CTA) and magnetic resonance angiography (MRA) are widely used for the diagnostic work-up in patients with suspected RAS. While CTA has demonstrated high accuracy for the detection of significant RAS in several studies,[23] its usefulness is somewhat limited by the risks associated with the use of the nephrotoxic iodinated contrast agents.[24] A recent meta-analysis[25] found that CTA and contrast-enhanced MRA (CE-MRA) were both significantly better than conventional non-contrast MRA (time-of-flight), ultrasonography, captopril renal scintigraphy, and the captopril test at identifying RAS using DSA as the gold standard. A large prospective multicenter study[26] suggested that CTA (sensitivity 64%) and MRA (sensitivity 62%) were not reproducible or sensitive enough to rule out RAS in hypertensive patients, although the specificity was felt adequate for detecting RAS (84% for MRA, 92% for CTA). The author's final conclusion[26] was that DSA still remains the diagnostic method of choice. In this study, each participating hospital was equipped with a state-of-the-art CT or MR scanner at that time (1998 to 2001). Given the rapid technological advances in MR and CT over the past 10 years, these results may be quite different if performed today, and a new multicenter study is warranted. One interesting difference between this study and most other published studies is a relatively high proportion of young patients with fibromuscular dysplasia (38%), a disease both MRA and CTA struggle to detect.[6]

A more recent MR-only meta-analysis[27] compiling 12 renal artery CE-MRA studies found a much higher accuracy for detecting significant RAS, with a reported sensitivity of 97% and specificity of 93%. Most of these patients, however, had a diagnosis of atherosclerotic RAS. Other studies[6,28–33] focusing on patients with fibromuscular dysplasia reported much poorer results for accurately detecting RAS.

Before January 2006, when Grobner[34] published the link between gadolinium-based contrast agents and nephrogenic systemic fibrosis (NSF) in patients suffering from severe renal insufficiency, MR imaging with gadolinium-based contrast agents was considered safe for use in patients with impaired renal function.[35] Given the frequent coexistence of renal parenchymal disease and RAS, a substantial number of the patients referred to MR imaging to rule out RAS are potentially at risk for developing NSF. Even if the pathogenesis of NSF is not yet fully understood, many centers have decided to apply new guidelines for administering gadolinium-based contrast agents, however these vary from hospital to hospital and country to country. Nonetheless, the aim of any MR examination, particularly a screening test, is to avoid administering gadolinium-based contrast agents to patients considered at risk for NSF.

Present guidelines suggest avoiding gadolinium chelates in the following conditions: acute or chronic severe renal insufficiency (glomerular filtration rate [GFR] <30 mL/min/1.73 m^2), acute renal insufficiency of any severity due to hepato-renal syndrome, in the perioperative liver transplantation period, and in patients on dialysis. Because patients referred to rule out RAS often have coexistent impaired renal function, obtaining GFR and clinical history is recommended before performing CE-MRA. The updated Food and Drug Administration (FDA) guidelines are available at www.fda.gov/cder/drug/infopage/gcca/default.htm.

In the clinical setting, renal MRA is typically performed after administration of gadolinium contrast material. Although CE-MRA has gained rapid clinical acceptance, one of the greatest strengths of MR imaging is the ability to use multiple contrast mechanisms to assess both renal and arterial morphology and perform functional measurements of arterial flow and parenchymal perfusion without administering potentially harmful contrast or exposing the patient to ionizing radiation. Furthermore, if renal MRA can be performed without using contrast material, this would save the approximately $40 to $80 cost of the contrast agent per examination. Finally, any MR technique has the inherent advantage of being less operator dependent than duplex ultrasonography. All of this explains why renal MRA is evolving into a first-line imaging modality for the evaluation of renovascular disease.

An ideal renal artery imaging study should answer the following questions:[6]

(1) Localization and number of arteries
(2) Characterization of arterial stenosis, including etiology of stenosis, localization, and poststenotic dilatation
(3) Hemodynamic and functional significance of the stenosis

(4) Further pathologies or variants that might have an influence on treatment planning

In this article, we focus on non-contrast MRA techniques for evaluating these questions. Time-of-flight (TOF), phase contrast (PC), steady-state free procession (SSFP), and arterial spin labeling (ASL) will each be discussed. Before performing any of these techniques, most MR studies to assess the kidneys and their arteries typically begin with a morphologic analysis of the kidneys including axial and/or coronal T_1- and T_2-weighted sequences to localize the kidneys, assess the kidney size and cortico-medullary differentiation, and detect mass lesions or collecting system abnormalities.

Time-of-Flight Magnetic Resonance Angiography

Time-of-flight MRA (TOF-MRA) is one of the earliest MRA techniques and one of the first successfully applied in the clinical environment.[36] TOF is a two dimensional (2D) or 3D gradient-echo technique that causes flow-related enhancement based on the inflow of unsaturated blood into a saturated image volume. Because the blood flowing into the volume has not been perturbed by the multiple slice-selective radiofrequency pulses exciting the volume of interest, it flows in with its full longitudinal magnetization, and is thus much brighter than the surrounding saturated stationary tissue within the volume. Selective inversion pulses can be placed on either side adjacent to

the volume of interest to allow directional suppression of the blood flow, eg, nulling venous inflow while arterial inflow remains bright. **Fig. 1** demonstrates a 2D TOF-MRA of the renal arteries. While very effective for neurovascular applications, particularly for the circle of Willis, TOF-MRA has not proven particularly useful for the evaluation of RAS because of several intrinsic artifacts. First, TOF-MRA is degraded by turbulence-induced signal loss in regions of stenosis, often leading to stenosis overgrading[37] and making accurate grading of a stenosis difficult. Second, vessels oriented along the image plane, particularly if flow is slow, become progressively saturated and lose signal—so-called "in-plane" saturation. This is a particular problem given the geometry of the renal arteries, where they typically arise from the aorta in a relatively axial plane. TOF-MRA is much better suited to carotid or peripheral arteries, where the vessels are generally perpendicular to the slice. Third, the technique is slow, with a set of 2D slices or a 3D volume requiring several minutes, causing breathing-related degradation or extremely long scan times for signal averaging. Finally, there is often poor visualization of the distal arterial segments, where flow is slow.[38] Past work with 3D renal TOF-MRA[37] demonstrated it to be a simple method for detecting stenoses (>50%) in the proximal main renal arteries, but unreliable for detecting stenoses more than 3 cm distal to the origin. A recent multicenter Phase III study (268 patients)[39] comparing TOF-MRA and CE-MRA for detecting RAS (using DSA as the gold standard)

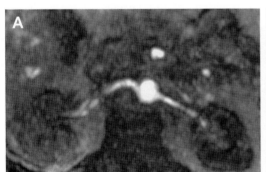
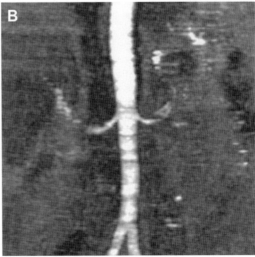

Fig. 1. Two-dimensional TOF nongadolinium MRA of the renal arteries in a 62-year-old female patient without renal artery stenosis. (A) Axial 2D TOF MRA and (B) MIP reformat from the 2D TOF MRA, 40 mm thickness. Note the slice step artifacts on the minimum intensity projection, and the poor visualization of the mid and distal renal arteries in general.

found the sensitivity of TOF-MRA to be only 28% to 33% among three readers compared with a sensitivity between 60% and 84% for CE-MRA. Specificity for TOF-MRA was 68% to 89% compared with 88% to 93% for CE-MRA, with TOF-MRA accuracy of 53% to 66% falling well short of CE-MRA accuracy of 80% to 87%. These numbers are comparable with older studies and clearly demonstrate that TOF-MRA is not an appropriate technique for the evaluation of renal artery disease.

Phase-Contrast Magnetic Resonance Angiography

Phase-contrast MRA (PC-MRA) is a non-contrast MRA technique that not only depicts the morphologic nature of a stenosis, but also allows direct quantitative evaluation of flow dynamics to help assess the hemodynamic significance of a RAS.[40] The basic principle of PC-MRA is that a "flow-encoding" magnetic gradient is applied causing moving spins to experience a phase shift proportional to their velocity. A standard PC-MRA sequence acquires one dataset per desired direction of velocity encoding (phase, frequency, slice), plus some sort of a phase reference data set, typically doing so in an interleaved fashion. The directional flow-encoding gradients cause protons moving in the flow-encoded direction to acquire a phase shift proportional to their velocity, and image phase maps are created where signal intensity represents velocity. Averaging data over the entire cardiac cycle yields a 2D or 3D map of average flow velocity, and can be used to visualize vascular structures, often with spectacular success.[41,42] Furthermore, PC-MRA can distinguish between arterial and venous flow based on the direction of flow. Unfortunately, the same phase-encoding gradients that provide velocity contrast can cause significant motion sensitivity and dephasing in regions of turbulence, with resultant signal loss. These regions of turbulence usually represent disease, thus significantly limiting phase contrast for accurate depiction of diseased vascular anatomy. This otherwise detrimental effect has been applied to advantage as an adjunct to renal CE-MRA, helping to classify the degree of stenosis as "hemodynamically significant" or not based on the presence of signal loss.[32] If the stenosis is evident on CE-MRA and has signal loss on PC-MRA, it can be graded as severe. But if there is no spin dephasing with PC-MRA, it can be graded as moderate and of questionable hemodynamic significance.[43] One study showed that severe PC-MRA dephasing was noted for RAS greater than 75%, whereas in lesions less than 75% there was minimal or no dephasing.[44] **Fig. 2**

demonstrates an example of a high-grade stenosis in a renal transplant artery.

Combining phase contrast with cardiac gating, a 2D velocity map can be obtained,[45] often called "quantitative" or "q" flow.[32] Examining a vessel in cross section, or any single voxel, flow maps are produced very similar in appearance to Doppler ultrasound. With sufficient temporal resolution (40 ms)[46] this technique is accurate for flow quantification, having found a particular niche in cardiac MR imaging.[47] Application of quantitative PC-MRA to renal MRA can help identify and grade stenotic lesions by evaluating their flow profiles and flow parameters. The characteristic flow profile of the normal renal artery shows an early systolic peak, which is most probably the result of an early capacitive inflow effect,[48] followed by an incision, a smaller midsystolic peak, and relatively continuous diastolic flow (**Fig. 3**). The early systolic peak is highly sensitive (but not specific) to arterial stenosis. Typical flow profile changes with RAS begin with loss of the early systolic peak (at 70% stenosis in animal models). As the degree of stenosis increases, the midsystolic peak decreases, as does mean flow.[41,49,50] Schoenberg and colleagues[32] used these findings to propose a 4-grade scale of RAS, which is illustrated in **Fig. 3**.

Steady-State Free Procession Magnetic Resonance Angiography

Three-dimensional steady-state free precession (SSFP) is the most promising non-contrast technique for renal MRA. SSFP, also termed balanced fast field echo, true-fast imaging with steady-state precession, or fast imaging employing steady-state acquisition, is a non-contrast bright blood pulse sequence that has proven to be extremely successful for cardiac CINE imaging and coronary MRA.[51–53] SSFP is well suited for non-contrast MRA, as it is intrinsically fast, high in signal-to-noise ratio (SNR), and flow compensated in all three axes—the latter because of the symmetric nature of the applied gradient pulses. Furthermore, and perhaps most importantly, there is inherently high blood signal intensity and high blood-to-soft tissue contrast, as signal intensity is proportional to the ratio of T2/T1.[54] Water and fat also have high signal with SSFP, as they both have a high T2/T1 ratio as well. High fat signal is the most concerning, as arteries (including renal) are often intimately surrounded by fat. This makes some form of fat suppression essential for SSFP MRA, and several variations for achieving this background suppression are detailed in the techniques described in later sections of this article. All described SSFP renal MRA variants share

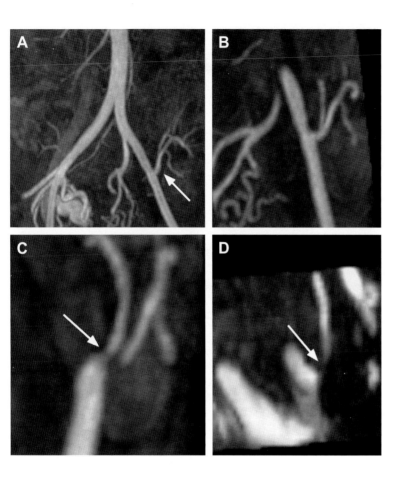

Fig. 2. CE-MRA (*A, B, C*) and PC-MRA (*D*) in a 36-year-old female patient with left-sided renal transplant and worsening renal function. The renal transplant artery can be clearly seen on the CE-MRA coronal MIP (*A*) (*arrow*). On different CE-MRA MIP projections (*B, C*), an early bifurcation of the renal artery is seen, with a short segment focal stenosis at the origin of the smaller arterial branch (*arrow on C*). A MIP from the PC-MRA in a similar projection (*D*) shows a large flow void in the same vessel consistent with a high-grade stenosis—likely a "kinked" vessel. Note also in (*A*) a right arteriovenous fistula with early drainage into the right external iliac vein in the previous cadaveric renal transplant.

being planned as a 3D axial slab centered over the renal arteries, and can be performed either breath-hold or free breathing (acquisition time of 15 seconds to several minutes). In addition, all have the potential for very high spatial resolution (on the order of 1.3×1.3 mm^2 in plane, making them as high as or higher in plane resolution than most CE-MRA techniques). A clinical example is presented in **Fig. 4**.

Five recent clinical studies[55–59] have demonstrated SSFP MRA to be excellent for non-contrast evaluation of RAS, with a uniform 100% sensitivity and 100% negative predictive value. Coenegrachts and colleagues[55] implemented a breath-hold 3D SSFP sequence with water selective excitation to evaluate 25 patients, using digital subtraction angiography as the gold standard. Selective saturation bands were placed over the kidneys and inferior vena cava to selectively suppress venous blood. Their group reported sensitivity, specificity, and positive/negative predictive values of 100%, 98%, 80%, and 100% respectively (RAS prevalence, 22%). Another recent study by Herborn and colleagues[56] compared a breath-hold 3D fat-suppressed SSFP with CE-MRA in 21 patients. No details of the fat-suppression technique

were provided. Although this study was limited in that only two high-grade stenoses were present, both were accurately detected (sensitivity, 100%), and specificity was reported to be 81%.

Our group[60] compared a free-breathing, navigator-gated, selective water excitation SSFP renal MRA sequence with CE-MRA in 40 patients, again using selective saturation bands over the kidneys and IVC. We obtained nearly identical sensitivity, specificity, and positive/negative predictive value to Coenegrachts and colleagues,[55] with values of 100%, 84%, 79%, and 100% (renal artery stenosis prevalence, 38%). While we did not claim SSFP to be superior in image quality to CE-MRA, the technique correctly classified all 20 renal arteries graded greater than 50% stenosis, and we suggested that the technique is well suited for ruling out RAS, particularly in cases of severe renal impairment where the use of contrast agent is contraindicated. Another work by our group[61] concluded that free-breathing navigator-gated SSFP was superior to breath-hold SSFP MRA, making the technique applicable to patients who cannot breath-hold.

Variants of this technique using cardiac triggering to make use of maximal inflow were

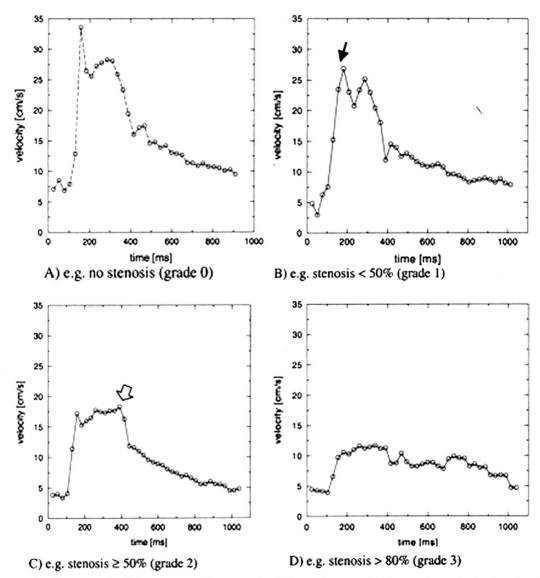

Fig. 3. (A–D) Time-resolved phase contrast flow curves for different degrees of RAS. A semiquantitative functional grading scheme can be applied based on distinct changes in the shape of the flow profile. Normal flow profiles (*upper left*) reveal a characteristic early systolic peak and a midsystolic maximum. Low-grade stenoses (*upper right*) demonstrate only partial loss of early systolic peak (*solid arrow*), whereas midsystolic peak is preserved. Moderate stenoses (*lower left*) display complete loss of early systolic peak and decreased midsystolic maximum (*open arrow*). High-grade stenoses (*lower right*) show a featureless flattened flow profile. (*Reprinted from* Schoenberg SO, Knopp MV, Londy F, et al. Morphologic and functional magnetic resonance imaging of renal artery stenosis: a multireader tricenter study. J Am Soc Nephrol 2002;13:158–69; with permission.)

introduced by Spuentrup[58] and Katoh and colleagues.[59] Spuentrup and colleagues[58] developed a free-breathing, navigator-gated, cardiac-triggered 3D SSFP projection MRA technique that acquired datasets with and without a 2D pencil beam inversion labeling pulse placed over the aorta. By subtracting the two datasets, inverted blood flowing in the renal arteries is accentuated, while static tissue and venous blood is suppressed. This group successfully applied the technique to eight healthy volunteers and seven patients suspected of RAS,[58] comparing the patients to CE-MRA. They obtained high spatial resolution, high-contrast renal MRAs with visualization of all renal artery stenoses (n = 7, presumed sensitivity of 100%), clearly depicting even branches embedded in the parenchyma.

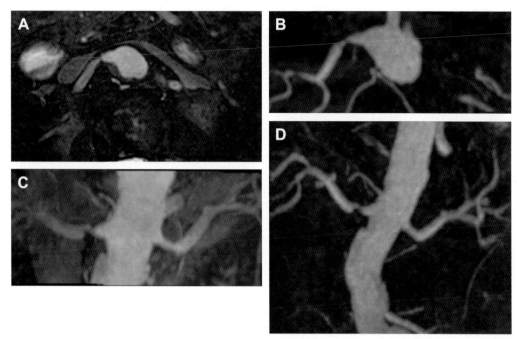

Fig. 4. Navigator gated SSFP MRA in a 71-year-old male with renal artery stenosis and worsening renal function, (*A*) SSFP source image, (*B*) the axial MIP CE-MRA, (*C*) SSFP coronal MIP, and (*D*) coronal MIP CE-MRA. A significant right renal artery stenosis is depicted by both sequences (62% by CE-MRA, 57% by SSFP), whereas both sequences agree on a nonsignificant left-sided renal artery stenosis (45% by CE-MRA, 42% by SSFP).

A somewhat similar SSFP technique not based on subtraction was introduced by Katoh and colleagues.[59] This study used a free-breathing navigator-gated SSFP sequence with a slice selective inversion prepulse (inversion delay 325 ms) and cardiac triggering to suppress background venous blood, renal parenchyma, and retroperitoneal tissue. By synchronizing to the ECG and applying the inversion pulse before forward systolic flow and timing the readout to occur after systolic inflow, noninverted blood enters the slice during the inversion delay and is bright, while the venous blood, renal parenchyma, and retroperitoneum remain suppressed (**Fig. 5**). This small study (eight healthy volunteers and eight patients) was compared with CE-MRA. The authors stated that all low-grade (n = 3) and high-grade (n = 2) stenoses were verified by CE-MRA or DSA, implying sensitivity and negative predictive value were 100%. A recent follow-up of this work compared SSFP MRA with CE-MRA in 30 patients, 11 of whom were positive for renal artery stenosis.[62] This study again showed 100% sensitivity, with specificity of 95% and 90% and accuracy of 92% and 96% respectively (two readers).

Taken together, these renal SSFP MRA studies screened a total of 131 patients for RAS, with a perfect 100% sensitivity and 100% negative predictive value as compared with DSA or CE-MRA. Reported

specificities ranged from 84% to 98%, which are quite acceptable for a screening test. Our group[60] showed a mean absolute value difference between SSFP and CE-MRA to be 10% ± 9%. We also showed moderate dependence of SSFP on inflow for signal intensity, meaning vessels with slow flow (including poststenotic regions) lose signal intensity. This can be seen distal to the stenosis in **Fig. 4**. This would likely also be the case for an even more inflow-dependent technique such as that described by Katoh and colleagues,[59] but this remains to be proven. If there is such signal loss, SSFP will likely overcall a RAS, again acceptable for a screening test in which the goal is to ultimately decrease the need for either gadolinium or iodinated contrast. Assuming a 20% RAS prevalence in the general screening population, and their (lowest of the group) specificity of 84%, we calculated that by screening for RAS with SSFP MRA and administering gadolinium contrast only in positive cases, this would decrease gadolinium administration by 67%.[60] This number would improve if specificity could be increased.

Based on these studies, we suggest breath-hold, or preferably navigator-gated SSFP MRA could be performed as the first-line MRA technique to rule out RAS in patients at risk of NSF. If the SSFP is negative for high-grade RAS (~50% or more), RAS has been excluded without using

A

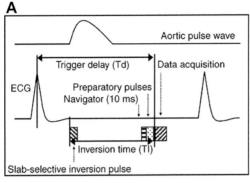

B

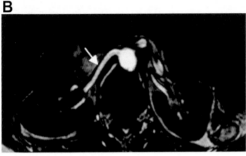

Fig. 5. (*A*) Schematic of the sequence elements for cardiac-triggered navigator-gated SSFP renal MRA. Trigger delay time (Td) was individually adjusted to apply the inversion prepulse before, and data acquisition after, the pulsatory wave. Using an inversion delay time of 325 ms, signal of the renal parenchyma and the venous blood were suppressed. The real-time navigator precedes the preparatory pulses, which are used to reach steady-state conditions. (*B*) Single-slice image demonstrating the effect of a slab-selective inversion pulse. The arrow is pointing to the right renal artery, which is clearly delineated. (*Reprinted from Katoh M, Bueker A, Stuber M, et al. Free-breathing renal MR angiography with steady-state free-precession (SSFP) and slab-selective spin inversion: initial results. Kidney Int 2004;66(3):1272–78; with permission.*)

gadolinium-based contrast agents. If the SSFP is positive, then further workup may be warranted (CE-MRA, DSA, CTA) to better define the stenosis and ensure it is not a false positive. Limitations do exist, most notably the very real possibility of excluding an accessory renal artery from the limited imaging volume and the uncertainty for how well the technique performs for more distal renal artery pathology such as fibromuscular dysplasia (FMD). Hence, it is probably premature to suggest SSFP renal MRA if the clinical concern is FMD or a pretransplant evaluation requiring recognition of all accessory renal arteries.

Arterial Spin Labeling

Arterial spin labeling (ASL) uses blood as an endogenous contrast agent in a fashion somewhat similar to TOF, and can be used to create vascular images or to semiquantitatively evaluate tissue perfusion. To perform ASL MRA, two images are obtained: the first image labels inflowing blood, typically with an excitation focused on the aorta, and the second (control) image does not label blood. The two images are then subtracted to create an MR angiogram. A cardiac-triggered version of ASL termed signal targeting with alternating radiofrequency (STAR) was applied to renal MRA back in 1995.[63] This was a 3D scheme combining echo planar imaging readouts and k-space segmentation. The authors examined 17 healthy patients, 3 potential renal donors, and 2 patients with suspected RAS, demonstrating excellent visualization of the renal arteries to the level of the intrarenal branch vessels. Although these are intriguing results, no further studies have been published with this technique.

All of the techniques discussed thus far have been used to depict vessel morphology and flow parameters in the larger arteries, but are unable to grade actual renal parenchymal damage, which is better evaluated by measuring renal parenchymal perfusion. Particularly in the early stages of renal disease, renal parenchymal blood flow itself must be quantified to grade renal damage. The kidneys are highly vascular organs, receiving 20% of the cardiac output. This high rate of perfusion is most accurately quantified through the bolus passage of contrast material,[50,64–66] but can also be semi-quantitatively evaluated without the use of contrast through a variant of the ASL technique.[67]

One method of ASL perfusion uses the flow-sensitive alternating inversion recovery method,[68] first described for the assessment of cerebral perfusion. This technique labels the image using nonselective, global inversion, thus inverting all the blood in the abdomen, particularly the aorta. The control image is acquired with selective inversion only (**Fig. 6**), such that the aorta is not inverted. After subtraction, the stationary tissue, which has been inverted in both sequences, subtracts out, leaving signal proportional to the amount of blood perfusing the kidneys during the inversion time. A single coronal slice can be obtained in a breath-hold.

This technique is noninvasive and does not use contrast agents, but has not reached broad clinical acceptance owing to the low signal-to-noise ratio and its susceptibility to artifacts (**Fig. 7**). Only limited studies have been published with patient data. One recent study demonstrated a significant qualitative agreement between ASL perfusion of the kidney and the relative signal distribution in renal scintigraphy, although they also concluded the

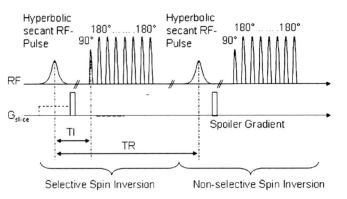

RF

G_{slice}

Hyperbolic secant RF-Pulse

90° 180° .... 180°

Hyperbolic secant RF-Pulse

90° 180° .... 180°

TI

TR

Spoiler Gradient

Selective Spin Inversion   Non-selective Spin Inversion

Fig. 6. Schematic timing diagram of the ASL pulse sequence. In the first step, only the slice plane containing the kidney is selectively inverted. In the second step, the entire abdomen is inverted. The inversion time is approximately 1200 ms during which time blood from the aorta enters the imaging slice. (*Reprinted from* Michaely HJ, Schoenberg SO, Ittrich C, Dikow R, Bock M, Guenther M. Renal disease: value of functional magnetic resonance imaging with flow and perfusion measurements. Invest Radiol 2004;39:698–705; with permission.)

ASL technique was marginal in terms of SNR, and contrast perfusion techniques, while more complex, were superior.[69] Nonetheless, this study attempted to classify renal disease based on a combination of phase-contrast flow profile and ASL renal perfusion. Using a two-branch classification tree, where mean flow greater than 354.5 mL/min was normal, and mean flow less than this combined with ASL "SNR" less than 7.31 was diseased, they achieved a sensitivity of 69%

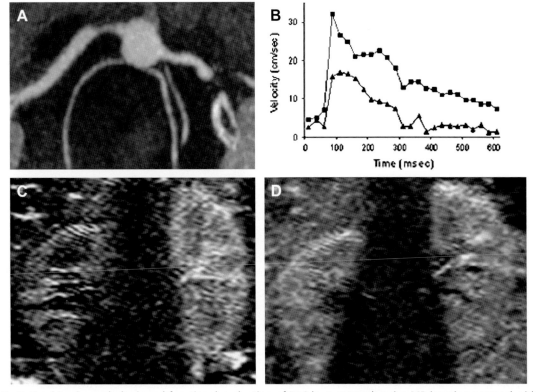

Fig. 7. Combined morphologic and functional evaluation of RAS by a comprehensive MR imaging protocol with 3D-Gd-MRA, phase contrast flow measurements, and ASL perfusion imaging. (*A*) MRA of a 52-year-old female patient with a right-side RAS of 60%. (*B*) MR CINE phase contrast flow measurement reveals a reduced flow profile of the affected renal artery (*triangles*), confirming a hemodynamically significant stenosis as suspected on MRA. (*C*) ASL perfusion-weighted image shows decreased signal intensity of the involved kidney. The signal-to-noise ratio of the affected kidney is 4.8 versus 8.6 of the healthy kidney. (*D*) The same kidney after stenting of the stenosed artery. Both kidneys appear equally intense, with a signal-to-noise ratio of 7.0 (formerly affected kidney) versus 7.5 (healthy kidney). (*Reprinted from* Michaely HJ, Schoenberg SO, Ittrich C, Dikow R, Bock M, Guenther M. Renal disease: value of functional magnetic resonance imaging with flow and perfusion measurements. Invest Radiol 2004;39:698–705; with permission.)

and specificity of 99% for detecting renal disease (a combination of RAS, FMD, and medical renal disease).

Perfusion measurements help to assess the impact of RAS on the parenchymal blood flow. If ASL and flow quantification were added to the MR protocol for evaluating renal artery disease, the information derived could potentially help characterize the degree of stenosis and underlying renal dysfunction. Furthermore, ASL perfusion measurements alone may help to establish a diagnosis for impaired renal function even in the absence of RAS.

SUMMARY

Although DSA and CE-MRA of the renal arteries compete for being the gold standard in evaluating RAS, non–contrast-enhanced MRA techniques are attracting more and more attention, particularly in light of NSF. We suggest breath-hold, or preferably navigator-gated SSFP MRA be performed as the first line MRA technique to rule out RAS in any patient felt to be at risk of NSF or having any other contraindication to gadolinium contrast. Adding MR flow and MR perfusion measurements to this protocol improves the grading of RAS and can potentially allow us to differentiate between RAS and renoparenchymal disease as the cause for renal impairment. As all the studies evaluating non–contrast-enhanced renal MRA had relatively small patient numbers with essentially all atherosclerotic disease, the experience with FMD is too limited to allow a detailed recommendation for this entity at this point. SSFP MRA is also not yet recommended for pretransplant evaluation, as the limited acquired imaging volume may miss important accessory renal arteries. Additional SSFP MRA studies in larger patient cohorts are necessary to obtain further data validating this promising technique.

REFERENCES

1. Derkx FH, Schalekamp MA. Renal artery stenosis and hypertension. Lancet 1994;344(8917):237–9.
2. Simon N, Franklin SS, Bleifer KH, et al. Clinical characteristics of renovascular hypertension. JAMA 1972;220(9):1209–18.
3. Wachtell K, Ibsen H, Olsen MH, et al. Prevalence of renal artery stenosis in patients with peripheral vascular disease and hypertension. J Hum Hypertens 1996;10(2):83–5.
4. Olin JW, Melia M, Young JR, et al. Prevalence of atherosclerotic renal artery stenosis in patients with atherosclerosis elsewhere. Am J Med 1990;88(1N):46N–51N.
5. Preston RA, Epstein M. Ischemic renal disease: an emerging cause of chronic renal failure and end-stage renal disease. J Hypertens 1997;15(12 Pt 1):1365–77.
6. Dellegrottaglie S, Sanz J, Rajagopalan S. Technology insight: clinical role of magnetic resonance angiography in the diagnosis and management of renal artery stenosis. Nat Clin Pract Cardiovasc Med 2006;3(6):329–38.
7. Tollefson DF, Ernst CB. Natural history of atherosclerotic renal artery stenosis associated with aortic disease. J Vasc Surg 1991;14(3):327–31.
8. Caps MT, Perissinotto C, Zierler RE, et al. Prospective study of atherosclerotic disease progression in the renal artery. Circulation 1998;98(25):2866–72.
9. Blum U, Krumme B, Flugel P, et al. Treatment of ostial renal-artery stenoses with vascular endoprostheses after unsuccessful balloon angioplasty. N Engl J Med 1997;336(7):459–65.
10. De Cobelli F, Venturini M, Vanzulli A, et al. Renal arterial stenosis: prospective comparison of color Doppler US and breath-hold, three-dimensional, dynamic, gadolinium-enhanced MR angiography. Radiology 2000;214(2):373–80.
11. Schoenberg SO, Bock M, Kallinowski F, et al. Correlation of hemodynamic impact and morphologic degree of renal artery stenosis in a canine model. J Am Soc Nephrol 2000;11(12):2190–8.
12. Isles CG, Robertson S, Hill D. Management of renovascular disease: a review of renal artery stenting in ten studies. QJM 1999;92(3):159–67.
13. Leertouwer TC, Gussenhoven EJ, Bosch JL, et al. Stent placement for renal arterial stenosis: where do we stand? A meta-analysis. Radiology 2000;216(1):78–85.
14. Beebe HG, Chesebro K, Merchant F, et al. Results of renal artery balloon angioplasty limit its indications. J Vasc Surg 1988;8(3):300–6.
15. Dorros G, Jaff M, Mathiak L, et al. Four-year follow-up of Palmaz-Schatz stent revascularization as treatment for atherosclerotic renal artery stenosis. Circulation 1998;98(7):642–7.
16. Watson PS, Hadjipetrou P, Cox SV, et al. Effect of renal artery stenting on renal function and size in patients with atherosclerotic renovascular disease. Circulation 2000;102(14):1671–7.
17. van Jaarsveld BC, Krijnen P, Pieterman H, et al. The effect of balloon angioplasty on hypertension in atherosclerotic renal-artery stenosis. Dutch Renal Artery Stenosis Intervention Cooperative Study Group. N Engl J Med 2000;342(14):1007–14.
18. Harden PN, MacLeod MJ, Rodger RS, et al. Effect of renal-artery stenting on progression of renovascular renal failure. Lancet 1997;349(9059):1133–6.
19. Desberg AL, Paushter DM, Lammert GK, et al. Renal artery stenosis: evaluation with color Doppler flow imaging. Radiology 1990;177(3):749–53.

20. Argalia G, Cacciamani L, Fazi R, et al. Utilizzo dell'ecoamplificatore nella diagnosi della stenosi dell'arteria renale a confronto con angio-RM [Contrast-enhanced sonography in the diagnosis of renal artery stenosis: comparison with MR-angiography]. Radiol Med (Torino) 2004;107(3):208–17 [in Italian].

21. Huot SJ, Hansson JH, Dey H, et al. Utility of captopril renal scans for detecting renal artery stenosis. Arch Intern Med 2002;162(17):1981–4.

22. De Scheerder I, De Man F, Herregods MC, et al. Intravascular ultrasound versus angiography for measurement of luminal diameters in normal and diseased coronary arteries. Am Heart J 1994;127(2):243–51.

23. Willmann JK, Wildermuth S, Pfammatter T, et al. Aortoiliac and renal arteries: prospective intraindividual comparison of contrast-enhanced three-dimensional MR angiography and multi-detector row CT angiography. Radiology 2003;226(3):798–811.

24. Lufft V, Hoogestraat-Lufft L, Fels LM, et al. Contrast media nephropathy: intravenous CT angiography versus intraarterial digital subtraction angiography in renal artery stenosis: a prospective randomized trial. Am J Kidney Dis 2002;40(2):236–42.

25. Vasbinder GB, Nelemans PJ, Kessels AG, et al. Diagnostic tests for renal artery stenosis in patients suspected of having renovascular hypertension: a meta-analysis. Ann Intern Med 2001;135(6):401–11.

26. Vasbinder GB, Nelemans PJ, Kessels AG, et al. Accuracy of computed tomographic angiography and magnetic resonance angiography for diagnosing renal artery stenosis. Ann Intern Med 2004;141(9):674–82 [discussion 682].

27. Tan KT, van Beek EJ, Brown PW, et al. Magnetic resonance angiography for the diagnosis of renal artery stenosis: a meta-analysis. Clin Radiol 2002;57(7):617–24.

28. Galanski M, Prokop M, Chavan A, et al. [Accuracy of CT angiography in the diagnosis of renal artery stenosis]. Rofo 1994;161(6):519–25 [in German].

29. Rieumont MJ, Kaufman JA, Geller SC, et al. Evaluation of renal artery stenosis with dynamic gadolinium-enhanced MR angiography. AJR Am J Roentgenol 1997;169(1):39–44.

30. Farres MT, Lammer J, Schima W, et al. Spiral computed tomographic angiography of the renal arteries: a prospective comparison with intravenous and intraarterial digital subtraction angiography. Cardiovasc Intervent Radiol 1996;19(2):101–6.

31. Kim TS, Chung JW, Park JH, et al. Renal artery evaluation: comparison of spiral CT angiography to intraarterial DSA. J Vasc Interv Radiol 1998;9(4):553–9.

32. Schoenberg SO, Knopp MV, Londy F, et al. Morphologic and functional magnetic resonance imaging of renal artery stenosis: a multireader tricenter study. J Am Soc Nephrol 2002;13(1):158–69.

33. Vasbinder GB, Maki JH, Nijenhuis RJ, et al. Motion of the distal renal artery during three-dimensional contrast-enhanced breath-hold MRA. J Magn Reson Imaging 2002;16(6):685–96.

34. Grobner T. Gadolinium—a specific trigger for the development of nephrogenic fibrosing dermopathy and nephrogenic systemic fibrosis? Nephrol Dial Transplant 2006;21(4):1104–8.

35. Kirchin MA, Runge VM. Contrast agents for magnetic resonance imaging: safety update. Top Magn Reson Imaging 2003;14(5):426–35.

36. Miyazaki T, Yamashita Y, Shinzato J, et al. Two-dimensional time-of-flight magnetic resonance angiography in the coronal plane for abdominal disease: its usefulness and comparison with conventional angiography. Br J Radiol 1995;68(808):351–7.

37. Loubeyre P, Revel D, Garcia P, et al. Screening patients for renal artery stenosis: value of three-dimensional time-of-flight MR angiography. AJR Am J Roentgenol 1994;162(4):847–52.

38. McCauley TR, Monib A, Dickey KW, et al. Peripheral vascular occlusive disease: accuracy and reliability of time-of-flight MR angiography. Radiology 1994;192(2):351–7.

39. Soulez G, Pasowicz M, Benea G, et al. Accuracy of Gadobenate dimeglumine-enhanced MR angiography in the evaluation of renal artery stenosis: comparison with unenhanced time-of-flight MR angiography versus digital subtraction angiography (DSA). Berlin: Proceedings of the International Society for Magnetic Resonance in Medicine; 2007.

40. Debatin JF, Ting RH, Wegmuller H, et al. Renal artery blood flow: quantitation with phase-contrast MR imaging with and without breath holding. Radiology 1994;190(2):371–8.

41. Schoenberg SO, Knopp MV, Bock M, et al. Renal artery stenosis: grading of hemodynamic changes with CINE phase-contrast MR blood flow measurements. Radiology 1997;203(1):45–53.

42. Schoenberg SO, Just A, Bock M, et al. Noninvasive analysis of renal artery blood flow dynamics with MR CINE phase-contrast flow measurements. Am J Physiol 1997;272(5 Pt 2):H2477–84.

43. Prince MR. Renal MR angiography: a comprehensive approach. J Magn Reson Imaging 1998;8(3):511–6.

44. Dong Q, Schoenberg SO, Carlos RC, et al. Diagnosis of renal vascular disease with MR angiography. Radiographics 1999;19(6):1535–54.

45. Pelc NJ, Herfkens RJ, Shimakawa A, et al. Phase contrast CINE magnetic resonance imaging. Magn Reson Q 1991;7(4):229–54.

46. Bock M, Schoenberg SO, Schad LR, et al. Interleaved gradient echo planar (IGEPI) and phase contrast CINE-PC flow measurements in the renal artery. J Magn Reson Imaging 1998;8(4):889–95.

47. Didier D. Assessment of valve disease: qualitative and quantitative. Magn Reson Imaging Clin N Am 2003;11(1):115–34, vii.

48. Kirchheim H. Effect of common carotid occlusion on arterial blood pressure and on kidney blood flow in unanesthetized dogs. Pflugers Arch 1969;306(2):119–34.

49. de Haan MW, van Engelshoven JM, Houben AJ, et al. Phase-contrast magnetic resonance flow quantification in renal arteries: comparison with 133Xenon washout measurements. Hypertension 2003;41(1):114–8.

50. Schoenberg SO, Rieger JR, Michaely HJ, et al. Functional magnetic resonance imaging in renal artery stenosis. Abdom Imaging 2006;31(2):200–12.

51. Kunz RP, Oellig F, Krummenauer F, et al. Assessment of left ventricular function by breath-hold CINE MR imaging: comparison of different steady-state free precession sequences. J Magn Reson Imaging 2005;21(2):140–8.

52. Foo TK, Ho VB, Marcos HB, et al. MR angiography using steady-state free precession. Magn Reson Med 2002;48(4):699–706.

53. Stuber M, Weiss RG. Coronary magnetic resonance angiography. J Magn Reson Imaging 2007;26(2):219–34.

54. Barkhausen J, Ruehm SG, Goyen M, et al. MR evaluation of ventricular function: true fast imaging with steady-state precession versus fast low-angle shot CINE MR imaging: feasibility study. Radiology 2001;219(1):264–9.

55. Coenegrachts KL, Hoogeveen RM, Vaninbroukx JA, et al. High-spatial-resolution 3D balanced turbo field-echo technique for MR angiography of the renal arteries: initial experience. Radiology 2004;231(1):237–42.

56. Herborn CU, Watkins DM, Runge VM, et al. Renal arteries: comparison of steady-state free precession MR angiography and contrast-enhanced MR angiography. Radiology 2006;239(1):263–8.

57. Alerci M, Braghetti A, Gallino A, et al. Free-breathing steady-state free precession (SSFP) MR angiography of the renal arteries without contrast agent: a prospective intraindividual comparison with high-spatial-resolution contrast-enhanced MR angiography. Washington, DC: Seattle; 2006.

58. Spuentrup E, Manning WJ, Bornert P, et al. Renal arteries: navigator-gated balanced fast field-echo projection MR angiography with aortic spin labeling: initial experience. Radiology 2002;225(2):589–96.

59. Katoh M, Buecker A, Stuber M, et al. Free-breathing renal MR angiography with steady-state free-precession (SSFP) and slab-selective spin inversion: initial results. Kidney Int 2004;66(3):1272–8.

60. Maki JH, Wilson GJ, Eubank WB, et al. Navigator-gated MR angiography of the renal arteries: a potential screening tool for renal artery stenosis. AJR Am J Roentgenol 2007;188(6):W540–6.

61. Maki JH, Wilson GJ, Eubank WB, et al. Steady-state free precession MRA of the renal arteries: breath-hold and navigator-gated techniques vs. CE-MRA. J Magn Reson Imaging 2007;26(4):966–73.

62. Wyttenbach R, Braghetti A, Wyss M, et al. Renal artery assessment with nonenhanced steady-state free precession versus contrast-enhanced MR angiography. Radiology 2007;245(1):186–95.

63. Wielopolski PA, Adamis M, Prasad P, et al. Breath-hold 3D STAR MR angiography of the renal arteries using segmented echo planar imaging. Magn Reson Med 1995;33(3):432–8.

64. Prasad PV, Priatna A. Functional imaging of the kidneys with fast MRI techniques. Eur J Radiol 1999;29(2):133–48.

65. Prasad PV, Cannillo J, Chavez DR, et al. First-pass renal perfusion imaging using MS-325, an albumin-targeted MRI contrast agent. Invest Radiol 1999;34(9):566–71.

66. Aumann S, Schoenberg SO, Just A, et al. Quantification of renal perfusion using an intravascular contrast agent (part 1): results in a canine model. Magn Reson Med 2003;49(2):276–87.

67. Williams DS, Detre JA, Leigh JS, et al. Magnetic resonance imaging of perfusion using spin inversion of arterial water. Proc Natl Acad Sci U S A 1992;89(1):212–6.

68. Kim SG. Quantification of relative cerebral blood flow change by flow-sensitive alternating inversion recovery (FAIR) technique: application to functional mapping. Magn Reson Med 1995;34(3):293–301.

69. Michaely HJ, Schoenberg SO, Ittrich C, et al. Renal disease: value of functional magnetic resonance imaging with flow and perfusion measurements. Invest Radiol 2004;39(11):698–705.

Diffusion-weighted MR Imaging of the Kidneys and the Urinary Tract

Sooah Kim, MD[a], Mohit Naik, MD[a], Eric Sigmund, PhD[b],
Bachir Taouli, MD[c],*

KEYWORDS
- MR imaging • Diffusion • Kidney • Renal neoplasm
- Renal function

Diffusion-weighted imaging (DWI) provides quantification of Brownian motion of water protons by calculating the apparent diffusion coefficient (ADC), and can be used for in vivo quantification of the combined effects of capillary perfusion and diffusion.[1] Diffusion contrast is based on the thermally driven random motion of molecules in tissue. Bulk fluids show a mean-squared displacement that grows linearly with time at a rate given by the ADC. In such free fluids, the diffusion coefficient is determined by molecular architecture, interactions, and temperature. In tissue, however, the protons' motion is hindered or restricted by different components such as cell membranes, cellular density, or macromolecules. This is manifested macroscopically by an ADC that is reduced from the bulk value. If the underlying tissue structure is ordered (such as the medullary tubules in the kidney), the ADC shows a corresponding anisotropy along different directions. If the tissue structure shows no preferred direction when averaged over the MR imaging resolution (such as in the renal cortex), the ADC will appear isotropic, although reduced from the bulk value. In all of these cases, the ADC (and other indices derived from them) serves as markers of the structural and functional state of the imaged tissue. Some examples include (1) anisotropic diffusion in white matter tissue in diffusion tensor imaging (DTI),[2] providing both quantitative biomarkers and qualitative fiber tractography information, and

(2) corticomedullary differentiation in the kidney due to the medulla's anisotropic tubules.[3] In general, the clinical implications of ADC change depend on the tissue under investigation; an anomalous rise in ADC can indicate increased edema, cystic changes, and necrosis; whereas an anomalous reduction in ADC might indicate ischemia, infection, or tumor. As such, diffusion measures should be taken in context with other imaging contrasts to ensure an accurate diagnosis. In DWI, the ADC is quantitatively measured through the application of a diffusion gradient, a magnetic field that spatially varies along a particular direction, which induces a variation in Larmor precession frequency among the spins.[4,5] Furthermore, the stochastic motion of the spins along this gradient causes an irreversible loss of phase coherence that reduces the total magnitude of the spin magnetization, ie, the MR signal. The rate of this decay as a function of an experimentally determined diffusion-weighting factor b determines the ADC. DWI incorporates this measurement into a spatially resolved scan. The most common method employed in clinical MRI scanners is bipolar-gradient diffusion preparation with single-shot echo-planar imaging (EPI) (Fig. 1).[6,7] This approach captures the diffusion contrast while minimizing both eddy current[8] and motion artifacts, but can be limited by susceptibility artifacts at high magnetic field. Many other DWI techniques[9–12] have been developed to

[a] Department of Radiology, New York University Medical Center, 560 First Avenue, New York, NY 10016, USA
[b] Department of Radiology, New York University Medical Center, Center for Biomedical Imaging, 660 First Avenue, New York, NY 10016, USA
[c] Department of Radiology, New York University Langone Medical Center, 560 First Avenue, New York, NY 10016, USA
* Corresponding author.
E-mail address: bachir.taouli@nyumc.org (B. Taouli).

Magn Reson Imaging Clin N Am 16 (2008) 585–596
doi:10.1016/j.mric.2008.07.006

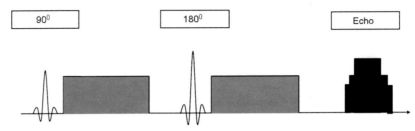

Fig. 1. Gradient scheme for the single shot echo planar imaging sequence with diffusion-sensitizing gradients (in *gray*) located on each side of the 180° pulse.

circumvent this problem, and may prove vital in the successful migration of DWI to the high- and ultra-high field platforms (3 T and above).

DIFFUSION ACQUISITION PARAMETERS FOR IMAGING THE KIDNEYS AND THE URINARY TRACT

Breath-hold or respiratory triggered (using a navigator echo) DWI is acquired before contrast injection using single-shot echoplanar imaging, with the suggested following parameters: axial or coronal acquisition, fat suppression, tridirectional gradients using the following b-values: 0 (used as reference), 400 (intermediate), and 800 (high) sec/mm^2. The choice of b-values is somehow arbitrary and depends on the equipment used. Lower b-values will generate higher ADC values, owing to the contribution of intravoxel incoherent motion effects other than diffusion (eg, perfusion or flow phenomena), as opposed to higher b-values, which will enable "pure" diffusion weighting, at the expense of lower residual signal. To reduce the effects of intravoxel incoherent motion, maximum b-values of 800 sec/mm^2 or greater are suggested whenever possible. We suggest a baseline b = 0 sec/mm^2 image (used as a reference) and intermediate b-value (for example, 400 sec/mm^2), which provides intermediate diffusion weighting with acceptable image quality, and a higher b-value (for example, b = 800 sec/mm^2), which provides higher diffusion weighting, free from perfusion and flow contamination. In addition, the use of three b-values provides a more precise ADC fit. The other parameters used in our protocol are as follows: repetition time 1800 to 2300 msec, time to echo min (65 to 68 msec), field of view 240 to 315 × 320 to 420 mm, matrix 180 × 192, slice thickness/gap 7/1.4 mm, number of averages 2 (breath-hold) or 4 (respiratory triggered acquisition), parallel imaging (acceleration factor 2), EPI factor 144 to 192, bandwidth 1302 Hz/pixel, acquisition time approximately 2 × 20 seconds to cover the whole kidneys (for the breath-hold acquisition), and at least 2 minutes for the respiratory triggered acquisition. We obtain pixel-based ADC maps

(integrating the three b-values) using a commercial workstation, ADC is calculated with a linear regression analysis of the function S = S$_0$ × exp (−b × ADC), where S is the SI after application of the diffusion gradient, and S$_0$ is the SI at b = 0 sec/mm^2.

DWI APPLICATIONS IN DIFFUSE RENAL DISEASE AND RENAL TRANSPLANT

There are several published studies that have investigated the use of DWI in normal kidneys,[3,13–19] for the assessment of diffuse renal disease,[16,20,21] renal artery stenosis,[22] renal infection,[23] urinary obstruction,[19] and renal transplants.[24]

The feasibility of DWI of the kidneys in healthy volunteers has been reported by several investigators. The reported ADC values of renal cortex and medulla vary considerably from study to study depending on the equipment and the sequence parameters, particularly the b-value,[13,15,16,20] with mean ADCs of normal kidney ranging from 1.63 to 5.76 × 10^{-3} mm^2/sec. In our experience, using b-values of 0 to 400 to 800 sec/mm^2, the mean ADC of normal cortex and medulla were 2.16 ± 0.37 and 1.90 ± 0.26 × 10^{-3} mm^2/sec, respectively (in 64 patients), with significantly higher ADC in the cortex ($P < .05$).

Murtz and colleagues[17] showed better ADC reproducibility when using a pulse trigger, with smaller standard deviation of ADC with a trigger compared with the acquisition without a trigger. Muller and colleagues[13] investigated the effect of hydration and anisotropic kidney diffusion using multiple b-values on 23 volunteers, and renal ADC values of dehydrated subjects were substantially increased with rehydration. Ries and colleagues[3] used diffusion tensor imaging to investigate the anisotropic diffusion in the normal kidney, and were able to demonstrate the anisotropic structure of the renal medulla, which had a higher fractional anisotropy (FA) compared with the cortex (0.39 ± 0.11 versus 0.22 ± 0.12, respectively).

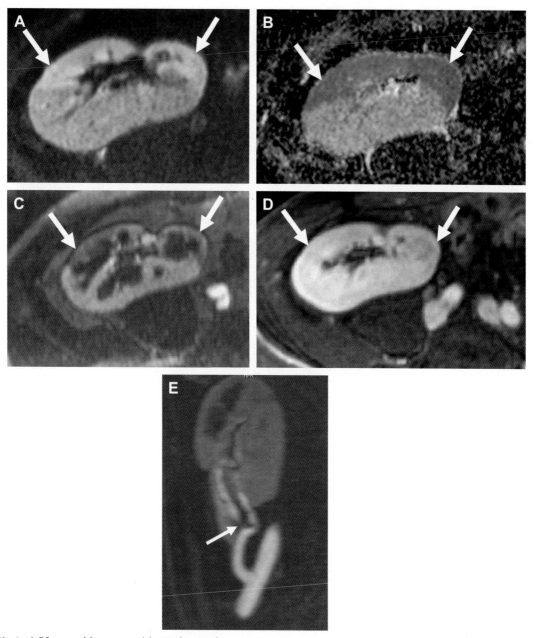

Fig. 2. A 56-year-old woman with renal transplant segmental ischemia caused by high-grade stenosis of the transplant renal artery. Axial single-shot echoplanar diffusion-weighted images demonstrate segmental restricted diffusion involving the anterior aspect of the transplant kidney (*arrows*) on images at b = 800 sec/mm² (*A*) and ADC map (*B*) compared with the remainder of the renal parenchyma. Axial contrast-enhanced fat suppressed T1-weighted images obtained at the corticomedullary (*C*) and nephrographic (*D*) phases demonstrate decreased perfusion in the corresponding area consistent with ischemia. Coronal reconstruction of MR angiography (*E*) demonstrates severe stenosis of the anterior branch of the transplant renal artery (*arrow*).

Several studies have shown the potential use of ADC as a marker of renal function, most studies showing lower ADC in kidney dysfunction. For example, Namimoto and colleagues[20] demonstrated that the ADC values in both the cortex and medulla in chronic renal failure (CRF) and acute renal failure (ARF) kidneys were significantly lower than those of normal kidneys. In the cortex, ADC values were above 1.8×10^{-3} mm²/sec in all normal kidneys (n = 32), ranging from 1.6 to 2.0×10^{-3} mm²/sec in all ARF kidneys (n = 8), and below 1.5×10^{-3} mm²/sec in 14 of 15 CRF

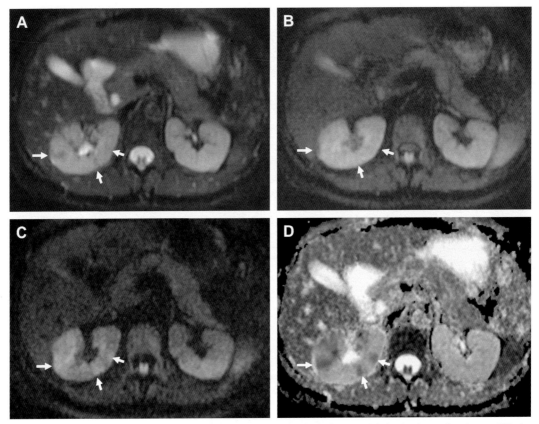

Fig. 3. A 63-year-old woman with acute pyelonephritis of the right kidney. Axial single shot echoplanar diffusion-weighted images demonstrate multifocal patchy lesions that are hypointense at b = 0 sec/mm² (*A*), isointense at b = 500 (*B*), and hyperintense at b = 1000 sec/mm² (*C*) compared with renal parenchyma (*arrows*). ADC map (*D*) shows low ADC (1.35 ± 0.4 × 10–3 mm²/sec for b = 0 to 500 to 1000 sec/mm², *arrows*) compared with the remainder of the normal parenchyma.

kidneys (using b-values of 0, 30, and 300 sec/mm²). In the medulla, there was considerable overlap in the ADC values of the normal and diseased kidneys. There was a linear correlation between ADC value and serum creatinine level in the cortex (r = 0.75) and a weak linear correlation in the medulla (r = 0.60). Thoeny and colleagues[19] have shown that ADC of cortex was higher than medulla in normal kidneys, as in our experience. In addition, the ADC values using all b-values were lower in chronic renal disease compared with normal kidneys, as well as in patients with pyelonephritis compared with the contralateral side, whereas patients with ureteral obstruction showed varying degrees of difference in all ADC values compared with the contralateral side. However, another study by Muller and colleagues[13] on ureteral obstruction in an animal model showed decreased ADC in ureteral obstruction.

Recently, Xu and colleagues[21] reported a positive correlation between ADC (measured with b-values of 0 and 500 sec/mm²) and the split glomerular filtration rate (GFR) in 55 patients (r = 0.709). The ADCs were significantly lower in impaired kidneys than in normal kidneys. The mean renal ADCs (× 10⁻³ mm²/sec) of the four groups (normal renal function, GFR > 40 mL/min/1.73 m²; mild renal impairment, GFR between 20 and 40 mL/min/1.73 m²; moderate renal impairment, GFR between 10 and 20 mL/min/1.73 m²; and severe renal impairment, GFR < 10 mL/min/1.73 m²) were 2.87 ± 0.11, 2.55 ± 0.17, 2.29 ± 0.10, and 2.20 ± 0.11, respectively.

Namimoto and colleagues[20] also evaluated the ADC values in seven kidneys with renal artery stenosis (RAS). In RAS, the ADC values in the cortex (1.5 × 10⁻³ mm²/sec) were significantly lower than those of the normal and the contralateral kidneys, but ADC values of medulla were slightly lower than normal but not significantly different. Recently, Yildririm and colleagues[22] compared the ADC values of 13 kidneys with RAS and 26 with normal renal arteries using multiple b-values, and found significant differences in mean ADC of kidneys

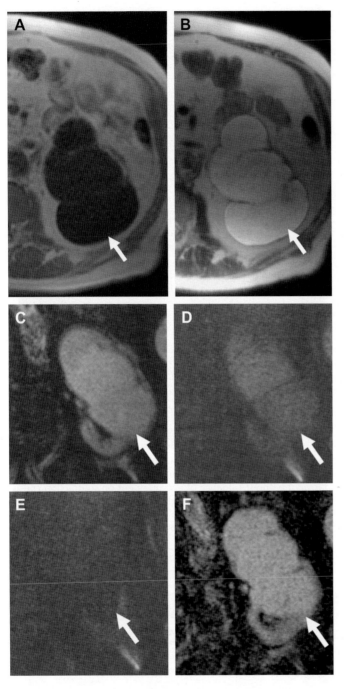

Fig. 4. A 83-year-old man with septated cyst of the left kidney. Axial breath-hold in-phase T1-weighted image (*A*) and breath-hold T2-weighted imaging (*B*) with a half-Fourier acquisition single shot turbo spin-echo sequence demonstrate a 13 cm partially septated cyst in the left kidney. Axial single-shot echoplanar diffusion-weighted images demonstrate a left renal mass that is hyperintense on diffusion-weighted MR image at b = 0 sec/mm^2 (*C*), with strong signal drop at b = 400 (*D*), and stronger at b = 800 sec/mm^2 (*E*). ADC map (*F*) shows high ADC (3.3 $\pm$ 0.15 10 mm^2/sec for b = 0 to 400 to 800 sec/mm^2).

using lower, average, and high b-values between two groups (average ADC 1.7 $\times$ 10^{-3} mm^2/sec for RAS versus 1.9 $\times$ 10^{-3} mm^2/sec for normal kidneys).

There are extremely limited data on the use of DWI in renal transplantation. The only available study by Thoeny and colleagues[19] was performed in normal-functioning kidney transplants and normal native kidneys. In their study, the ADCs of native kidneys were significantly higher in the cortex than in the medulla, whereas the ADCs of the transplant kidneys were almost identical in the medulla and the cortex, while the perfusion fraction (measured with smaller b-values) showed greater variation. The perfusion fraction reflects microcirculation of blood and movement in

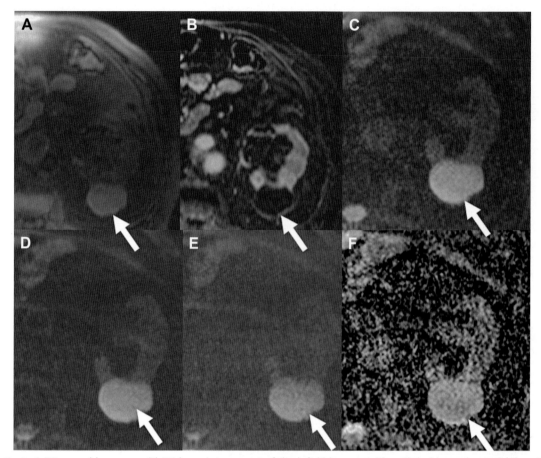

Fig. 5. A 74-year-old woman with T1 hyperintense cyst of the left kidney. Axial breath-hold unenhanced (*A*) and contrast-enhanced subtracted (*B*) fat-suppressed T1-weighted interpolated spoiled gradient recalled echo images show a 3-cm T-1 hyperintense left renal mass (*arrows*) without evidence of enhancement on subtraction consistent with a benign cyst. Axial single-shot echoplanar imaging diffusion-weighted images demonstrate a right renal mass (*circles*) that is hyperintense on diffusion-weighted MR image at b = 0 sec/mm^2 (*C*), b = 50 (*D*), and at b = 500 sec/mm^2 (*E*) compared with renal parenchyma. ADC map (*F*) shows high ADC (3.90 ± 0.6 × 10^{-3} mm^2/sec).

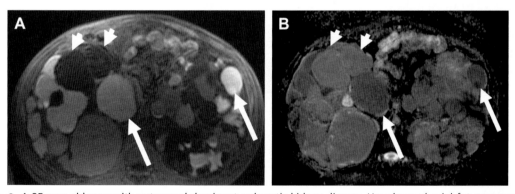

Fig. 6. A 35-year-old man with autosomal dominant polycystic kidney disease. Unenhanced axial fat-suppressed T1-weighted gradient echo image (*A*) shows variable signal intensity of the renal cysts because of interval hemorrhage or proteinaceous contents. ADC map obtained from axial single-shot echoplanar diffusion-weighted using b-values of 0 and 400 sec/mm^2 (*B*) shows relatively decreased ADC in some of the cysts with higher signal intensity on precontrast T1-weighted image (*long arrows*) compared with simple cysts (*small arrows*).

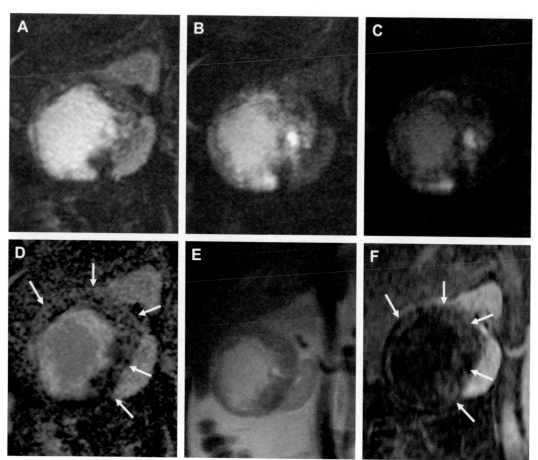

Fig. 7. A 43-year-old man with papillary renal cell carcinoma of the right kidney. Large 10 cm centrally cystic and peripherally solid right renal mass demonstrated on coronal single-shot echoplanar diffusion-weighted images at b = 0 (*A*), b = 400 (*B*), and b = 800 sec/mm² (*C*), ADC map (*D*), coronal T2-weighted image with a half-Fourier acquisition single-shot turbo spin-echo sequence (*E*) and subtracted postcontrast coronal reformatted T1-weighted image (*F*). The ADC was lower in the solid portion compared with the central cystic portion (1.10 vs. 1.75×10^{-3} mm²/sec).

predefined structures, such as tubular flow and glomerular filtration in the kidneys. The corticomedullary difference was relatively small and was not significantly different in the transplanted kidneys. This suggests that perfusion fraction is influenced predominantly by factors other than blood perfusion, such as tubular flow. There are no reports on the utility of DWI for the diagnosis of posttransplant complications, such as vascular complications (stenosis, thrombosis, and infarction), acute tubular necrosis, and rejection. Validation of DWI is needed in renal transplants with histopathologic correlation, given the noninvasive nature of diffusion measurement, performed without gadolinium injection.

Based on our experience, DWI could be used to demonstrate acute renal transplant infarction (**Fig. 2**), and to diagnose acute pyelonephritis (**Fig. 3**).

DWI FOR THE CHARACTERIZATION OF FOCAL RENAL LESIONS

The diagnosis of renal neoplasm is usually based on the presence of enhancement on CT or MR imaging, and image subtraction has been shown to be superior to signal intensity measurement for the diagnosis of renal cell carcinoma (RCC).[25] DWI provides qualitative and quantitative information on tissue characterization without the need for gadolinium administration, and there is a strong need for alternatives to gadolinium-enhanced sequences for renal lesion characterization for the patients at risk for nephrogenic systemic fibrosis (NSF).[26–28] However, there are limited studies on the application of DWI for the assessment of renal masses.[29–32] Solid or malignant lesions generally have lower ADC with restricted diffusion

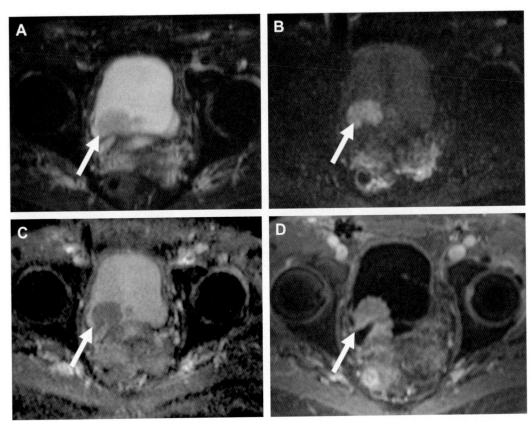

Fig. 8. Papillary urothelial carcinoma of the bladder located at the right ureterovesicular junction. The tumor is hypointense on axial single-shot echoplanar diffusion-weighted image at b = 0 sec/mm^2 (A), and hyperintense at b = 500 sec/mm^2 compared with urine (B) (arrow). The mass has restricted diffusion with lower ADC compared with urine as seen on the ADC map (C) (arrow). The mass demonstrates intense enhancement on contrast-enhanced image (D) (arrow).

compared with benign or cystic lesions, since the motion of water molecules is restricted in tissues with a high cellular density associated with numerous intact cell membranes (eg, tumor tissue), which act as barriers to motion of water molecules.

Cova and colleagues[30] applied DWI using b-values 0 and 500 sec/mm^2 for 20 focal renal lesions and compared ADC values between lesions and normal renal parenchyma: mean ADC in simple cysts (n = 13) was 3.65 ± 0.09 × 10^{-3} mm^2/sec, which was significantly higher than normal renal parenchyma (mean 2.19 ± 0.17 × 10^{-3} mm^2/sec). Solid benign and malignant tumors (three RCCs, one oncocytoma, and three angiomyolipomas [AMLs]) showed a mean ADC value of 1.55 ± 0.20 × 10^{-3} mm^2/sec, ranging between 1.28 ± 0.11 and 1.83 ± 0.14 ×10^{-3} mm^2/sec, significantly lower than normal renal parenchyma. In another study from the same group (using the same b-values), Squillaci and colleagues[29] also demonstrated lower ADC values in solid renal tumors (n = 19, including 12 RCCs) compared

with simple cysts (n = 20): 1.7 ± 0.48 versus 3.65 ± 0.09 × 10^{-3} mm^2/sec. Yoshikawa and colleagues[31] evaluated a total of 67 renal lesions (including 12 RCCs, ADC = 2.49 ± 0.72, AMLs [n = 8] 1.81 ± 0.41, cysts [n = 42] 3.82 ± 0.39, complicated cysts [n = 5] 2.78 ± 0.71 [b = 0 to 600 sec/mm^2]), and found similar results as in the previously mentioned studies[29,30]: ADCs of renal cysts were significantly higher than those of RCCs (3.82 ± 0.39 versus 2.49 ± 0.72 × 10^{-3} mm^2/sec). They found, however, no significant difference between ADCs of RCC versus complicated cysts and renal parenchyma. Recently, Zhang and colleagues[32] reported the use of DWI in solid and partially cystic renal masses (in 25 patients) using b-values of 0, 500, and 1000 sec/mm^2. Their ADC measurement method consisted first by putting large regions of interest fitting the whole lesion, and then by segmenting lesions into necrotic/cystic and solid components based on contrast-enhanced imaging. Their findings extended those reported previously (high ADC in

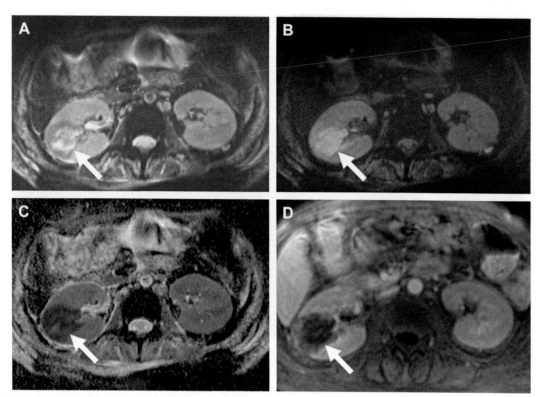

Fig. 9. A 39-year-old woman with renal abscess, a false positive of diffusion-weighted imaging. Axial single-shot echoplanar diffusion-weighted images demonstrate a hyperintense lesion with peripheral hypointense rim at b = 0 sec/mm^2 (A), the lesion is hyperintense at b = 400 sec/mm^2 (B) compared with renal parenchyma. ADC map (C) shows low ADC (1.28 ± 0.33 × 10^{-3} mm^2/sec) compared with normal parenchyma. Axial post-contrast fat-suppressed T1-weighted image obtained at the nephrographic phase (D) demonstrates a necrotic lesion with peripheral rim enhancement consistent with a renal abscess, which was subsequently confirmed by surgical drainage.

simple cysts compared with neoplasms), with the addition of finding lower ADC values in cystic/necrotic portions of neoplasms compared with simple cysts: 2.21 ± 0.63 versus 3.26 ± 061 (P < .05). However, none of the previously mentioned studies have evaluated the accuracy of DWI for renal mass characterization.

We have been using DWI systematically since 2005, and based on our experience, we believe that renal lesions can be accurately characterized with DWI, however with lower sensitivity and specificity compared with contrast-enhanced sequences. For diagnosing RCC, the AUC (area under the curve) sensitivity and specificity were 0.856, 85.7% and 80.3%, respectively for DWI (using ADC ≤ 1.92 × 10^{-3} mm^2/sec for b = 0 to 400 to 800 sec/mm^2), compared with 0.944, 100% and 88.6% for contrast-enhanced sequences (based on 99 lesions in 62 patients).

The distribution of ADC values (mean ± SD, × 10^{-3} mm^2/sec) was as follows: simple cysts (category I from the Bosniak classification)[33] (highest ADC 2.78 ± 0.45), category II (2.47 ± 0.64)

(Figs. 4–6), oncocytomas (1.91 ± 0.97), category IIF (1.85 ± 0.71), category III-IV (1.83 ± 0.85), solid RCCs (1.41 ± 0.61), and angiomyolipomas (AMLs) (0.74 ± 0.45).[34]

As in prior studies, we found RCCs (**Fig. 7**) and AMLs to have the lowest ADCs. Cystic RCCs may have higher ADC values than solid tumors due to their cystic components. The decreased ADC in AMLs can be explained by the muscular and fat components restricting diffusion.

Another interesting finding in our series was the possibility of characterizing solid neoplasms with DWI: oncocytomas having higher ADC than solid RCCs (1.91 ± 0.97 versus 1.54 ± 0.69, P < .01). Moreover, papillary RCCs demonstrated lower ADC compared with nonpapillary RCCs (mostly clear cell RCCs): 1.12 ± 0.18 versus 1.62 ± 0.73 × 10^{-3} mm^2/sec (using b-values of 0 to 400 to 800 sec/mm^2).

We have also shown that T1 hyperintense cysts (which include proteinaceous and hemorrhagic cysts) have slightly lower ADC compared with simple cysts, probably related to a T2 effect, and

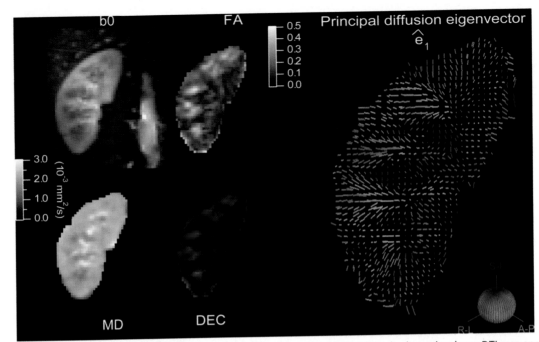

Fig.10. Diffusion tensor imaging (DTI) in a normal kidney at 3 T. Breath-hold single-shot echoplanar DTI sequence with b = 0 and 500 s/mm², using diffusion gradients in six directions. DEC and e1 maps are color coded according to standard RGB directional reference (lower right). The b0 map shows normal corticomedullary differentiation. The MD map shows slightly lower ADC in the medulla than in the surrounding cortex. Dramatic contrast between cortex and medulla appears in the FA map, where the anisotropic microstructure of the medullary tubules induces high FA values. Finally, the DEC and eigenvector maps confirm the radial orientation of the diffusion tensor in the medullary compartments, where the tubules point toward the urinary collection system at the center of the kidney. b0, T2-weighted reference image; MD, mean diffusivity (ADC map); FA, fractional anisotropy map; DEC, direction encoded color map; e1, principal diffusion eigenvector (length weighted by FA).

to restricted diffusion in hemorrhage or high protein component as described in brain hematomas.[35] However, the ADCs of T1 hyperintense benign cysts were still higher than those of T1 hyperintense RCCs: 2.50 ± 0.53 versus 1.75 ± 0.57, $P < .0001$.[36]

DWI FOR DETECTION AND FUNCTIONAL EVALUATION OF BLADDER CANCER

Bladder cancer is the most common cancer of the urinary tract, with an estimated 68,810 new cases and 14,100 deaths expected to occur in 2008.[37] Urothelial carcinoma is the most common tumor constituting over 90% of cancers.

Clinically, over 80% of patients with bladder cancer present with hematuria, either macroscopic or microscopic. All patients with macroscopic hematuria and those patients with microscopic hematuria where a benign cause has been excluded, require urologic workup. Current guidelines recommend direct evaluation of the bladder with cystoscopy and imaging evaluation of the upper tract.

DWI could be used both for detection and functional evaluation of bladder cancer, however there are extremely limited data on the subject.[38,39] Our recent experience with DWI for assessment of bladder cancer is very promising.[40] Bladder neoplasms have restricted diffusion, and are therefore easily detected in the background urine using intermediate and high b-values, with increased conspicuity (**Fig. 8**). Thus, DWI may be considered as an alternative to gadolinium contrast in patients with chronic renal insufficiency where there is increased concern for NSF.

We also demonstrated a significant correlation of ADC and normalized ADC (ADC tumor/ADC urine) with tumor grade and stage (r −0.83, $P < .001$). Normalized ADC had a sensitivity, specificity, and accuracy of 100% for prediction of tumor stage of III or higher (for a threshold nADC ≤ 0.46).

LIMITATIONS OF DWI

There are several limitations to the technique that will delay its widespread use: the ADC values are highly dependent on the parameters and the scanner used, thus the need for standardization of acquisition parameters and postprocessing methods between centers. More data are needed for the correlation between DWI and histopathology, and for its use as a predictor of treatment response. Another limitation is the lack of sensitivity and specificity of ADC measurement for the diagnosis of neoplasm, as ADC can be decreased in renal abscesses (**Fig. 9**), and falsely elevated in cystic RCCs. And last but not least, there is a need for improving image quality, for example using a combination of 3T, parallel imaging, and a navigator echo acquisition.

FUTURE DIRECTIONS

To be validated as a biomarker of treatment response, studies correlating ADC changes with response to treatment are needed (for example, post local ablation of RCC, and post neoadjuvant therapy in bladder cancer). Histogram analysis of ADC values is also worth investigating in heterogeneous cystic renal lesions. Another interesting application is the use of diffusion tensor imaging, which has the potential to shade light on the microstructure of the cortex and medulla (**Fig. 10**).

SUMMARY

In conclusion, DWI has shown promise for the assessment of focal and diffuse renal disease as well as in bladder cancer, with multiple potential applications. Advantages of DWI include the ability to characterize focal renal lesions, and the prediction of stage and grade of bladder cancer. The ability to perform DWI without intravenous gadolinium is also a major advantage of DWI. However, more supporting data comparing DWI to contrast-enhanced imaging and pathology are needed.

REFERENCES

1. Le Bihan D. Diffusion/perfusion MR imaging of the brain: from structure to function. Radiology 1990; 177:328–9.
2. Basser PJ. Inferring microstructural features and the physiological state of tissues from diffusion-weighted images. NMR Biomed 1995;8:333–44.
3. Ries M, Jones RA, Basseau F, et al. Diffusion tensor MRI of the human kidney. J Magn Reson Imaging 2001;14:42–9.
4. Callaghan PT. Principles of nuclear magnetic resonance microscopy. Oxford (United Kingdom): Oxford University Press; 1993. p. 492.
5. Hahn EL. Spin echoes. The Physical Review 1950; 80(4):580–94.
6. Stehling MK, Turner R, Mansfield P. Echo-planar imaging—magnetic-resonance-imaging in a fraction of a second. Science 1991;254:43–50.
7. Feinberg DA, Jakab PD. Tissue perfusion in humans studied by Fourier velocity distribution, line scan, and echo-planar imaging. Magn Reson Med 1990; 16:280–93.
8. Reese TG, Heid O, Weisskoff RM, et al. Reduction of eddy-current-induced distortion in diffusion MRI using a twice-refocused spin echo. Magn Reson Med 2003;49:177–82.
9. Nolte UG, Finsterbusch J, Frahm J. Rapid isotropic diffusion mapping without susceptibility artifacts: whole brain studies using diffusion-weighted single-shot STEAM MR imaging. Magn Reson Med 2000;44:731–6.
10. Bastin ME, Le Roux P. On the application of a non-CPMG single-shot fast spin-echo sequence to diffusion tensor MRI of the human brain. Magn Reson Med 2002;48:6–14.
11. Pipe JG, Farthing VG, Forbes KP. Multishot diffusion-weighted FSE using PROPELLER MRI. Magn Reson Med 2002;47:42–52.
12. Miller KL, Pauly JM. Nonlinear phase correction for navigated diffusion imaging. Magn Reson Med 2003;50:343–53.
13. Muller MF, Prasad PV, Bimmler D, et al. Functional imaging of the kidney by means of measurement of the apparent diffusion coefficient. Radiology 1994;193:711–5.
14. Siegel CL, Aisen AM, Ellis JH, et al. Feasibility of MR diffusion studies in the kidney. J Magn Reson Imaging 1995;5:617–20.
15. Ichikawa T, Haradome H, Hachiya J, et al. Diffusion-weighted MR imaging with single-shot echo-planar imaging in the upper abdomen: preliminary clinical experience in 61 patients. Abdom Imaging 1999; 24:456–61.
16. Fukuda Y, Ohashi I, Hanafusa K, et al. Anisotropic diffusion in kidney: apparent diffusion coefficient measurements for clinical use. J Magn Reson Imaging 2000;11:156–60.
17. Murtz P, Flacke S, Traber F, et al. Abdomen: diffusion-weighted MR imaging with pulse-triggered single-shot sequences. Radiology 2002;224:258–64.
18. Chow LC, Bammer R, Moseley ME, et al. Single breath-hold diffusion-weighted imaging of the abdomen. J Magn Reson Imaging 2003;18:377–82.
19. Thoeny HC, De Keyzer F, Oyen RH, et al. Diffusion-weighted MR imaging of kidneys in healthy volunteers and patients with parenchymal diseases: initial experience. Radiology 2005;235:911–7.
20. Namimoto T, Yamashita Y, Mitsuzaki K, et al. Measurement of the apparent diffusion coefficient in diffuse renal disease by diffusion-weighted echo-planar MR imaging. J Magn Reson Imaging 1999; 9:832–7.

21. Xu Y, Wang X, Jiang X. Relationship between the renal apparent diffusion coefficient and glomerular filtration rate: preliminary experience. J Magn Reson Imaging 2007;26:678–81.

22. Yildirim E, Kirbas I, Teksam M, et al. Diffusion-weighted MR imaging of kidneys in renal artery stenosis. Eur J Radiol 2008;65:148–53.

23. Chan JH, Tsui EY, Luk SH, et al. MR diffusion-weighted imaging of kidney: differentiation between hydronephrosis and pyonephrosis. Clin Imaging 2001;25:110–3.

24. Thoeny HC, Zumstein D, Simon-Zoula S, et al. Functional evaluation of transplanted kidneys with diffusion-weighted and BOLD MR imaging: initial experience. Radiology 2006;241:812–21.

25. Hecht EM, Israel GM, Krinsky GA, et al. Renal masses: quantitative analysis of enhancement with signal intensity measurements versus qualitative analysis of enhancement with image subtraction for diagnosing malignancy at MR imaging. Radiology 2004;232:373–8.

26. Grobner T. Gadolinium—a specific trigger for the development of nephrogenic fibrosing dermopathy and nephrogenic systemic fibrosis? Nephrol Dial Transplant 2006;21:1104–8.

27. Sadowski EA, Bennett LK, Chan MR, et al. Nephrogenic systemic fibrosis: risk factors and incidence estimation. Radiology 2007;243:148–57.

28. Boyd AS, Zic JA, Abraham JL. Gadolinium deposition in nephrogenic fibrosing dermopathy. J Am Acad Dermatol 2007;56:27–30.

29. Squillaci E, Manenti G, Di Stefano F, et al. Diffusion-weighted MR imaging in the evaluation of renal tumours. J Exp Clin Cancer Res 2004;23:39–45.

30. Cova M, Squillaci E, Stacul F, et al. Diffusion-weighted MRI in the evaluation of renal lesions: preliminary results. Br J Radiol 2004;77:851–7.

31. Yoshikawa T, Kawamitsu H, Mitchell DG, et al. ADC measurement of abdominal organs and lesions using parallel imaging technique. AJR Am J Roentgenol 2006;187:1521–30.

32. Zhang J, Tehrani YM, Wang L, et al. Renal masses: characterization with diffusion-weighted MR imaging—a preliminary experience. Radiology 2008; 247:458–64.

33. Israel GM, Bosniak MA. MR imaging of cystic renal masses. Magn Reson Imaging Clin N Am 2004;12: 403–12, v.

34. Taouli B, Thakur R, Mannelli L, et al. Diffusion-weighted MR imaging for characterization of renal lesions: comparison with contrast-enhanced MR imaging. Radiology; in press.

35. Silvera S, Oppenheim C, Touze E, et al. Spontaneous intracerebral hematoma on diffusion-weighted images: influence of T2-shine-through and T2-blackout effects. AJNR Am J Neuroradiol 2005;26: 236–41.

36. Kim S, Jain M, Harris AB, et al. Characterization of T1 hyperintense renal lesions: performance of diffusion-weighted MR imaging compared to contrast-enhanced MR imaging. Radiology, in press.

37. Jemal A, Siegel R, Ward E, et al. Cancer statistics, 2008. CA Cancer J Clin 2008;58:71–96.

38. Matsuki M, Inada Y, Tatsugami F, et al. Diffusion-weighted MR imaging for urinary bladder carcinoma: initial results. Eur Radiol 2007;17:201–4.

39. Yoshida S, Masuda H, Ishii C, et al. Initial experience of functional imaging of upper urinary tract neoplasm by diffusion-weighted magnetic resonance imaging. Int J Urol 2008;15:140–3.

40. Naik M, Hardie A, Chandarana H, et al. Diffusion-weighted imaging for detection and staging of urothelial neoplasms. ISMRM proceedings, 2008.

Assessment of Renal Function with Dynamic Contrast-Enhanced MR Imaging

Louisa Bokacheva, PhD[a],*, Henry Rusinek, PhD[a],
Jeff L. Zhang, PhD[a], Vivian S. Lee, MD, PhD, MBA[b]

KEYWORDS

- Dynamic contrast-enhanced MR imaging
- MR renography • Gadolinium chelates • Renal function
- Renal blood flow • Glomerular filtration rate
- Tracer kinetic modeling

The primary functions of the kidneys are to filter and excrete metabolic waste products and maintain homeostasis by regulating acid-base balance, blood pressure, and fluid volume. Assessment of renal function is often required in radiologic diagnosis, mainly for assessment of renal insufficiency, renovascular disease, renal transplants, and abdominal trauma. Noninvasive tests of renal function also can be helpful in longitudinal and translational studies.

Several noninvasive tests of renal function have been developed. These include measurements of serum creatinine level and endogenous creatinine clearance, renal scintigraphy and contrast-enhanced CT. These methods, however, have serious drawbacks. Creatinine indicators are imprecise and depend on body mass and age and cannot assess a single-kidney function. Renal scintigraphy requires radioactive tracers and provides little information about the kidney anatomy. CT has excellent spatial resolution, but exposes the patient to radiation and potentially nephrotoxic contrast agents.

MR imaging provides highly detailed anatomic information and has shown a great promise in noninvasive assessment of the renal function.[1–4] Dynamic contrast-enhanced MR imaging of the kidney, or MR renography, monitors the transit of contrast materials, typically gadolinium chelates, through the intrarenal regions, the renal cortex, the medulla, and the collecting system (**Fig. 1**). Most gadolinium contrast agents are cleared by glomerular filtration and pass from the renal vasculature into the renal tubules while enhancing the signal of the renal tissues. Typically, the kidney enhancement shows the following stages: (1) bolus arrival in the large vessels; (2) cortical enhancement (20–30 seconds after administration of contrast) that mostly reflects the contrast within renal vasculature (**Fig. 1**B); (3) medullary enhancement that usually occurs about a minute later and is dominated by the contrast in renal tubules (**Fig. 1**C); and (4) enhancement of the collecting system several minutes afterward (**Fig. 1**D). By analyzing the enhancement of the renal tissues as a function of time (**Fig. 2**), one can determine such clinically important single-kidney parameters as the renal blood flow (RBF), glomerular filtration rate (GFR), and cortical and medullary blood volumes.[5]

The most widely used gadolinium contrast agent is gadopentetate dimeglumine (Gd-DTPA).[6] It is freely filtered by the glomerulus and is neither reabsorbed nor secreted by the renal tubules, which makes it a suitable marker of glomerular filtration. Until recently, gadolinium contrast agents have been considered safe for all patients. In the past

[a] Department of Radiology, New York University School of Medicine, 660 First Avenue, New York, NY 10016, USA
[b] Department of Radiology, New York University Langone Medical Center, 560 First Avenue, New York, NY 10016, USA
* Corresponding author.
E-mail address: louisa.bokacheva@nyumc.org (L. Bokacheva).

Magn Reson Imaging Clin N Am 16 (2008) 597–611
doi:10.1016/j.mric.2008.07.001
1064-9689/08/$ – see front matter © 2008 Elsevier Inc. All rights reserved.

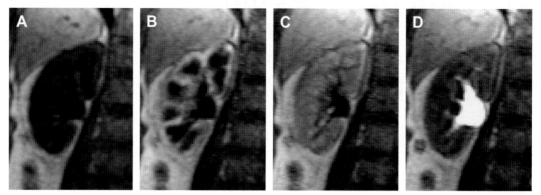

Fig. 1. Representative MR renography images of the right kidney of a 65-year-old woman with normal kidney function showing progressive enhancement of kidney tissue (injected dose 4 mL of Gd-DTPA at 2 mL/s; three-dimensional FLASH, TR/TE/FA = 2.84/1.05/12 degrees, voxel volume $1.7 \times 1.7 \times 2.5$ mm^3). (A) Unenhanced. (B) Maximum cortical enhancement. (C) Maximum medullary enhancement. (D) Collecting system enhancement.

few years, however, these contrast agents have been linked with the risk of developing nephrogenic systemic fibrosis, a debilitating and potentially fatal condition that affects patients with renal insufficiency (with total GFR<30 mL/min/1.73m^2).[7,8] So far, about 260 cases of nephrogenic systemic fibrosis have been reported worldwide.[9,10] MR renography should be performed with caution in patients with decreased renal function, and whenever possible such patients should be studied with alternative, contrast-free methods.

The MR renography studies performed to date have accumulated a wealth of physiologic and methodologic information relevant for dynamic studies of the kidneys and other abdominal organs. Several excellent reviews of functional renal imaging using MR imaging have been published by Huang and colleagues,[11] Michoux and colleagues,[12] Prasad,[13] and Michaely and colleagues.[14] This article provides an update of the recent developments in T1-weighted, gadolinium-enhanced MR renography and quantification of renal perfusion and filtration based on MR renography data.

MR RENOGRAPHY: KEY STEPS

Numerous MR renography studies have been reported in the past few years. Although there is no consensus regarding the optimal procedure, MR renography examination usually consists of the following steps: (1) acquisition of dynamic image series, (2) image postprocessing for motion correction and tissue segmentation, (3) quantification of contrast concentration, and (4) analysis of the concentration versus time data leading to

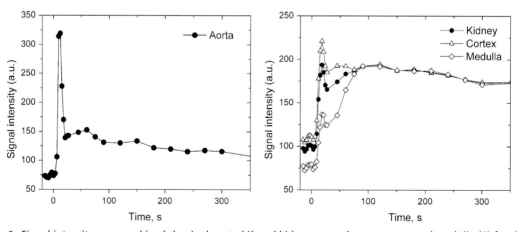

Fig. 2. Signal intensity measured in abdominal aorta (A) and kidney parenchyma, cortex, and medulla (B) for the same patient as in Fig. 1. Rapid first-pass signal changes in aorta and kidneys are sampled every 3 seconds during the first 30 seconds. The whole kidney, cortical, and medullary signal intensity curves show sharper peaks caused by renal vasculature followed by broader peaks caused by the contrast in the renal tubules.

derivation of renal functional parameters. These steps are discussed next.

Acquisition

Current MR renography studies typically use T1-weighted, gradient recalled echo sequences. Three-dimensional acquisitions provide continuous whole-kidney coverage and enable assessment of the whole-kidney function, but require longer acquisition times. Two-dimensional images can be acquired with higher temporal and spatial resolution but sample only selected slices. Also, two-dimensional acquisition of a limited number of slices precludes the use of spatial alignment (see later) because there is some anteroposterior renal motion (ie, perpendicular to the customary coronal acquisition plane).

Although most of the published work has been done at 1 to 1.5 T, higher field (3 T) offers better signal-to-noise ratio.[15] The flip angle is usually selected to maximize signal-to-noise ratio and the contrast between the enhanced and unenhanced kidney tissues.[16,17] This approach favors lower flip angles. For example, for gradient recalled echo sequence with repetition time TR = 3 milliseconds, the cortical signal with unenhanced T1 = 1000 milliseconds is estimated to be about three times higher at flip angle of 12 degrees than at 40 degrees. For an expected maximum cortical contrast concentration of 0.4 mM, the contrast between the enhanced and unenhanced cortical signals is 2.3 times higher for 12 degrees than for 40 degrees. The downside of using lower flip angles is the strong nonlinearity of signal with gadolinium concentration. As an alternative, the flip angle may be chosen to maximize the range and accuracy of the linear relationship between signal and concentration.[18,19]

One of the greatest challenges in quantitative functional imaging is the measurement of the signal in arterial blood, which plays the role of arterial input required by most tracer kinetic models. The arterial signal is usually sampled in the abdominal aorta and may be affected by the flow-related artifacts. To minimize these effects, imaging can be done in the coronal plane,[16,17] or magnetic preparation (saturation or inversion) can be added to axial acquisitions.[20–25]

After collecting several unenhanced images for a reliable estimate of baseline signal, dynamic images are acquired every few seconds during free breathing, during separate breath-holds, or as a combination of both. Rapid changes of blood and tissue signal intensities during the first-pass enhancement are best captured during breath-holding, whereas slower-changing subsequent stages may be acquired with quiet breathing or respiratory triggering.[17,25] Parallel imaging may be used to improve temporal resolution of MR renography, especially for imaging of the rapid signal changes during the first-pass perfusion, but may provide decreased image quality and is most suitable for imaging when high signal-to-noise ratio is expected.[26] The temporal resolution used in published MR renography studies varies from 1 second during the first-pass phase to 60 seconds during later (excretion) stages. In experiments on healthy volunteers performed with 1-second resolution, Michaely and colleagues[27] have shown that the temporal resolution of at least 4 seconds is required to achieve 10% precision in estimates of renal perfusion and filtration rates. Parameters describing the plasma and tubular volumes proved to be more tolerant to temporal resolution and require 9 second sampling interval to reach 10% precision. Note, however, that estimating the precision of renal functional parameters is a complex task, because the precision depends on many factors, including contrast dose and injection rate, arterial sampling scheme, and the choice of the model for parameter identification.

The total acquisition time of MR renography series is 3 to 10 minutes with longer time needed to characterize more distal portions of the nephrons. Shorter acquisition time (20–30 seconds) is sufficient for estimates of renal perfusion, intermediate acquisition time of 2 to 5 minutes for assessment of the filtration and tubular properties, and the longest acquisition time is required for characterization of the collecting system. In healthy volunteers, Michaely and colleagues[27] estimated that acquisition time of at least 35 seconds is required to characterize plasma flow, acquisition time of 85 seconds is needed for plasma volume, 230 seconds for tubular flow, and 255 seconds is needed for tubular volume characterization with precision of 10% or better. Longer acquisition times are needed in patients with decreased renal plasma flow (RPF) and GFR.

T1-mapping is sometimes performed before MR renography to determine the unenhanced T1 values of the renal tissue for quantification of contrast concentration (**Fig. 3**). Because three-dimensional T1-mapping within one breath-hold is technically challenging, this measurement is frequently done on a single representative slice through the kidney. Available T1 measurement methods include dual flip gradient echo angle technique,[17] conventional inversion recovery methods,[28] inversion-recovery prepared low-flip angle TrueFISP,[29] the Look-Locker method,[30] and T1 fast acquisition relaxation mapping.[31]

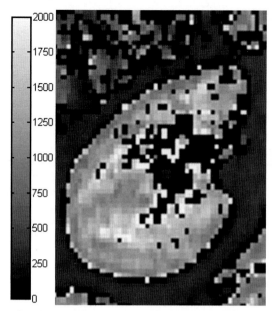

Fig. 3. Kidney T_1-map measured with single breath-hold, segmented, inversion-recovery prepared TrueFISP with flip angle of 10 degrees.[29] Cortical T_1 is about 1050 ms and medullary T_1 is about 1400–1500 ms. T_1 was set to zero in voxels where fitting failed or yielded T_1 above 2000 ms.

Contrast Dose

Many groups use standard doses of gadolinium for MR renography (0.1–0.2 mmol/kg). There is considerable evidence, however, that lower contrast doses do not compromise the precision of renal functional parameters. Using Monte Carlo simulations, the authors' group determined the relationship between the contrast dose and the precision of renography-derived GFR.[32] According to this analysis, injected doses of Gd-DTPA above approximately 1.5 to 2 mmol do not result in increased precision of GFR (Fig. 4). The highest GFR precision is achieved at approximately 0.02 mmol/kg dose in normal patients, and approximately 0.025 mmol/kg in patients with decreased renal function. Several studies demonstrated the feasibility of MR renography with ultra-low doses (ie, doses that are up to 10 times lower than the standard ones), and showed that these doses help to avoid the susceptibility effects associated with concentrated gadolinium in renal medulla and collecting system.[33,34]

Quantification of Contrast Concentration

Kinetic modeling requires that the MR renography signal be converted into gadolinium concentration. This conversion presents a challenge because in addition to contrast concentration, MR signal intensity varies with the pulse sequence parameters; the precontrast relaxation times; and in the case of blood, the flow velocity.[33] Moreover, the relationship between signal and concentration is in general nonlinear. At higher contrast concentrations, the susceptibility may cause the signal intensity to decrease with increasing concentration.

The simplest approach is to express gadolinium concentration as the relative enhancement

$$[Gd] = k\frac{S(t) - S(0)}{S(0)} \tag{1}$$

where $S(0)$ and $S(t)$ are the baseline (at time $t = 0$) and the contrast-enhanced ($t > 0$) signal intensities, respectively. The tissue-dependent constant k can be derived from phantom measurements. As the concentration increases, however, this linear relationship is associated with progressively increasing errors.

Gadolinium concentration can also be computed from analytic expressions of signal intensity. For example, the spoiled gradient echo signal intensity is given by[35]

$$S(t) = S_0 \sin\alpha \frac{1 - e^{-R_1(t)TR}}{1 - \cos\alpha \cdot e^{-R_1(t)TR}} \tag{2}$$

where S_0 is the equilibrium signal, α is the flip angle, TR is the repetition time, and $R_1 = 1/T_1$ is the longitudinal relaxation rate. Equation 2 can be solved for $R_1(t)$, enabling [Gd] to be derived from the relationship:

$$R_1(t) = R_1(0) + [Gd]r_1 \tag{3}$$

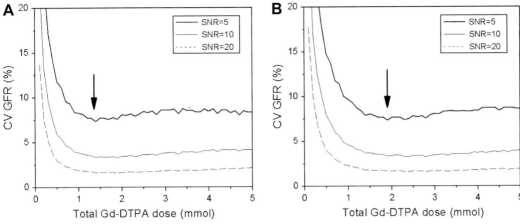

Fig. 4. The effect of gadolinium dose on precision of GFR measurement with MR renography. Coefficient of variation (CV) of GFR was estimated by Monte Carlo simulations for normal (*A*) and diseased (*B*) kidney versus the total injected dose. Arrows indicate the minimum of CV. (*Data from* Rusinek H, Lee VS, Johnson G. Optimal dose of Gd-DTPA in dynamic MR studies. Magn Reson Med 2001;46(2):312–6.)

where $R_1(0)$ is the longitudinal relaxation rate of tissue before contrast injection and r_1 is the specific relaxivity of the contrast agent. The specific relaxivity of a contrast agent required by equation 3 may depend on the surrounding medium,[36] and in vivo measurements of relaxivities are particularly challenging. Specific relaxivities of commonly used contrast agents were recently measured at different fields; temperatures; and in different media (water, saline, plasma, whole blood).[37,38] The resulting relaxivities were somewhat lower than the previously used values. Rohrer and colleagues[37] found for Gd-DTPA at 1.5 T and 37°C, $r_1 = 4.1$ (mmol/L)$^{-1}$ s^{-1} in plasma and 4.3 (mmol/L)$^{-1}$ s^{-1} in whole blood. At 3 T and 37°C, the plasma r_1 was decreased to 3.7 (mmol/L)$^{-1}$ s^{-1}. Pintaske and colleagues[38] obtained similar values, also for Gd-DTPA at 37°C in plasma: at 1.5 T r_1 was 3.9 (mmol/L)$^{-1}$ s^{-1}, and at 3 T r_1 decreased to 3.3 (mmol/L)$^{-1}$ s^{-1}.

Alternatively, the relationship between the signal intensity and T1, denoted $f(T_1)$, may be determined empirically by imaging a gadolinium-doped water phantom, either imaged separately or together with the subject.[20,21,25,39] The tissue signal intensity is assumed to be proportional to $f(T_1)$ scaled by a numerical factor g, which depends on system gain, coil sensitivity, and patient habitus:

$$S = g \cdot f(T_1) \qquad (4)$$

The coefficient g can be found from a pair of closely matched signal and T1 measurements (eg, acquired before the injection of contrast). The authors have shown that for a three-dimensional fast low angle shot (FLASH) sequence the phantom-derived $f(T_1)$ dependence is similar to

this relationship in human tissues (**Fig. 5**).[39] Compared with the concentrations determined by direct T1-mapping, concentrations calculated from in vivo MR renography signal intensity measurements agreed on average within 13% ($r = 0.99$) up to 1.4 mM when the phantom-based conversion method was used, whereas the relative enhancement conversion progressively underestimated the concentrations above 0.8 mM by 20% or more.

Signal calibrations with static phantoms do not account for all variations of the signal intensity,

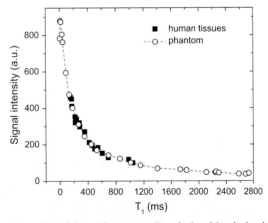

Fig. 5. Signal intensity versus T_1 relationship derived from imaging a gadolinium-doped water phantom and in vivo human tissues.[29] The signal versus T1 dependence in the phantom and human tissues seems to be similar. (*Adapted from* Bokacheva L, Rusinek H, Chen Q, et al. Quantitative determination of Gd-DTPA concentration in T1-weighted MR renography studies. Magn Reson Med 2007;57:1012–8; with permission.)

because of rapid flow in large blood vessels. The inflow of fresh blood with fully polarized spins causes the flow-related signal enhancement, which may result in incorrect arterial concentration and errors in renal functional parameters. To account for inflow effects, Ivancevic and colleagues[40] performed signal intensity versus concentration measurements at varying flow velocity in flow phantoms and applied this calibration to renal perfusion imaging. The calibration had a particularly strong effect on the concentration at the bolus peak. In the phantom, the bolus peak concentration obtained with static calibration was 3.2 times higher than the flow-corrected value, which was not significantly different from the directly measured concentration. In axial fast gradient echo acquisitions performed in patients, without the flow correction, the peak aortic concentration measured at systole was 2.5 times larger than at diastole. When flow-corrected conversion was used, the difference between systolic and diastolic measurements became insignificant. The discrepancy between systolic and diastolic measurements of the bolus peak concentration was reduced from 180% ± 37% with static calibration to 21% ± 15% with flow correction.

Coronal acquisitions may help minimize the inflow effect. As an alternative, some groups have investigated the use of population-based arterial curves.[41–43] Parker and colleagues[41] derived an average aortic curve from 67 MR imaging examinations of 23 cancer patients and obtained 40% narrower confidence intervals in repeated intraindividual measurements of perfusion parameters than with the individually measured arterial input. Wang and colleagues[42] reported an excellent correlation ($r > 0.99$) and no significant differences between perfusion parameters derived with individually measured and averaged arterial input functions sampled in femoral arteries of patients with osteosarcomas. This approach may be more successful with relatively uniform populations.

Image Analysis

MR renography image postprocessing typically consists of image coregistration and segmentation. Coregistration involves spatial aligning of the renal images at different time points [44–46], and segmentation is often required to identify the anatomic subregions of the kidney. The demands for image segmentation depend on the method of analysis. Some groups use renal cortex and others also use renal medulla signal to derive measures of renal function from MR renography. Whole kidney data are the simplest do obtain.

Absence of reliable image analysis software is one of the factors that limit implementation of MR renography in clinical practice. Segmentation may simply involve manual drawing of regions of interest.[17,20,21] Manual segmentation, however, is tedious, time-consuming, and requires anatomic expertise. Moreover, if only small subregions are sampled, the total renal volume required for GFR and RPF estimates remains unknown and the resulting enhancement curves may not be representative of the entire organ. Alternatively, using automated or semiautomated algorithms, the entire kidney may be segmented from the surrounding tissues and collecting system, and the renal parenchyma may be further divided into cortex and medulla (**Fig. 6**).[5,47–50]

A semiautomated tissue segmentation algorithm developed by Boykov and colleagues[51] enables segmentation of MR renography images into cortex, medulla, and collecting system regions based on an interactive graph cuts approach. Rusinek and colleagues[52] assessed the accuracy and precision of segmentation with this algorithm applied to simulated and in vivo data in comparison with manual segmentation performed by experienced readers. The semiautomatic segmentation produced a slight systematic oversegmentation of cortex at the expense

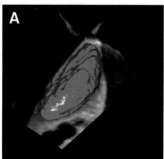 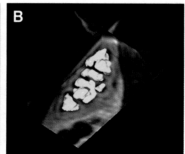 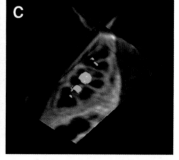

Fig. 6. Three-dimensional renderings and orthogonal views of renal tissue segmented using level sets algorithm of Song and colleagues.[47] (*A*) Whole kidney. (*B*) Medulla. (*C*) Renal pelvis.

of medulla (volume errors of about 10% in the cortex and 21% in the medulla relative to their true volumes). The precision of the segmentation was on average 5% in the cortex and 7% in the medulla. RPF and GFR derived from these data using a tracer kinetic model were determined with clinically acceptable accuracy and precision (both below 10% for RPF and below 15% for GFR). The processing time was reduced from 2 to 3 hours required for manual processing to about 21 minutes per kidney using semiautomatic segmentation.

As an alternative to tissue segmentation, a voxel-by-voxel analysis has also been applied to MR renography.[19,24,25] With this approach, the signal intensity in each voxel is traced across all time points and analyzed with an appropriate method. This approach provides local information about the kidney function and usually eliminates the need for a separate segmentation step, but is more computationally intense and more susceptible to misregistration errors and signal noise than segmentation-based analysis. Also, voxel-based analysis does not evaluate the whole-kidney function, unless followed by further processing steps.

RENAL PERFUSION QUANTIFICATION: CLINICAL APPLICATIONS

Assessment of renal perfusion is helpful in several renal diseases: for assessment of renal artery stenosis (RAS) and in renal transplant dysfunction (chronic ischemic nephropathy, drug nephropathy). Several methods have been used to quantify the renal perfusion from MR renography, such as the upslope method, semiquantitative parametric methods, deconvolution methods, and various compartmental models. It has to be noted, however, that low-molecular-weight contrast agents, such as Gd-DTPA (molecular weight 590 d), quickly leak from the bloodstream into the extracellular extravascular space and may provide incorrect estimates of perfusion. More accurate perfusion measurements may be obtained using intravascular contrast agents described in the next section.

The upslope method has been initially devised by Peters and colleagues[53] for nuclear medicine and adapted for MR imaging. It is based on a simplified picture of contrast behavior akin to microspheres: the tracer flowing into the kidney is assumed to remain in the kidney vasculature. This "inflow only" approximation is valid until the contrast begins to flow from the renal vasculature into the renal tubules. RBF can be found as the maximum slope of the kidney curve divided by the peak arterial concentration:

$$RBF = \frac{\text{maxslope }(K(t))}{\max(A(t))} \tag{5}$$

Montet and colleagues[23] used the upslope method to estimate the cortical RBF from dynamic MR imaging in nine rabbits. Reference RBF values were measured in the renal artery using an ultrasound flow probe. Experiments were performed at baseline and after a modification of the RBF by an intervention, either by mechanical RAS (ipsilateral to the flow probe) or administration of hyperosmolar agents (injections of dopamine or angiotensin II, or colloid infusion). The results demonstrated the benefits of taking into account the arterial input as opposed to using the maximum upslope of the kidney concentration curve alone as a measure of renal perfusion. The ultrasound RBF measurements correlated considerably better with the absolute RBF estimates ($r = 0.80$) than the maximum upslope of the kidney curve ($r = 0.53$).

Valée and colleagues[22] applied the upslope method to quantifying RBF in 27 subjects with normal kidneys, well-functioning renal transplants, and kidneys with RAS and renal failure. For functioning kidneys, the average blood flow was found to be 2.54 ± 1.16 mL/min/g in the cortex and 1.08 ± 0.50 mL/min/g in the medulla. In transplanted kidneys both cortical and medullary flows were increased by 30% to 40% compared with native kidneys. Compared with all functioning kidneys (native and transplant), cortical and medullary flows were 50% to 60% lower in kidneys with RAS and 70% to 80% lower in patients with renal failure.

Pedersen and colleagues[54] compared the upslope estimates of RBF in rats subjected to either unilateral renal artery occlusion or partial ureteral obstruction against rats in which the left ureter was dissected 1 hour before MR imaging (sham-operated). Normalized to the intact side, RBF on operated side was the lowest in kidneys with arterial occlusion (0.35 ± 0.02); slightly higher in kidneys with obstructed ureters (0.40 ± 0.03); and the highest in sham-operated kidneys (0.49 ± 0.01).

The advantage of the upslope method is its simplicity, whereas its main drawback is the need to measure the maximum of the arterial concentration, which is unreliable. The limited amount of data used for analysis, usually the first 20 to 30 seconds after injection, makes it more susceptible to errors, especially at low temporal resolution. The inflow-only approximation may be invalid in well-perfused kidneys beyond the first few seconds after the bolus arrival.

Feasibility of semiquantitative, parametric evaluation of patients with renal artery stenosis (RAS) was reported by Michaely and colleagues.[24] The two-dimensional data were acquired with saturation-recovery TurboFLASH sequence at 1-second temporal resolution for at least 4 minutes. High-resolution MR angiography served as the reference technique for detection and grading of RAS. Kidney enhancement curves were fitted with an empiric expression that consisted of a gamma variate function to describe the first-pass perfusion and a double-exponential function to describe the filtration. Four curve parameters were derived from voxel-by-voxel fitting: (1) time to peak, (2) mean transit time (MTT), (3) maximum upslope, and (4) maximum signal intensity. Significant differences were observed in maximum upslope, MTT, and time to peak between the combined group of normal and low-grade RAS versus the high-grade RAS, but kidneys without RAS and those with low-grade RAS could not be distinguished. MTT and time to peak correlated strongly ($r = 0.96$), and time to peak and maximum upslope showed moderate negative correlation ($r = -0.6$). Highly significant, but moderate correlations were found between all four parameters and serum creatinine (r approximately 0.4–0.5). Maximum upslope voxel maps enabled detection of segmental perfusion deficits in three kidneys in areas confirmed to be ischemic by biopsy.

Deconvolution approach to calculation of renal perfusion and filtration was used by Hermoye and colleagues.[21] MR renography experiments were performed in six rabbits with a saturation-prepared turbo field echo sequence at 1.1-second temporal resolution. After phantom-based conversion, the arterial input was numerically deconvolved from the cortical curve. The resulting cortical impulse response function was expected to exhibit three peaks corresponding to the contrast passing sequentially through the glomeruli, proximal convoluted tubules, and distal tubules. The vascular and the proximal tubules peaks were fitted by a sum of two gamma variate functions. The fractional plasma volume and the vascular MTT were determined from the area under the curve and the washout rate of the vascular curve. The renal perfusion was found as the ratio of fractional plasma volume to MTT and correlated well with the results of the upslope method ($r = 0.9$). As expected for numerical deconvolution, the errors in RPF and other parameters were shown to increase dramatically with noise level. At 5% noise, the error in RPF was about 20% relative to the ideal value, and at 10% it increased to about 50%.

The feasibility of voxel-based deconvolution analysis of MR renography in human kidneys was demonstrated by Dujardin and colleagues.[19] The perfusion parameters were determined in 14 volunteers and 1 transplant patient using inversion-recovery prepared TurboFLASH sequence. A flip angle of 50 degrees was used to improve the linearity of the signal versus concentration. The arterial input function was numerically deconvolved from the renal curves to determine the impulse response function in every voxel. The maximum of the impulse response function, the area under the impulse response function curve, and the ratio of the integral to the maximum were respectively interpreted as RBF, renal volume of distribution, and MTT. The average shape of observed impulse response function was similar to that obtained by Hermoye and colleagues.[21] In native kidneys RBF was 1.6 mL/min/mL and ranged from 0.8 and 4.5 mL/min/mL. Cortical RBF was found to be three times higher than the medullary RBF. Both the perfusion and the cortex-to-medulla ratio were lower than those reported elsewhere.[55,56] This underestimation was attributed to deconvolution errors, dispersion of the aortic bolus, and the inflow artifact in the aorta.

A two-compartment model proposed by Annet and colleagues,[20] in which the concentration in renal vascular compartment is determined by dispersion and delay of the aortic bolus, enables calculation of vascular volume and RBF (**Fig. 7**). The experiments of Annet and colleagues,[20] however, focused on assessing renal filtration, and perfusion estimates were not reported.

The reviewed results suggest that both semiquantitative and fully quantitative measures of perfusion can be useful in assessment of renal function. Semiquantitative parameters, such as the time to peak and maximum upslope, are usually robust and easy to assess, but have limited physiologic interpretation and cannot always be compared across different patients. The quantitative perfusion methods include simple inflow models, compartmental models, and deconvolution methods. The upslope method is simple, but relies on the initial part of the first-pass peak, which often contains just few data points, and on the inflow-only approximation, which may not be valid in the kidney beyond the first few seconds after the bolus arrival. The numerical deconvolution methods are sensitive to noise, more so than the compartmental models. All of the quantitative methods require measurements of the arterial input function, which may be unreliable because of sampling errors and inflow artifacts. Because the arterial input function is usually sampled in the aorta, the dispersion and delay of the bolus

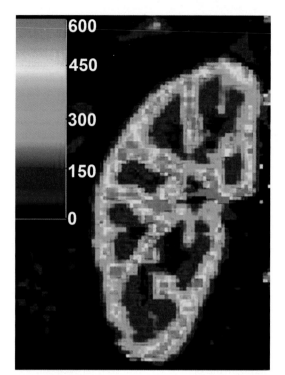

Fig. 7. Perfusion map calculated with two-compartment model of Annet and colleagues[20] in a normally functioning kidney. The units of the color bar are mL/min/100 mL. The regions of extremely high flow (*red*) are likely to reflect the renal vessels.

confounds the modeling. As a result, renal perfusion estimates are highly sensitive to the variations of the arterial input. Comparisons of the MR renography–derived perfusion against other established methods are needed.

Renal Perfusion Imaging using Intravascular Contrast Agents

Unlike the low-molecular-weight contrast agents, such as Gd-DTPA, which quickly distribute over the interstitial space, the so-called "intravascular contrast agents" stay in the bloodstream for a considerably longer time. Because these agents have not yet been approved for clinical use, data mostly from animal experiments are available, although few human studies also have been reported.

Prasad and colleagues[57] reported perfusion measurements using MS-325 (EPIX Medical, Cambridge, Massachusetts), a gadolinium-based intravascular contrast agent that binds to serum albumin in plasma. Protein binding reduces leakage of contrast out of the vasculature and increases the half-life of contrast in plasma. Pigs with surgically induced RAS were injected with MS-325 and imaged with turbo-FLASH sequence,

and cortical blood flow and MTT were estimated from the first-pass perfusion data using the upslope method. The resulting perfusion measurements agreed well with the reference microsphere experiments (258 mL/100 g/min versus 198 mL/100 g/min, respectively), but neither indicated any significant reduction in cortical perfusion over 5 weeks after surgery, which may be attributed to the ability of the kidney to regulate blood flow.

Aumann and colleagues[55] used the intravenous ultrasmall particle iron oxide contrast agent NC100150 to measure perfusion in eight dogs with ultrasound flow probes implanted at the origin of the left renal artery. This agent is cleared from blood by reticuloendothelial system and is not at all filtered by the kidney. As a result, the kidney enhancement reflects only perfusion and is free from the effects of filtration and excretion. Dynamic imaging was performed with a T2*-weighted FLASH sequence (TR/TE/FA=15/6/12 degrees, temporal resolution 1.92 seconds), and ultrasound flow measurement was done immediately before and after the MR imaging measurement. Voxel-based renal perfusion yielded RBF of 524 ± 47 mL/min/100 g versus the ultrasound-measured value of 403 ± 72 mL/min/100 g with moderate correlation ($r = 0.71$). The renal blood volume was found to be 27 ± 3.6 mL/100 g and the MTT was 3.4 ± 0.5 seconds. The MR imaging perfusion measurements overestimated both the blood flow and the blood volume compared with generally accepted values.

In a subsequent study, Schoenberg and colleagues[56] applied a similar measurement technique and the same contrast agent to dogs with surgically induced RAS and in humans with long-standing RAS. The baseline RBF in dogs was 496 mL/min/100 g and remained almost unchanged for stenosis up to 50% and decreased to 379 mL/min/100 g at stenosis of 80%. At further reduction of renal artery diameter to above 90%, RBF dropped to 151 mL/min/100 g. In human kidneys with parenchymal damage caused by RAS, RBF was considerably lower than in normal kidneys (166 mL/min/100 g versus 379 mL/min/100 g, respectively), whereas the blood volume was slightly lower in kidneys with RAS than in normal ones.

GLOMERULAR FILTRATION RATE

A variety of methods have been proposed for quantification of renal filtration, ranging from simpler upslope models, to more complex compartmental models (**Fig. 8**). These models share some common assumptions. The kidney is usually represented as a combination of at least two

A

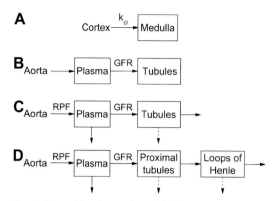

Fig. 8. Tracer kinetic renal models for GFR calculation: (A) Baumann-Rudin model. (B) Patlak-Rutland model. (C) Two-compartment models of Annet and colleagues[20] and Buckley and colleagues.[17] (D) Three-compartment models of Lee and colleagues[5] and Zhang and colleagues.[63] Aorta, cortex, and medulla are concentrations in blood and renal tissues; plasma, tubules, proximal tubules, and loops of Henle are intra-renal compartments; solid arrows, flow of contrast; dashed arrows, flow of contrast-free fluid.

homogeneous compartments, vascular and tubular, and GFR is found as the flow of contrast from the vascular into the tubular compartment.

Baumann and Rudin[58] proposed an inflow-only model in which the contrast flows from cortex to medulla with the rate given by the filtration coefficient (**Fig. 8A**). The cortex plays the role of the vascular compartment, and the medulla that of the tubular compartment. The outflow of contrast from the medulla is ignored. In experiments on rats, Laurent and colleagues[59] have shown that the filtration coefficient correlated with GFR measured by inulin clearance ($r = 0.75$). A related model has been recently proposed by Zhang and colleagues.[60] Both Baumann-Rudin and Zhang models have an attractive property of not requiring the arterial input function.

Adapted from cerebral perfusion, the Patlak-Rutland method has been applied for GFR calculations. This method is based on a two-compartment model, in which the outflow from the second, tubular compartment is ignored (**Fig. 8B**). In its traditional graphical implementation, the ratio of kidney K(t) to aortic concentration Ao(t) is plotted versus the ratio of the integral of Ao(t) to Ao(t). GFR is found as the slope of the linear regression to this curve and the vascular volume fraction as its intercept. Resulting GFR depends on the choice of the time interval used in computing the linear regression. In MR renography experiments on healthy volunteers and using slower contrast injections, Hackstein and colleagues[61] found that GFR values determined from the interval of 30 to

90 seconds correlated best with reference measurements. This interval coincides with the uptake of contrast by the renal tubules in a normal kidney (see **Fig. 1**). The correlation of Patlak-Rutland GFRs with the reference improved considerably at higher contrast doses and reached $r = 0.83$ at 16 mL of Gd-DTPA (in commercially available 500-mM dilution). This finding suggests that the Patlak-Rutland method may not be optimal for low-dose MR renography experiments or for protocols that provide a lower number of acquisitions within the tubular uptake interval.

Buckley and colleagues[17] compared GFRs estimated with the Patlak-Rutland method and its extension, a two-compartment model (inspired by the widely used cancer perfusion models[62]) in which the outflow from the tubules is accounted for (**Fig. 8C**). Both methods were applied to 35 patients with atherosclerotic renovascular disease. Dynamic three-dimensional images were acquired with gradient recalled echo sequence during free breathing at 4.5-second temporal resolution for up to 3.5 minutes. Data were extracted from a region of interest drawn around the kidney parenchyma on a single mid-coronal slice. Arterial input was measured in the abdominal aorta. Single-kidney GFR values obtained by both methods correlated significantly with the reference GFRs measured by ^{51}Cr-EDTA clearance and renal scintigraphy: Spearman correlation coefficient was $\rho = 0.81$ for Patlak-Rutland and $\rho = 0.71$ for the extended model. The extended model overestimated GFR by almost 100%, whereas the Patlak-Rutland method overestimated them by about 30%. Such overestimation may be caused by the use of a single mid-kidney slice, in which the volume fraction of medulla is higher than in peripheral slices. The subjects' mean global reference GFR was only 35 mL/min, which suggests severely decreased renal function. In such patients, the kidney uptake is low and slow, and the interval of 3.5 minutes may not be sufficient to characterize the outflow from the tubules, which may cause unreliable fitting with the compartmental model.

Higher GFR values produced by a compartmental model relative to the Patlak-Rutland model were first observed by Annet and colleagues.[20] Experimenting on rabbits, this group analyzed the cortical concentration curves with the Patlak-Rutland method and a two-compartment model that accounts for tubular outflow and the spread of the bolus in the renal vasculature (see **Fig. 8C**). Unlike Buckley and colleagues,[17] GFR obtained from Annet's model underestimated the reference GFR measured by[51] Cr-EDTA clearance. The extended model correlated better with reference GFRs ($r = 0.82$) than the Patlak-Rutland method ($r = 0.74$). The relationship between the two methods was similar to that found by Buckley and colleagues[17] (ie, lower GFRs were obtained with the Patlak-Rutland method compared with the extended model). The latter is likely caused by neglecting the outflow in the Patlak-Rutland method.

Similar results were obtained by Sourbron and colleagues[25] in 15 healthy volunteers, whose MR renography images were analyzed voxel-wise with both the Patlak-Rutland model and the two-compartment model similar to that of Annet and colleagues.[20] Both cortical and whole-kidney perfusion and filtration flows were determined. In agreement with Annet and colleagues[20] and Buckley and colleagues,[17] the full inflow-outflow model applied to whole-kidney data provided higher rates of perfusion (229 mL/min/100 mL) and filtration (31 mL/min/100 mL) than the Patlak-Rutland model (210 mL/ min/100 mL and 24 mL/min/100 mL, respectively). Cortical data provided higher perfusion, but lower filtration flow values (340 and 21 mL/min/100 mL with compartmental model; 331 and 15 mL/min/100 mL with the Patlak-Rutland model).

A three-compartment model proposed by the authors' group[5] makes use of separate cortical and medullary curves derived from segmented three-dimensional kidney images (**Fig. 8D**). Each tissue is thought to include the contributions from two compartments: a shared vascular compartment and a tubular compartment, proximal tubules in the cortex, and loops of Henle in the medulla. As in other renal models, the concentration in abdominal aorta provides the input function and is used to infer the concentration in the vascular compartment from which the contrast passes into the proximal tubules and then into the loops. Besides RPF and GFR, this model also yields cortical and medullary vascular volume fractions and fractions of contrast-free flow reabsorbed in proximal tubules and loops. Applied to three-dimensional MR renography data of 10 patients (20 kidneys) imaged using three-dimensional FLASH (TR/TE/FA = 2.84/1.05/12 degrees), the model produced GFRs in good correlation with the reference measurements from 99mTc-DTPA clearance and scintigraphy ($r = 0.84$; or $r = 0.93$ without one outlier kidney with multiple renal cysts) and a slight underestimation of GFR. As estimated by Monte Carlo simulations, for 5% concentration noise, the errors in RPF and GFR were approximately 10% and 5%, respectively, for a well-functioning kidney, and slightly lower for a dysfunctional kidney. The errors were below 12% for vascular volumes, but much higher in reabsorbed fractions (23%–30% in healthy case and over 300% in dysfunctional kidney). The model was also shown to provide robust estimates of GFR for different widths of aortic inputs.

To account for noninstantaneous mixing of contrast, Zhang and colleagues extended this model by considering a minimum transit time that is required for tracer to traverse each compartment into a model based on the same arrangement of compartments as the previous model (see **Fig. 8D**).[63] The model provides seven free parameters, including RPF, GFR, minimum transit times, and MTTs. Zhang's model yields significantly better curve fits: the average relative root mean square error was 11.6% versus 15.5% obtained by the model of Lee and colleagues.[5] Importantly, the model of Zhang and colleagues[60] provided substantially more reliable fitting of the data from dysfunctional kidneys (**Fig. 9**). Despite the higher number of parameters, their stability in the presence of the data noise was also improved, with errors in both RPF and GFR lower than 3% for both well-functioning and diseased kidneys. There was a good correlation of model-derived GFRs against radionuclide measurements ($r = 0.82$; or r = 0.92 without the outlier kidney) similar to that obtained with Lee and colleagues[5] model, although the GFR values were more strongly underestimated (on average by 41% versus 34% by Lee and colleagues[5] model) (**Fig. 10**).

Glomerular Filtration Rate Quantification from Clearance Measurements

Choyke and colleagues[1] compared GFR measured from clearance of 99mTc-DTPA (GFR$_{Tc}$) with GFR determined from clearance of Gd-DTPA (GFR$_{Gd}$) in 90 patients based on three urine and blood samples calculated using the standard clearance equation

$$GFR_{contrast} = \frac{F \cdot U}{P} \tag{6}$$

where F is the urine flow rate, and U and P are the concentrations of contrast in urine and plasma, respectively. The concentrations of Gd-DTPA in urine and plasma were determined by measurements of the T1 values of both fluids using nuclear MR spectrometer and an experimentally derived relationship to convert T1 into Gd-DTPA concentration. The correlation of GFR$_{Gd}$ and GFR$_{Tc}$ was high ($r = 0.94$) and the coefficient of variation of their differences was only 3.6%. A similar study was performed by Ros and colleagues[2] to determine GFR from plasma clearance of Gd-DTPA with MR angiography and MR renography. Again, the correlation between GFR$_{Gd}$ and GFR$_{Tc}$ was

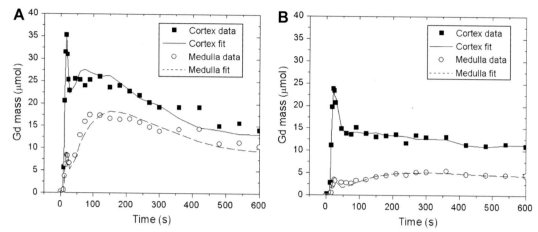

Fig. 9. Gadolinium residue (mass) in the cortex and medulla of a functioning kidney (*A*) and a diseased kidney (*B*) fitted by the three-compartment model of Zhang and colleagues.[63] Cortical and medullary residues are considerably lower in diseased kidney (*B*) than in the functioning kidney (*A*), but Zhang's model provides good curve fits in both cases. (*Adapted from* Zhang JL, Rusinek H, Bokacheva L, et al. Functional assessment of the kidney from MR and CT renography: impulse retention approach to a multicompartment model. Magn Reson Med 2008;59:278–88; with permission.)

found to be high ($r = 0.98$) and the standard error was 3.85 mL/min.

Boss and colleagues[64] measured GFR by capturing the clearance of gadobutrol from kidney and liver tissues of healthy volunteers over a long period of time (70 minutes) using a navigator-gated turbo-FLASH sequence. The rate of exponential decrease of MR imaging signal intensity with time is equal to the ratio of GFR and extracellular fluid volume, with the latter estimated from the weight and height of the subjects. The best estimates of GFR were obtained from measurements between 40 and 65 minutes after the injection of contrast, as compared with the simultaneous measurements of iopromide clearance from plasma, and were found to be within 5.9 ± 14.6 mL/min from the reference values. The mean half-life time of gadobutrol in renal cortex was found to be 92.6 ± 23.7 minutes. This approach to measurements of GFR has a number of limitations, such as the long imaging time and resulting susceptibility to motion artifacts, the reliance on the subject's height and weight to estimate the extracellular fluid volume, and inability to provide the differential renal function.

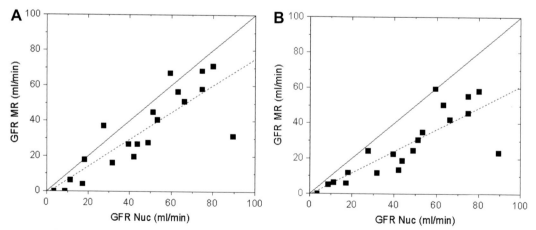

Fig. 10. Single-kidney GFRs obtained from the same data using models of Lee and colleagues[5] (*A*) and Zhang and colleagues[63] (*B*) versus the GFR values from the same-day nuclear medicine measurements. Both models underestimate GFR, especially Zhang's model, but provide comparable correlations with radionuclide measurements. The linear regressions (*dashed lines*) are $y = 0.76x - 1.14$ ($r = 0.84$) (*A*) and $y = 0.61x - 0.32$ ($r = 0.82$) (*B*). Solid lines are the identity lines.

LIMITATIONS AND FUTURE DIRECTIONS

MR renography suffers from several limitations. One fundamental limitation of MR renography is the decrease of signal-to-noise ratio with decreasing kidney function, because the uptake of contrast in diseased kidneys is reduced compared with normal kidneys. MR renography studies of diseased kidneys may not be able to provide as much information as those of well-functioning kidneys. Determination of physiologic parameters from MR renography data requires several steps, including acquisition, image analysis, signal-to-concentration conversion, and tracer kinetic modeling. Each of these steps may contribute errors to the final results. Currently, there is no agreement regarding the best acquisition and analysis schemes. The tools for image analysis of dynamic data must be improved. Tracer kinetic models for analysis of renal data provide varying results despite many shared assumptions and these variations have not been reconciled. Most tracer kinetic models require measurements of arterial input function, which requires acquisitions with high temporal resolution and may suffer from inflow artifacts. Studies verifying MR renography–derived kidney parameters against reference measurements are scarce.

Future work includes overcoming these challenges and designing optimal protocols and tools for comprehensive analysis of MR renography data, including coregistration, segmentation, and voxel-based modeling. Shared solutions to these challenges may pave the way for multicenter studies to validate MR renography and establish its use in the clinical setting.

SUMMARY

Quantitative evaluation of renal function, most importantly perfusion and filtration, is often required for diagnosis and monitoring of vascular diseases, hypertension, obesity, diabetes, renal transplantation, and obstruction of the urinary tract. In research settings, MR renography has been shown to provide excellent anatomic detail and functional information in a single examination. MR renography has been researched since the late 1990s and particularly actively in the past few years when the imaging technology has matured to provide dynamic acquisitions with adequate spatial resolution and temporal resolution of a few seconds. Numerous studies reported measurements of renal perfusion and filtration with promising results. The results tend to vary greatly among groups and are difficult to compare because there is little agreement regarding the

optimal experimental technique. Also in need of improvement are the image analysis tools for post-processing of large dynamic datasets. Greater understanding of the analytic methods, such as tracer kinetic models, is essential, as are the validation studies comparing the MR renography–derived functional parameters with those determined by established measurement techniques. Nevertheless, recent developments in MR renography are highly encouraging and it is hoped will lead to a consensus methodology. The implementation of MR renography in clinical practice has been hindered, however, because of the recently established connection between exposure to gadolinium contrast agents and developing nephrogenic systemic fibrosis in patients with renal insufficiency. Such patients may be evaluated using MR renography enhanced with macrocyclic contrast agents or by contrast-free methods, such as arterial spin labeling and blood oxygenation level dependent imaging.

With the development of reliable methods, MR imaging can become a one-stop modality that combines morphologic assessment with quantitative functional measures. Although further research is clearly needed to develop a clinically useful strategy, MR renography has the potential to become the leading diagnostic method for renal disease.

REFERENCES

1. Choyke PL, Austin HA, Frank JA, et al. Hydrated clearance of gadolinium-DTPA as a measurement of glomerular filtration rate. Kidney Int 1992;41:1595–8.
2. Ros PR, Gauger J, Stoupis C, et al. Diagnosis of renal artery stenosis: feasibility of combining MR angiography, MR renography, and gadopentetate-based measurements of glomerular filtration rate. AJR Am J Roentgenol 1995;165(6):1447–51.
3. Szolar DH, Preidler K, Ebner F, et al. Functional magnetic resonance imaging of human renal allografts during the post-transplant period: preliminary observations. Magn Reson Imaging 1997;15(7):727–35.
4. Wolf GL, Hoop B, Cannillo JA, et al. Measurement of renal transit of gadopentetate dimeglumine with echo-planar MR imaging. J Magn Reson Imaging 1994;4(3):365–72.
5. Lee VS, Rusinek H, Bokacheva L, et al. Renal function measurements from MR renography and a simplified multicompartmental model. Am J Physiol Renal Physiol 2007;292:F1548–59.
6. Knopp MV, Balzer T, Esser M, et al. Assessment of utilization and pharmacovigilance based on spontaneous adverse event reporting of gadopentetate dimeglumine as a magnetic resonance contrast

agent after 45 million administrations and 15 years of clinical use. Invest Radiol 2006;41(6):491–9.

7. Sadowski EA, Bennett LK, Chan MR, et al. Nephrogenic systemic fibrosis: risk factors and incidence estimation. Radiology 2007;243(1):148–57.

8. Grobner T. Gadolinium: a specific trigger for the development of nephrogenic fibrosing dermopathy and nephrogenic systemic fibrosis? Nephrol Dial Transplant 2006;21(4):1104–8.

9. Kuo PH. Gadolinium-containing MRI contrast agents: important variations on a theme for NSF. J Am Coll Radiol 2008;5(1):29–35.

10. DeHoratius DM, Cowper SE. Nephrogenic systemic fibrosis: an emerging threat among renal patients. Semin Dial 2006;19(3):191–4.

11. Huang AJ, Lee VS, Rusinek H. Functional renal MR imaging. Magn Reson Imaging Clin N Am 2004;12:469–86.

12. Michoux N, Vallée J-P, Pechère-Bertschi A, et al. Analysis of contrast-enhanced MR images to assess renal function. MAGMA 2006;19:167–79.

13. Prasad PV. Functional MRI of the kidney: tools for translational studies of pathophysiology of renal disease. Am J Physiol Renal Physiol 2006;290(5):F958–74.

14. Michaely HJ, Herrmann KA, Nael K, et al. Functional renal imaging: nonvascular renal disease. Abdom Imaging 2007;32(1):1–16.

15. Michaely HJ, Kramer H, Oesingmann N, et al. Intraindividual comparison of MR-renal perfusion imaging at 1.5 T and 3.0 T. Invest Radiol 2007;42(6):406–11.

16. Lee VS, Rusinek H, Noz M, et al. Dynamic three-dimensional MR renography for the measurement of single kidney function: initial experience. Radiology 2003;227:289–94.

17. Buckley DL, Shurrab A, Cheung CM, et al. Measurement of single kidney function using dynamic contrast-enhanced MRI: comparison of two models in human subjects. J Magn Reson Imaging 2006;24:1117–23.

18. Hackstein N, Heckrodt J, Rau WS. Measurement of single-kidney glomerular filtration rate using a contrast-enhanced dynamic gradient-echo sequence and the Rutland-Patlak plot technique. J Magn Reson Imaging 2003;18:714–25.

19. Dujardin M, Sourbron S, Luypaert R, et al. Quantification of renal perfusion and function on a voxel-by-voxel basis: a feasibility study. Magn Reson Med 2005;54(4):841–9.

20. Annet L, Hermoye L, Peeters F, et al. Glomerular filtration rate: assessment with dynamic contrast-enhanced MRI and a cortical-compartment model in the rabbit kidney. J Magn Reson Imaging 2004;20:843–9.

21. Hermoye L, Annet L, Lemmerling P, et al. Calculation of the renal perfusion and glomerular filtration rate from the renal impulse response obtained with MRI. Magn Reson Med 2004;51:1017–25.

22. Vallée JP, Lazeyras F, Khan HG, et al. Absolute renal blood flow quantification by dynamic MRI and Gd-DTPA. Eur Radiol 2000;10(8):1245–52.

23. Montet X, Ivancevic MK, Belenger J, et al. Noninvasive measurement of absolute renal perfusion by contrast medium-enhanced magnetic resonance imaging. Invest Radiol 2003;38(9):584–92.

24. Michaely HJ, Schoenberg SO, Oesingmann N, et al. Renal artery stenosis: functional assessment with dynamic MR perfusion measurements-feasibility study. Radiology 2006;238:586–96.

25. Sourbron SP, Michaely HJ, Reiser MF, et al. MRI-measurement of perfusion and glomerular filtration in the human kidney with a separable compartment model. Invest Radiol 2008;43(1):40–8.

26. Michaely HJ, Kramer H, Oesingmann N, et al. Semiquantitative assessment of first-pass renal perfusion at 1.5 T: comparison of 2D saturation recovery sequences with and without parallel imaging. AJR Am J Roentgenol 2007;188(4):919–26.

27. Michaely HJ, Sourbron SP, Buettner C, et al. Temporal constraints in renal perfusion imaging with a 2-compartment model. Invest Radiol 2008;43(2):120–8.

28. Hahn E. An accurate nuclear magnetic resonance method for measuring spin-lattice relaxation times. Physiol Rev 1949;76:145–6.

29. Bokacheva L, Huang AJ, Chen Q, et al. Single breath-hold T1 measurement using low flip angle TrueFISP. Magn Reson Med 2006;55(5):1186–90.

30. Look D, Dr L. Time saving in measurement of NMR and EPR relaxation times. Rev Sci Instrum 1970;41:250–1.

31. Chen Z, Prato FS, McKenzie C. T1 fast acquisition relaxation mapping (T1-FARM): an optimized reconstruction. IEEE Trans Med Imaging 1998;17(2):155–60.

32. Rusinek H, Lee VS, Johnson G. Optimal dose of Gd-DTPA in dynamic MR studies. Magn Reson Med 2001;46(2):312–6.

33. Taylor J, Summers PE, Keevil SF, et al. Magnetic resonance renography: optimisation of pulse sequence parameters and Gd-DTPA dose, and comparison with radionuclide renography. Magn Reson Imaging 1997;15(6):637–49.

34. Lee VS, Rusinek H, Johnson G, et al. MR renography with low-dose gadopentetate dimeglumine: feasibility. Radiology 2001;221(2):371–9.

35. Haacke EM, Brown RW, Thompson MR, et al. Fast imaging in the steady state: physical principles and sequence design. New York: Wiley-Liss; 1999. p. 451-67.

36. Stanisz GJ, Henkelman RM. Gd-DTPA relaxivity depends on macromolecular content. Magn Reson Med 2000;44(5):665–7.

37. Rohrer M, Bauer H, Mintorovitch J, et al. Comparison of magnetic properties of MRI contrast media

solutions at different magnetic field strengths. Invest Radiol 2005;40(11):715–24.

38. Pintaske J, Martirosian P, Graf H, et al. Relaxivity of gadopentetate dimeglumine (Magnevist), gadobutrol (Gadovist), and gadobenate dimeglumine (MultiHance) in human blood plasma at 0.2, 1.5, and 3 Tesla. Invest Radiol 2006;41(3):213–21.

39. Bokacheva L, Rusinek H, Chen Q, et al. Quantitative determination of Gd-DTPA concentration in T1-weighted MR renography studies. Magn Reson Med 2007;57:1012–8.

40. Ivancevic MK, Zimine I, Montet X, et al. Inflow effect correction in fast gradient-echo perfusion imaging. Magn Reson Med 2003;50(5):885–91.

41. Parker GJ, Roberts C, Macdonald A, et al. Experimentally-derived functional form for a population-averaged high-temporal-resolution arterial input function for dynamic contrast-enhanced MRI. Magn Reson Med 2006;56(5):993–1000.

42. Wang Y, Huang W, Panicek DM, et al. Feasibility of using limited-population-based arterial input function for pharmacokinetic modeling of osteosarcoma dynamic contrast-enhanced MRI data. Magn Reson Med 2008;59(5):1183–9.

43. Yankeelov TE, Lepage M, Chakravarthy A, et al. Integration of quantitative DCE-MRI and ADC mapping to monitor treatment response in human breast cancer: initial results. Magn Reson Imaging 2007;25(1):1–13.

44. Giele EL, de Priester JA, Blom JA, et al. Movement correction of the kidney in dynamic MRI scans using FFT phase difference movement detection. J Magn Reson Imaging 2001;14(6):741–9.

45. Gerig G, Kikinis R, Kuoni W, et al. Semiautomated ROI analysis in dynamic MR studies. Part I: image analysis tools for automatic correction of organ displacements. J Comput Assist Tomogr 1991;15(5):725–32.

46. Yim PJ, Marcos HB, Choyke PL, et al. Registration of time-series contrast enhanced magnetic resonance images for renography. Proceedings of the 14th IEEE Symposium on Computer-Based Medical Systems (CMBS): 2001:516–20.

47. Song T, Lee VS, Rusinek H, et al. Four dimensional MR image analysis of dynamic renography. Conf Proc IEEE Eng Med Biol Soc 2006;1:3134–7.

48. Yuksel SE, El-Baz A, Farag AA, et al. A kidney segmentation framework for dynamic contrast enhanced magnetic resonance imaging. Journal of Vibration and Control 2007;13(9–10):1505–16.

49. Ali AM, Farag AA, Ell-Baz AS. Graph cuts framework for kidney segmentation with prior shape constraints. Med Image Comput Comput Assist Interv Int Conf Med Image Comput Comput Assist Interv 2007;10(Pt 1):384–92.

50. de Priester JA, den Boer JA, Giele EL, et al. MR renography: an algorithm for calculation and correction of cortical volume averaging in medullary renographs. J Magn Reson Imaging 2000;12:453–9.

51. Boykov Y, Lee V, Rusinek H, et al. Segmentation of dynamic N-D data sets via graph cuts using Markov models. Proceedings of the 16th Annual Meeting of ISMRM. Toronto, Canada, May 3–9, 2008.

52. Rusinek H, Boykov Y, Kaur M, et al. Performance of an automated segmentation algorithm for 3D MR renography. Magn Reson Med 2007;57:1159–67.

53. Peters AM, Gunasekera RD, Henderson BL, et al. Noninvasive measurement of blood flow and extraction fraction. Nucl Med Commun 1987;8(10):823–37.

54. Pedersen M, Shi Y, Anderson P, et al. Quantitation of differential renal blood flow and renal function using dynamic contrast-enhanced MRI in rats. Magn Reson Med 2004;51(3):510–7.

55. Aumann S, Schoenberg SO, Just A, et al. Quantification of renal perfusion using an intravascular contrast agent (part 1): results in a canine model. Magn Reson Med 2003;49(2):276–87.

56. Schoenberg SO, Aumann S, Just A, et al. Quantification of renal perfusion abnormalities using an intravascular contrast agent (part 2): results in animals and humans with renal artery stenosis. Magn Reson Med 2003;49(2):288–98.

57. Prasad PV, Cannillo J, Chavez DR, et al. First-pass renal perfusion imaging using MS-325, an albumin-targeted MRI contrast agent. Invest Radiol 1999;34(9):566–71.

58. Baumann D, Rudin M. Quantitative assessment of rat kidney function by measuring the clearance of the contrast agent Gd(DOTA) using dynamic MRI. Magn Reson Imaging 2000;18:587–95.

59. Laurent D, Poirier K, Wasvary J, et al. Effect of essential hypertension on kidney function as measured in rat by dynamic MRI. Magn Reson Med 2004;47:127–34.

60. Zhang JL, Rusinek H, Chen Q, et al. Assessment of renal function using MR renography without aortic input information. In: Proceedings of the 16th Annual Meeting of ISMRM. Toronto, Canada; 2008. p. 456.

61. Hackstein N, Kooijman H, Tomaselli S, et al. Glomerular filtration rate measured using the Patlak plot technique and contrast-enhanced dynamic MRI with different amounts of gadolinium-DTPA. J Magn Reson Imaging 2005;22(3):406–14.

62. Tofts PS, Brix G, Buckley DL, et al. Estimating kinetic parameters from dynamic contrast-enhanced T(1)-weighted MRI of a diffusable tracer: standardized quantities and symbols. J Magn Reson Imaging 1999;10(3):223–32.

63. Zhang JL, Rusinek H, Bokacheva L, et al. Functional assessment of the kidney from MR and CT renography: impulse retention approach to a multicompartment model. Magn Reson Med 2008;59:278–88.

64. Boss A, Martirosian P, Gehrmann M, et al. Quantitative assessment of glomerular filtration rate with MR gadolinium slope clearance measurements. Radiology 2007;242:783–90.

Blood Oxygen Level-Dependent MR Imaging of the Kidneys

Lu-Ping Li, PhD[a,b], Sarah Halter, BA[a],
Pottumarthi V. Prasad, PhD[a,b],*

KEYWORDS

- BOLD • Kidney • MR imaging • Oxygenation
- Blood flow • Renal failure

Renal oxygenation status is receiving greater attention from both the scientific and clinical communities.[1–3] In most organs, regional oxygen tension (pO_2) closely follows the level of regional blood flow, because oxygen consumption is relatively constant. But this is not true in the kidney, where active tubular reabsorption demands more oxygen consumption whenever filtration and blood flow rise together.[4] The renal arterio-venous oxygen gradient is remarkably constant over a wide range of normal blood flows. For the purposes of function and oxygen supply, the mammalian kidney can be considered to be made of two separate organs: the cortex and medulla.[4] The flow of blood to the renal cortex normally supplies oxygen far in excess of its metabolic needs. By contrast, blood flow to the renal medulla is parsimonious. In addition, oxygen diffuses from the arterial to venous *vasa recta*, and the process of generating an osmotic gradient by active reabsorption of sodium requires a large amount of oxygen. All of these combined results in a poorly oxygenated medulla. A noninvasive method to evaluate this heterogeneous distribution of oxygen availability within the kidney is highly desirable. Blood oxygenation level-dependent (BOLD) MR imaging has been shown to be useful in evaluating intrarenal oxygenation status both in animal models and in human beings. This article provides an overview of the BOLD MR imaging method and reviews current state-of-the-art technique implementations and applications.

RENAL MEDULLARY HYPOXIA AND ITS CONSEQUENCES

Intrarenal oxygenation is an important determinant in renal pathophysiology, both in acute[5–7] and chronic settings.[2,3,8] It is now well established that the renal medulla functions at a significantly low ambient pO_2 (<20 mm Hg), lower compared with even systemic venous blood ($\sim$40 Hg mm). This is a consequence of lower blood flow to the medulla and the counter current arrangement of blood vessels permitting oxygen diffusion from the arterial to venous *vasa recta*. At the same time, the medullary thick ascending limbs are responsible for the generation of an osmotic gradient by active reabsorption of sodium, a process that requires a large amount of oxygen. A limited oxygen supply and heavy demand results in the renal medulla operating at extremely low levels of pO_2, making it vulnerable to hypoxic injury.[1]

Compromised renal perfusion (ischemic acute renal failure) and nephrotoxins are responsible for most episodes of acute renal failure.[5] Inadequate blood flow can be the result of renal artery stenosis, occlusion, or intrarenal small vessel lesions, such as atherosclerosis, atheroemboli, or vasculitis.[9] The functional integrity of microvasculature depends on the proper balance between vasoconstrictive and vasodilatory factors. Damage to the endothelium or alteration in endothelial function can result in local vasoconstriction because of increased production of

This work supported in part by a grant from the National Institutes of Health, DK-53221 (to P.V.P.).

[a] Center for Advanced Imaging, Department of Radiology, Evanston Northwestern Healthcare, Walgreen Building, Suite G507, 2650 Ridge Avenue, Evanston, IL 60201, USA
[b] Feinberg School of Medicine, Northwestern University, 303 East Chicago Avenue, Chicago, IL 60611, USA
* Corresponding author.
E-mail address: pprasad@enh.org (P.V. Prasad).

Magn Reson Imaging Clin N Am 16 (2008) 613–625
doi:10.1016/j.mric.2008.07.008

vasoconstrictive substances, such as endothelin, or decreased production of vasodilatory substances, such as nitric oxide. Alterations in endothelial cell function can be important in the local loss of autoregulation that occurs in ischemic renal failure.[10] Nephrotoxicity, caused by substances like iodinated contrast or nonsteroidal anti-inflammatory drugs, is thought to be caused by acute alterations in renal blood flow.[5] Renal hypoxia also plays a key role in the initiation and progression of chronic kidney disease.[2,3,8] A combination of microvascular changes and differences in oxygen consumption lead to enhanced hypoxia in the chronic setting.

BOLD MR IMAGING: A METHOD FOR NONINVASIVE EVALUATION OF INTRARENAL OXYGENATION

Most data on renal hypoxia have been based on invasive microelectrode techniques in rodent models.[11–15] Other methods include histologic staining based on pimonidazole,[16–18] electron paramagnetic resonance,[19,20] or fluorine-19 MR imaging using a fluorinated blood substitute.[21,22] To date, none of these are considered viable for human applications.

BOLD MR imaging uses the paramagnetic properties of deoxyhemoglobin to acquire images sensitive to local tissue oxygen concentration. As the deoxyhemoglobin concentration in blood increases, the T_2^* relaxation time of the protons decreases and more dephasing occurs in the surrounding tissues.[23] This produces measurable signal loss in areas of increased deoxyhemoglobin concentration. BOLD MR imaging has been used extensively in organs, such as the brain.[24–27] Changes in oxygen saturation of Hb associated with changes in blood pO_2 are most marked at low levels of pO_2.[28] This makes BOLD MR imaging ideally suited for oxygenation measurements in the renal medulla, where pO_2 is normally in the range of 15 mm Hg to 20 mm Hg.[1,29]

RENAL BOLD MR IMAGING ACQUISITION TECHNIQUES

Single-shot echo planar (EP) imaging is the technique commonly used for functional brain imaging and is readily applicable to the abdomen.[30,31] However, EP imaging has a high sensitivity to magnetic susceptibility differences, resulting in image distortions, signal loss, and limited spatial resolution. While spatial resolution and image quality may be compromised, EP imaging offers high temporal resolution. It may be advantageous for applications where fast changes are expected and when R_2^* mapping is not necessary.

A multiple gradient-recalled-echo (mGRE) sequence is currently the most widely used for renal BOLD MR imaging.[32] The mGRE technique provides R_2^* (= $1/T_2^*$) maps with improved signal to noise ratio (SNR), spatial resolution, and image quality compared with the EP imaging method. The two-dimensional (2D) mGRE technique acquires multiple gradient echoes (typically 8–16) following each excitation pulse, resulting in 8 to 16 images with different echo times (TE) to be used to fit for R2*. For optimal SNR, the maximum TE should be approximately equal to the T_2^* value of interest (in this case, the medulla). At 1.5T, medullary T_2^* is approximately 50 ms, and at 3T it is approximately 25 ms. In other words, maximum TE should be about 50 ms at 1.5T and 25 ms at 3T. With a repetition time (TR) of 50 ms to 100 ms, entire acquisition can be obtained within a breath-hold interval. A three-dimensional (3D) implementation has been shown to achieve full kidney coverage within a breath-hold time.[33,34] The benefit of a 3D technique is the increased SNR when compared with 2D mGRE with sequential multislice acquisition with comparable spatial coverage.

Selective water excitation technique avoids any potential chemical shift artifacts and amplitude modulations because of different phase accumulations between water and fat on GRE images.[35] This technique eliminates fat signals and avoids confusion between renal sinus fat and medulla on the R_2^* maps.[32] However, the selective excitation pulses increase scan time,[36] and it may not be necessary when regions of interest are defined based on the anatomic template.[32]

RENAL BOLD MR IMAGING DATA ANALYSIS

In functional brain MR imaging, T_2^* (= $1/R_2^*$)-weighted signal intensity (SI) is used for analysis. This is primarily because of the fact that the observed differences are small (typically <5% change in SI during activation). While changes in SI can be translated to changes in R_2^* (ΔR_2^* = ΔSI /TE), measurement of R_2^* is not performed routinely. R_2^* changes have been estimated to be on the order of 0.5 s^{-1} at 1.5T.[37] In the kidneys, ΔR_2^* in the medulla are typically 5 s to 10 s^{-1} and high temporal resolution is not a necessity. So, calculation of R_2^* is desirable to compare two measurements from different time points or different subjects. On the other hand, SI will depend on the scanner settings and potentially could be different, even within the same subject scanned at different time points. With EP imaging, one has to acquire images with different TEs. Because the bulk susceptibility effects scale with echo times, R_2^* mapping is usually not attempted and region of interest analysis is performed to calculate regional R_2^*.

R_2^* can be calculated as the slope of the straight line fit to Ln (SI) versus TE data,[30] or by fitting the SI versus TE data to a single decaying exponential function. By calculating R_2^* pixel by pixel, an R_2^* map can be generated. Regions of interest defined on the anatomic template can be used for estimation of R_2^* in the renal medulla and cortex. Areas affected by susceptibility artifacts (eg, **Fig. 1**) should be excluded. Artifacts because of bulk susceptibility differences appear dark, even on the low TE images, and show up very bright on the R_2^* maps.

Some investigators prefer to use a color scale to display R_2^* maps.[38–40] While they provide some advantages in terms of visualization, there is no fundamental difference in terms of information content. Use of standardized color bars would be necessary for comparison purposes.

Advantage of High-Field Strength

The potential advantage of high-field strength for MR imaging is that it increases the SNR and spatial resolution.[41] Signal changes because of BOLD effects also scale with magnetic field strength. However, chemical shift, susceptibility, flow, and patient motion artifacts can also increase at higher field strengths.[42,43]

Recent studies have demonstrated the advantage of 3T for renal BOLD MR imaging compared

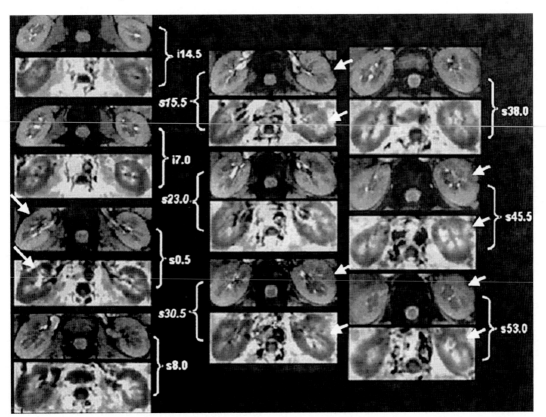

Fig. 1. Images obtained with the mGRE sequence in one representative healthy subject. Ten pairs of baseline anatomic (*top*) and R_2^* (*bottom*) images from different slices covering the entire kidney. The anatomic image is usually the first image of the series of 16 GRE images. The R_2^* map was obtained by fitting the signal intensity versus TE data to a single decaying exponential function. Note that in the R_2^* map, the medulla appears brighter than the cortex, implying a higher R_2^* value in the medulla, which in turn implies higher deoxyhemoglobin content or less tissue oxygenation. The arrows point to obvious bulk susceptibility-induced artifacts, probably because of the presence of bowel gas in close proximity. The MR imaging parameters used in this scan were TR/TE/flip angle/BW/FOV=65/7~40.1ms/30/62.5kHz/36cm at 3T with matrix size 256×256 and 0.75 phase FOV. (*From* Li LP, Vu AT, Li BS, et al. Evaluation of intrarenal oxygenation by BOLD MRI at 3.0 T. J Magn Reson Imaging 2004;20(5):902; with permission.)

with 1.5T.[33,44] The cortico-medullary contrast on the R_2^* map is significantly improved at 3T, with no evidence of increased level of bulk susceptibility artifacts (see **Fig. 1**). The magnitude of the baseline renal medullary R_2^* at 3T (37.4 ± 1.2 Hz) is roughly twice as large as that at 1.5T (21.8 ± 1.2 Hz) (**Fig. 2**).[44] Similarly, changes in R2* after pharmacologic maneuvers resulted in roughly twice the response at 3T compared with 1.5T.[33,44]

Validation of Renal BOLD MR Imaging for Evaluation of Intrarenal Oxygenation

Preliminary validation of the renal BOLD MR imaging measurements were performed by comparing previously published data in rat kidneys using invasive microelectrodes[11] to observe trends, such as response to furosemide versus acetazolamide.[30,32] Acetazolamide is a diuretic similar to furosemide, but acts on a cortical portion of the nephron, and thus has minimal effect on medullary oxygen consumption. There have also been reports comparing BOLD MR imaging with simultaneously acquired measurements using invasive electrodes in the contralateral kidneys of swine.[45] By varying the inspired gas ratio (oxygen to nitrogen), investigators observed a linear relationship

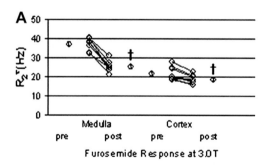

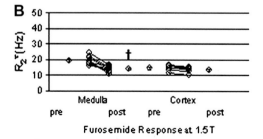

† implies $p < 0.05$ by paired two tailed Students t-test.

Fig. 2. (*A*) Summary of individual changes in medullary and cortical R_2^* after furosemide in healthy young volunteers at 3T. (*B*) Similar data obtained at 1.5T in a different group of healthy young subjects. (*From* Li LP, Vu AT, Li BS, et al. Evaluation of intrarenal oxygenation by BOLD MRI at 3.0 T. J Magn Reson Imaging 2004;20(5):903; with permission.)

between R_2^* and pO_2 as measured by the electrodes ($r = 0.67$ and 0.73 in medulla and cortex, respectively). Using this relationship, Simon-Zoula and colleagues[46] converted their R_2^* measurements in human kidneys and estimated the pO_2 of 42 mm Hg in the medulla and 50 mm Hg in cortex. However, it should be noted that such calibration is strictly valid only for the kidneys in which the simultaneous measurements were obtained.

Reproducibility of Renal BOLD MR Imaging Measurements

One important aspect of validation is reproducibility. Simon-Zoula and colleagues[46] have reported on short-term reproducibility of renal R_2^* measurements. Three identical measurements on three axial and three coronal slices of right and left kidneys were performed with a 5-minute break in between. Subjects were moved from the scanner and a subsequent BOLD scan performed with a complete new calibration. The mean R_2^* values determined in medulla and cortex showed no significant differences over three repetitions and low intrasubject coefficients of variation (3% and 4% in medulla and cortex, respectively). Only a minor influence of slice orientation was observed. The investigators also point out a 3% difference between left and right kidneys, which is within their reproducibility variation. In renal transplants, the reproducibility over 65 days was found to be similar.[47] Long-term reproducibility (81–272 days) in renal R_2^* measurements were shown to be within approximately 12% based on a coefficient of variance analysis.[48] These observations support the feasibility of performing sequential studies in the same subject: for example, with a different pharmacologic maneuver.

RENAL BOLD MR IMAGING APPLICATIONS
Physiologic and Pharmacologic-Induced Changes in Intrarenal Oxygenation

BOLD MR imaging is most effective in monitoring changes induced by pharmacologic and physiologic maneuvers.[30,32,49–53] The most widely applied maneuver is administration of furosemide.[33,44,52] **Figs. 3** and **4** are related and will be described in the same part of this article. **Fig. 3** illustrates the differences in R_2^* map before and after administration of furosemide. **Fig. 4**[33] shows the temporal response in R_2^*, both in cortex and medulla, following administration of furosemide in a representative subject. This clearly points to the sensitivity of the technique to follow changes in renal oxygenation. Waterload is another simple and effective maneuver to acutely

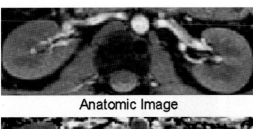

Anatomic Image

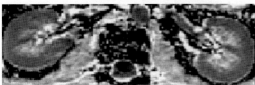

Pre-furosemide R_2* Map

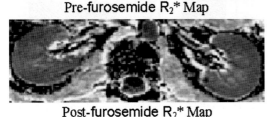

Post-furosemide R_2* Map

Fig. 3. Representative images obtained with the mGRE sequence in a healthy subject before and after furosemide administration. The top is the anatomic image of the kidney (first image of the series of 16 GRE images); the middle is the before-furosemide R_2* map; the bottom is the after-furosemide R_2* map obtained at the same slice location. The windowing was held constant for both the maps. Note that the medulla appears much brighter than the cortex on the before-furosemide R_2* map, but looks close to isointense compared with the cortex on the after-furosemide R_2* map, implying improved oxygenation on the latter. (*From* Li LP, Vu AT, Li BS, et al. Evaluation of intrarenal oxygenation by BOLD MRI at 3.0 T. J Magn Reson Imaging 2004;20(5):903; with permission.)

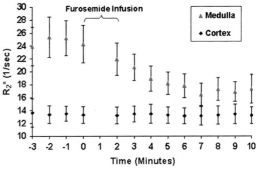

Fig. 4. The R_2* values as a function of time obtained in one representative subject. The first four points represent the mean baseline R_2* values. Zero on the time axis represents the time of furosemide administration. The error bars represent the standard deviation of the pixel data for all of the regions of interest used to determine a single time-point. Note that the cortical R_2* remain relatively constant over the entire acquisition period, whereas medullary R_2* approaches that of the cortex after administration of furosemide. (*From* Tumkur S, Vu A, Li L, et al. Evaluation of intrarenal oxygenation at 3.0 T using 3-dimensional multiple gradient-recalled echo sequence. Invest Radiol 2006;41(2):183; with permission.)

change medullary oxygenation.[34,49,53] The observed improvement in medullary oxygenation (lower R_2*) has been shown to be related to endogenous prostaglandin production.[34,49] This maneuver has also been shown to differentiate responses in the elderly (**Fig. 5**)[49] and diabetics[53] compared with healthy young subjects.

Vasoactive substances influence intrarenal oxygenation and, thus, could be monitored using BOLD MR imaging. Chronic infusions of angiotensin II have been shown to diminish renal perfusion[54] and are therefore expected to reduce renal oxygenation. This was recently confirmed by the BOLD MR imaging measurement in healthy subjects where angiotensin II caused a shortening of BOLD T_2* in the renal cortex.[31] Sodium nitroprusside and norepinephrine, although of equal potency concerning blood pressure responses, did not alter the renal BOLD signal, probably because of autoregulation. Angiotensin II is known to override the autoregulation.

Nitric oxide (NO) is a soluble gas that is continuously synthesized by the endothelium[55] and has a wide range of biologic properties, including relaxation of vascular tone. In rat kidneys, administration of L-NAME (Nitro-L-arginine methyl ester, a nitric oxide synthase inhibitor) resulted in further increase in medullary R_2*, suggesting enhanced hypoxia.[56] Interestingly, such an increase was absent in a genetic model of hypertension[56] and was shown to be restored when treated with an antioxidant.[57] Preliminary data in a small number of healthy young human subjects with NO synthase have been reported.[58]

Several pharmaceuticals are known to adversely influence renal hemodynamics and, subsequently, affect renal oxygenation. Because renal hypoxia is implicated in the development of drug-induced renal failure, monitoring the effects of these drugs would help for a better understanding of the pathophysiology, and therefore help in developing appropriate methods to clinically manage acute renal failure. Contrast medium-induced nephropathy (CIN) is a well-known cause of acute renal failure, but the development of CIN remains poorly understood.[59] Iodinated contrast-medium iopromidum produced an increase in medullary and cortical R_2* values in human beings 20 minutes after administration.[60]

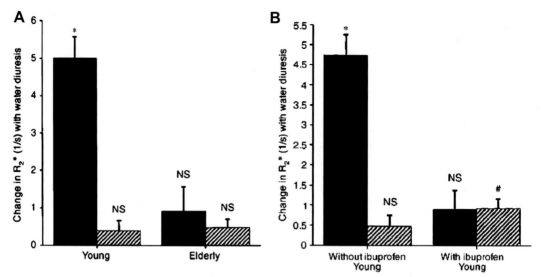

Fig. 5. (*A*) Comparison of changes in R_2* in response to waterload in nine young and nine elderly subjects. (*B*) Comparison of changes in R_2* in response to waterload in six young subjects with and without cyclooxygenase inhibition with ibuprofen. Columns are mean ± SEM. Filled column, medulla; diagonal striped column, cortex; NS, not significant, * implies $P < .01$; # implies $P < .02$. (*From* Prasad PV, Epstein FH. Changes in renal medullary pO_2 during water diuresis as evaluated by blood oxygenation level-dependent magnetic resonance imaging: effects of aging and cyclooxygenase inhibition. Kidney Int 1999;55(1):296–7; with permission.)

Calcineurin inhibitors, cyclosporine microemulsion (CsA-ME), and tacrolimus are currently the most widely used baseline immunosuppressants for prevention of acute rejection following kidney transplantation. However, their use is associated with acute and chronic toxicity. A significant reduction in medullary R_2* values (suggesting improvement in oxygenation) was observed 2 hours after CsA-ME administration in healthy subjects.[60] This is in apparent contradiction to the previously reported decrease in renal blood flow related to afferent arteriolar vasoconstriction.[61] However, the study also suggested reduction in glomular filtration rate (GFR) and it is possible that there is an associated reduction in oxygen consumption related to reduced sodium reabsorption in the medulla. Tacrolimus had no significant effect on R_2* values for the medulla or cortex in healthy subjects,[60] even though the nephrotoxic effects are known to be similar to CsA. Further studies are necessary to fully evaluate the significance of these observations.

Nonsteroidal anti-inflammatory drugs (NSAID) are the most commonly used medicines to reduce ongoing inflammation, pain, and fever.[62] Chronic use is known to be associated with gastrointestinal, renal, and even cardiac effects.[63,64] NSAIDs block the synthesis of vasodilatory prostaglandins and reduce renal perfusion.[1] Indomethacin has been shown to reduce medullary oxygenation by microelectrodes[65] and BOLD MR imaging[50] in rat

kidneys; however, it did not induce a significant change in renal medullary R_2* in healthy subjects.[60] This might indicate that a single dose of indomethacin, as routinely prescribed, does not significantly influence renal oxygenation in human beings. Similarly, another common NSAID, ibuprofen, did not change baseline renal medullary and cortical R_2*.[52] However, administration of ibuprofen (and similarly naproxen) significantly reduced the response to waterload.[34,49] This may suggest that use of a provocative maneuver, such as waterload, may be necessary to evaluate the effects of prostaglandin inhibition.

Renal BOLD MR Imaging in Disease

Renal artery stenosis (RAS) is a common cause of ischemia, and thus has consequences to intrarenal oxygenation. Juillard and colleagues[66] used a well-designed preclinical model to test if BOLD can detect the presence of renal hypoxia induced by RAS. They found that R_2* relaxivity increased continuously and progressively in parallel with the decrease in renal blood flow in response to increasing levels of stenosis, suggesting evolving hypoxia in both the medulla and cortex. The investigators offered the following concluding remarks: "new functional tools, such as BOLD, capable of detecting ischemia and characterizing patterns of intra-renal oxygen levels, may assist in identifying patients that would be more likely to benefit from therapeutic procedures." Alford and colleagues[67] also documented an increase in R_2^* following acute occlusion of renal artery. Contralateral kidney showed no such change. They also demonstrated that the R_2^* returned to baseline values upon releasing the occlusion. Recently, Textor and colleagues[68] reported on measurements in human subjects with RAS. In normal-sized kidneys downstream of high-grade renal arterial stenoses, R_2^* was elevated at baseline (suggesting enhanced hypoxia) and fell after administration of furosemide. This was true even when the GFR was significantly reduced.

These results are supported by previous reports of preserved cortical tissue volume in poststenotic kidneys, despite reduced function as measured by isotope renography.[69] These in turn may suggest that GFR might be recoverable for such cases and that nonfiltering kidney tissue represents a form of "hibernation" in the kidney, with the potential for restoring kidney function after restoring blood flow.[69] On the other hand, atrophic kidneys beyond totally occluded renal arteries demonstrated low levels of R_2^* (improved oxygenation) that did not change after furosemide.[68] This may suggest nonfunctioning kidney with limited or no oxygen consumption. The article also includes an example where a kidney with multiple arteries showed different R_2^* values in regions supplied by a stenosed renal artery. Given the recent concerns with nephrogenic systemic fibrosis,[70–73] use of contrast-enhanced MR angiography and evaluation of GFR in subjects with compromised renal function need additional caution. Noncontrast methods, such as BOLD MR imaging, may provide important alternative techniques for investigating vascular compromise and renal functional status.

Unilateral ureteral obstruction

Pedersen and colleagues[45] demonstrated changes on BOLD MR imaging in a pig model of unilateral ureteral obstruction (UUO). Twenty-four hours of UUO was associated with an increased R_2^* in the cortex and a decreased R_2^* in the medulla, as compared with the baseline indicating that pO_2 levels were reduced in the cortex and increased in the medulla during and after release of obstruction. A similar result was observed by Thoeny and colleagues[74] in 10 patients with a distal unilateral urethral calculus. All patients had significantly lower medullary and cortical R_2^* values in the obstructed kidney than in the nonobstructed kidney. The increase in oxygen content in the medulla may be because of a decrease in oxygen consumption as a result of reduced GFR in the obstructed kidney. R_2^* in the obstructed kidneys

were also significantly lower than the kidneys of healthy subjects.

Diabetes mellitus

Renal involvement in diabetes mellitus is the main cause of end-stage renal failure and a leading cause of morbidity and mortality in diabetic patients.[75] Renal hypoxia has long been a suspect in the development of renal failure from diabetes mellitus. A recent animal study using invasive microelectrodes has shown that the pO_2 in chronic diabetic rats is decreased throughout the renal parenchyma.[76] Ries and colleagues[77] observed in an animal model that the diabetic kidney showed significantly lower oxygenation levels in the renal medulla when compared with a control group using BOLD MR imaging at 5 days after induction. A similar study[78] with BOLD MR imaging, along with invasive blood flow and oxygenation measurement by optical fiber probes, showed that the pO_2 was considerably lower in diabetic rats after 2, 5, 14, and 28 days following induction of diabetes when compared with control rats. No blood flow changes were observed in both diabetes and normal groups over this time period, suggesting that the reduced oxygenation was related to increased consumption, probably related to hyperfiltration. Furthermore, there was a significant and progressive decrease in the renal oxygenation by fiber-optic probe in diabetic animals compared with the control group over time. The increase in the BOLD signal was also progressive, with the highest increase observed with the 28-day group for both renal medulla and cortex.

BOLD MR imaging has also been used to evaluate diabetic human subjects. A study of 18 human subjects (nine healthy nondiabetics and nine with mild, controlled diabetes)[53] showed that in the healthy subjects, water-diuresis led to a significant increase in the oxygenation of the renal medulla, but not in the diabetic patients as evaluated by BOLD MR imaging. These results suggest that even patients with mild diabetes already show signs of renal injury long before the onset of symptoms that usually accompany kidney disease, and a likely deficiency in the synthesis of endogenous vasodilator substances, like prostaglandin or NO.

BOLD MR imaging may provide important insight into the pathophysiology of renal injury at early stages in diabetes, and allow for means to evaluate novel drug interventions, especially those targeting renal hypoxia.

Hypertension

The kidney is believed to play a role in the pathogenesis of essential hypertension.[79,80] In particular, reduced renal medullary blood flow is thought to be one of the important factors in the development of the disease.[81] Animal studies have shown that medullary blood flow is decreased in hypertension and, more importantly, that reduced medullary blood flow is sufficient to produce hypertension.[82]

A study using BOLD MR imaging techniques showed that medullary R_2^* increased significantly in control rats in response to NO synthase inhibition, while hypertensive rats exhibited a minimal change.[56] The baseline R_2^* in hypertensive rats were found to be comparable to post-L-NAME values in controls, suggesting a basal deficiency of NO in hypertension rats.[56] This observation was consistent with previous reports based on invasive blood flow measurement.[83–89]

Tempol (4-hydroxy-2,2,6,6-tetramethyl piperidinoyl) is a superoxide scavenger and is known to improve NO bioavailability. Short- and long-term administration of tempol has been shown to increase medullary blood flow in hypertension rats by 35% to 50% and reduce mean arterial pressure (MAP) by 20 mm Hg compared, with untreated hypertension rats as evaluated by invasive technique.[90–93] Tempol showed no effect on the R_2^* in normal rats but significantly decreased in hypertensive rats evaluated by BOLD MR imaging[57] The degree of R_2^* changes is in qualitative agreement with the observed medullary blood flow and MAP changes induced by tempol administration assessed by invasive measurement.[90]

These studies, combined with the report on angiotensin II,[31] support a role for BOLD MR imaging in the understanding of pathophysiology of hypertension, and potentially play a role in the evaluation of novel drug interventions.

Renal allografts

Kidney transplantation allows patients with end-stage renal disease to lead close to normal lives. However, graft dysfunction is a major concern and early characterization of the underlying cause of graft dysfunction is important. Delayed treatment can lead to the irreversible loss of nephrons and hasten graft loss over time.[94,95] Allograft rejection and acute tubular necrosis (ATN) are two important causes of early kidney allograft dysfunction, and it is difficult to discriminate between them by regular clinical tests. Percutaneous transplant biopsy is the most effective method, but it has risks, such as bleeding, kidney rupture, and rarely, graft loss.[96,97] Developing a noninvasive method may be highly desirable. Several groups have evaluated the feasibility of BOLD MR imaging in patients with renal allografts.

Thoeny and colleagues[47] compared the BOLD index between transplanted kidney and the native kidney in healthy volunteers. The medullary R_2^* was found to be lower in transplant patients than in healthy volunteers ($P < .004$), implying a relatively improved oxygenation in transplanted kidney. This could be explained as the result of reduced tubular fractional reabsorption of sodium and increased blood flow because of allograft denervation. The investigators believe that these observations may also be influenced by the time of the study following transplantation.

Sadowski and colleagues[98] evaluated 20 patients who had recently received renal transplants in an attempt to obtain preliminary data on potential differences between normal functioning transplants and those experiencing acute rejection and ATN. Six patients had clinically normal functioning transplants, eight had biopsy-proved rejection, and six had biopsy-proven ATN. Their results showed that R_2^* measurements in the medullary regions of transplanted kidneys with acute rejection were significantly lower than those in normally functioning transplants or transplants with ATN. It is also suggested that using a threshold R_2^* value of 18 s^{-1}, acute rejection could be differentiated from normal function and ATN in all cases. The investigators comment, "this is important because if MR imaging can help exclude acute rejection, a substantial number of percutaneous transplant biopsies could be avoided. Furthermore, clinicians weigh their concern that acute rejection is actually present against the risks of percutaneous biopsy. Patients are often watched over a period of time so that trends in laboratory values can be evaluated before a decision is made to proceed with biopsy. Having a noninvasive means of determining the presence of acute rejection could allow patients to be evaluated without the concerns associated with percutaneous biopsy. This, in turn, would lead to an increase in the screening of patients and, potentially, earlier detection of kidney transplant rejection." Similar findings were reported by a more recent study in a much larger number of subjects ($n = 82$), including biopsy-proven acute rejection and ATN (**Fig. 6**).[40]

Djamali and colleagues[99] applied BOLD-MR imaging to discriminate different types of rejection early after kidney transplantation. Twenty-three patients underwent imaging in the first 4 months after transplant. Five had normal functioning transplants and 18 had biopsy-proven acute allograft dysfunction, acute tubular necrosis, and acute rejection, including borderline rejection ($n = 3$), IA rejection ($n = 4$), IIA rejection ($n = 6$), and C4d(+) rejection ($n = 9$). Their results in general agreed with those of Sadowski and colleagues[98] in that medullary R_2^* levels were higher (increased local deoxyhemoglobin concentration) in normal

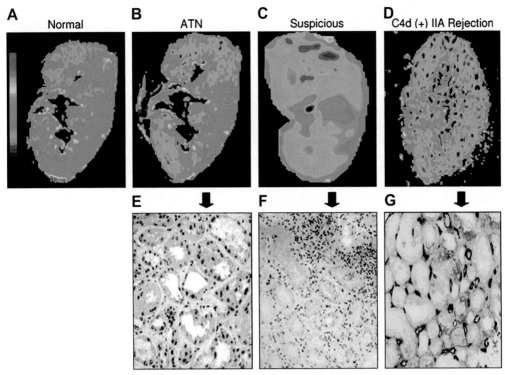

Fig. 6. BOLD-MR color R_2^* map of coronal sections and corresponding histopathologic findings. (*A–D*) Color R_2^* maps in the coronal planes of normal kidney allograft and transplants with acute dysfunction. Blue represents the lowest R_2^* value (lowest deoxyhemoglobin concentration), and green, yellow, and red show increasing R_2^* values. Color map scale is similar in all figures. (*E–G*) Pathology sections (20× magnification) of the corresponding kidney with ATN (*E*), suspicious for rejection (*F*) and C4d (+) IIA rejection (*G* with insert). (*From* Djamali A, Sadowski EA, Samaniego-Picota M, et al. Noninvasive assessment of early kidney allograft dysfunction by blood oxygen level-dependent magnetic resonance imaging. Transplantation 2006;82(5):624; with permission.)

functioning allografts (24.3/s ± 2.3) compared with acute rejection (16.6/s ± 2.1) and ATN (20.9/s ± 1.8) ($P < .05$). There was no statistically significant difference in cortical R_2^*. Medullary R_2^* was the lowest in acute rejection with a vascular component (ie, IIA and C4d (+) compared with IA and "borderline" rejection). Receiver operator characteristic curve analyses suggested that medullary R_2^* and medullary-cortical ratio could accurately discriminate acute rejection in the early posttransplant period.

Chronic allograft nephropathy (CAN) is the leading cause of kidney transplant failure.[100] A better understanding of CAN's pathogenesis may lead to the development of strategies to prevent or delay its development or progression. Djamali and colleagues[38] used BOLD MR imaging to evaluate patients with CAN and looked for correlations with other conventional biomarkers of oxidative stress. Similar to previous reports on acute rejection, subjects with CAN showed lower medullary and cortical R_2^* values. More importantly, they observed that intrarenal oxygenation as evaluated

by BOLD MR imaging showed a high level of correlation with serum and urine biomarkers of oxidative stress. They concluded, "this pilot study is provocative in suggesting that oxygenation patterns are different in CAN and, moreover, are strongly associated with oxidative stress. Our therapeutics to date have not used oxygen delivery as an outcome of therapy, but it may well be the case that optimal tissue oxygenation, not hypoxia nor hyperoxia, is a target of therapy. The association in CAN between aberrant kidney oxygenation and oxidative stress is important and may provide leads as to how to slow loss of transplant function."

RENAL BOLD MR IMAGING: LIMITATIONS

Several limitations of BOLD MR imaging technique have to be considered. BOLD signal depends more on field inhomogeneity contributions and can be influenced by oxygen supply, oxygen consumption, blood flow,[25,101] blood volume,[25,101] hematocrit,[102] and pO_2.[103] Moreover, changes in the oxygen-hemoglobin dissociation curve may be influenced by factors such as pH and temperature.[104] In addition, R_2^* is influenced by the vessel geometry and applied pulse-sequence parameters. Therefore, the absolute magnitude of R_2^* are less reliable in practice than the relative changes observed. For the same reason, a direct calibration of R_2^* versus pO_2 has to be viewed with caution.

Susceptibility artifacts caused by bowel gas[105] are sometimes marked, and at times lead to non-interpretable observations. Motion artifacts because of breathing should also be carefully monitored. Use of a respiratory monitor could minimize errors because of improper breath holding.

Because hydration status can significantly influence the renal BOLD MR imaging measurements, it is preferred to perform studies following 12-hour fasting (overnight). This would facilitate combining data from different individual subjects and comparison of different groups of subjects.

SUMMARY

BOLD MR imaging is an endogenous contrast mechanism and allows for rapid, noninvasive means to assess intrarenal oxygenation both in animal models and human beings. To-date, the method has been shown to be reproducible within and across several laboratories throughout the world. The technique is most efficacious in evaluating physiologic or pharmacologic maneuvers that can influence renal oxygenation status. This may have important applications in understanding renal physiology and pathophysiology, and in turn lead to the development of novel interventional strategies. The technique has been shown to be of value in characterizing disease that can potentially influence patient management: for example, identifying kidneys that may be amenable to functional recovery by restoring blood flow in cases with renal artery stenosis, and distinguishing between acute rejection from acute tubular necrosis in renal transplants. In a recent editorial, Drs. Wang and Yeh[106] comment, "the assessment of renal oxygenation could potentially provide insights into early derangements of renal physiology and function before the onset of irreversible renal injury." They further conclude, "BOLD MRI imaging promises to become an important tool for monitoring renal oxygenation in various clinical scenarios."

REFERENCES

1. Brezis M, Rosen S. Hypoxia of the renal medulla—its implications for disease. N Engl J Med 1995; 332(10):647–55.

2. Norman JT, Fine LG. Intrarenal oxygenation in chronic renal failure. Clin Exp Pharmacol Physiol 2006;33(10):989–96.

3. Eckardt KU, Bernhardt WM, Weidemann A, et al. Role of hypoxia in the pathogenesis of renal disease. Kidney Int Suppl 2005;(99):S46–51.

4. Epstein FH, Agmon Y, Brezis M. Physiology of renal hypoxia. Ann N Y Acad Sci 1994;718:72–81 [discussion: 81–2].

5. Thadhani R, Pascual M, Bonventre JV. Acute renal failure. N Engl J Med 1996;334(22):1448–60.

6. Rosenberger C, Rosen S, Heyman SN. Renal parenchymal oxygenation and hypoxia adaptation in acute kidney injury. Clin Exp Pharmacol Physiol 2006;33(10):980–8.

7. Heyman SN, Fuchs S, Brezis M. The role of medullary ischemia in acute renal failure. New Horiz 1995; 3(4):597–607.

8. Nangaku M. Chronic hypoxia and tubulointerstitial injury: a final common pathway to end-stage renal failure. J Am Soc Nephrol 2006;17(1):17–25.

9. Bonventre JV. Mechanisms of ischemic acute renal failure. Kidney Int 1993;43(5):1160–78.

10. Conger JD, Robinette JB, Schrier RW. Smooth muscle calcium and endothelium-derived relaxing factor in the abnormal vascular responses of acute renal failure. J Clin Invest 1988;82(2):532–7.

11. Brezis M, Agmon Y, Epstein FH. Determinants of intrarenal oxygenation. I. Effects of diuretics. Am J Physiol 1994;267(6 Pt 2):F1059–62.

12. Brezis M, Heyman SN, Epstein FH. Determinants of intrarenal oxygenation. II. Hemodynamic effects. Am J Physiol 1994;267(6 Pt 2):F1063–8.

13. Dinour D, Brezis M. Effects of adenosine on intrarenal oxygenation. Am J Physiol 1991;261(5 Pt 2): F787–91.

14. Brezis M, Heyman SN, Dinour D, et al. Role of nitric oxide in renal medullary oxygenation. Studies in isolated and intact rat kidneys. J Clin Invest 1991; 88(2):390–5.

15. Heyman SN, Rosen S, Fuchs S, et al. Myoglobinuric acute renal failure in the rat: a role for medullary hypoperfusion, hypoxia, and tubular obstruction. J Am Soc Nephrol 1996;7(7): 1066–74.

16. Rosenberger C, Goldfarb M, Shina A, et al. Evidence for sustained renal hypoxia and transient hypoxia adaptation in experimental rhabdomyolysis-induced acute kidney injury. Nephrol Dial Transplant 2008;23(4):1135–43.

17. Rosenberger C, Khamaisi M, Abassi Z, et al. Adaptation to hypoxia in the diabetic rat kidney. Kidney Int 2008;73(1):34–42.

18. Tanaka T, Kato H, Kojima I, et al. Hypoxia and expression of hypoxia-inducible factor in the aging kidney. J Gerontol A Biol Sci Med Sci 2006;61(8): 795–805.

19. Swartz HM, Clarkson RB. The measurement of oxygen in vivo using EPR techniques. Phys Med Biol 1998;43(7):1957–75.

20. Gallez B, Jordan BF, Baudelet C, et al. Pharmacological modifications of the partial pressure of oxygen in murine tumors: evaluation using in vivo EPR oximetry. Magn Reson Med 1999; 42(4):627–30.

21. Hunjan S, Zhao D, Constantinescu A, et al. Tumor oximetry: demonstration of an enhanced dynamic mapping procedure using fluorine-19 echo planar magnetic resonance imaging in the Dunning prostate R3327-AT1 rat tumor. Int J Radiat Oncol Biol Phys 2001;49(4):1097–108.

22. Xia M, Kodibagkar V, Liu H, et al. Tumour oxygen dynamics measured simultaneously by near-infrared spectroscopy and 19F magnetic resonance imaging in rats. Phys Med Biol 2006; 51(1):45–60.

23. Thulborn KR, Waterton JC, Matthews PM, et al. Oxygenation dependence of the transverse relaxation time of water protons in whole blood at high field. Biochim Biophys Acta 1982;714(2):265–70.

24. Blatow M, Nennig E, Durst A, et al. fMRI reflects functional connectivity of human somatosensory cortex. Neuroimage 2007;37(3):927–36.

25. Shen Q, Ren H, Duong TQ. CBF, BOLD, CBV, and CMRO(2) fMRI signal temporal dynamics at 500-msec resolution. J Magn Reson Imaging 2008; 27(3):599–606.

26. Fukunaga M, Horovitz SG, de Zwart JA, et al. Metabolic origin of BOLD signal fluctuations in the absence of stimuli. J Cereb Blood Flow Metab 2008.

27. Herrmann CS, Debener S. Simultaneous recording of EEG and BOLD responses: a historical perspective. Int J Psychophysiol 2008;67(3):161–8.

28. Cherniack NS, Altose MG, Kelsen SG. Gas exchange and gas transport. In: Physiology. St Louis (MO): C.V. Mosby Company; 1988.

29. Brezis M, Rosen S, Silva P, et al. Renal ischemia: a new perspective. Kidney Int 1984;26(4):375–83.

30. Prasad PV, Edelman RR, Epstein FH. Noninvasive evaluation of intrarenal oxygenation with BOLD MRI. Circulation 1996;94(12):3271–5.

31. Schachinger H, Klarhofer M, Linder L, et al. Angiotensin II decreases the renal MRI blood oxygenation level-dependent signal. Hypertension 2006;47(6):1062–6.

32. Prasad PV, Chen Q, Goldfarb JW, et al. Breath-hold R2* mapping with a multiple gradient-recalled echo sequence: application to the evaluation of intrarenal oxygenation. J Magn Reson Imaging 1997; 7(6):1163–5.

33. Tumkur S, Vu A, Li L, et al. Evaluation of intrarenal oxygenation at 3.0 T using 3-dimensional multiple gradient-recalled echo sequence. Invest Radiol 2006;41(2):181–4.

34. Tumkur SM, Vu AT, Li LP, et al. Evaluation of intra-renal oxygenation during water diuresis: a time-resolved study using BOLD MRI. Kidney Int 2006; 70(1):139–43.

35. Wehrli FW, Perkins TG, Shimakawa A, et al. Chemical shift-induced amplitude modulations in images obtained with gradient refocusing. Magn Reson Imaging 1987;5(2):157–8.

36. Thomasson D, Purdy D, Finn JP. Phase-modulated binomial RF pulses for fast spectrally-selective musculoskeletal imaging. Magn Reson Med 1996; 35(4):563–8.

37. Bandettini PA, Wong EC, Jesmanowicz A, et al. Spin-echo and gradient-echo EPI of human brain activation using BOLD contrast: a comparative study at 1.5 T. NMR Biomed 1994;7(1–2): 12–20.

38. Djamali A, Sadowski EA, Muehrer RJ, et al. BOLD-MRI assessment of intrarenal oxygenation and oxidative stress in patients with chronic kidney allograft dysfunction. Am J Physiol Renal Physiol 2007;292(2):F513–22.

39. Zuo CS, Rofsky NM, Mahallati H, et al. Visualization and quantification of renal R2* changes during water diuresis. J Magn Reson Imaging 2003;17(6): 676–82.

40. Han F, Xiao W, Xu Y, et al. The significance of BOLD MRI in differentiation between renal transplant rejection and acute tubular necrosis. Nephrol Dial Transplant 2008;23(8):2666–72.

41. Edelstein WA, Glover GH, Hardy CJ, et al. The intrinsic signal-to-noise ratio in NMR imaging. Magn Reson Med 1986;3(4):604–18.

42. Yang Y, Gu H, Zhan W, et al. Simultaneous perfusion and BOLD imaging using reverse spiral scanning at 3T: characterization of functional contrast and susceptibility artifacts. Magn Reson Med 2002;48(2):278–89.

43. Gonen O, Gruber S, Li BS, et al. Multivoxel 3D proton spectroscopy in the brain at 1.5 versus 3.0 T: signal-to-noise ratio and resolution comparison. AJNR Am J Neuroradiol 2001;22(9):1727–31.

44. Li LP, Vu AT, Li BS, et al. Evaluation of intrarenal oxygenation by BOLD MRI at 3.0 T. J Magn Reson Imaging 2004;20(5):901–4.

45. Pedersen M, Dissing TH, Morkenborg J, et al. Validation of quantitative BOLD MRI measurements in kidney: application to unilateral ureteral obstruction. Kidney Int 2005;67(6):2305–12.

46. Simon-Zoula SC, Hofmann L, Giger A, et al. Non-invasive monitoring of renal oxygenation using BOLD-MRI: a reproducibility study. NMR Biomed 2006;19(1):84–9.

47. Thoeny HC, Zumstein D, Simon-Zoula S, et al. Functional evaluation of transplanted kidneys with diffusion-weighted and BOLD MR imaging: initial experience. Radiology 2006;241(3):812–21.

48. Li LP, Storey P, Pierchala L, et al. Evaluation of the reproducibility of intrarenal R2* and DeltaR2* measurements following administration of furosemide and during waterload. J Magn Reson Imaging 2004;19(5):610–6.

49. Prasad PV, Epstein FH. Changes in renal medullary pO2 during water diuresis as evaluated by blood oxygenation level-dependent magnetic resonance imaging: effects of aging and cyclooxygenase inhibition. Kidney Int 1999;55(1):294–8.

50. Prasad PV, Priatna A, Spokes K, et al. Changes in intrarenal oxygenation as evaluated by BOLD MRI in a rat kidney model for radiocontrast nephropathy. J Magn Reson Imaging 2001;13(5):744–7.

51. Priatna A, Epstein FH, Spokes K, et al. Evaluation of changes in intrarenal oxygenation in rats using multiple gradient-recalled echo (mGRE) sequence. J Magn Reson Imaging 1999;9(6):842–6.

52. Epstein FH, Prasad P. Effects of furosemide on medullary oxygenation in younger and older subjects. Kidney Int 2000;57(5):2080–3.

53. Epstein FH, Veves A, Prasad PV. Effect of diabetes on renal medullary oxygenation during water diuresis. Diabetes Care 2002;25(3):575–8.

54. Hall JE, Granger JP. Renal hemodynamic actions of angiotensin II: interaction with tubuloglomerular feedback. Am J Physiol 1983;245(2):R166–73.

55. Palmer RM, Ashton DS, Moncada S. Vascular endothelial cells synthesize nitric oxide from L-arginine. Nature 1988;333(6174):664–6.

56. Li L, Storey P, Kim D, et al. Kidneys in hypertensive rats show reduced response to nitric oxide synthase inhibition as evaluated by BOLD MRI. J Magn Reson Imaging 2003;17(6):671–5.

57. Li LP, Li BS, Storey P, et al. Effect of free radical scavenger (tempol) on intrarenal oxygenation in hypertensive rats as evaluated by BOLD MRI. J Magn Reson Imaging 2005;21(3):245–8.

58. Li LP, Pierchala L, Prasad P, editors. Effect of nitric oxide inhibitor on intrarenal R2* measurements in humans. ISMRM 12th Scientific Meeting and Exhibition. Kyoto, Japan, 2004.

59. Persson PB, Hansell P, Liss P. Pathophysiology of contrast medium-induced nephropathy. Kidney Int 2005;68(1):14–22.

60. Hofmann L, Simon-Zoula S, Nowak A, et al. BOLD-MRI for the assessment of renal oxygenation in humans: acute effect of nephrotoxic xenobiotics. Kidney Int 2006;70(1):144–50.

61. Klein IH, Abrahams A, van Ede T, et al. Different effects of tacrolimus and cyclosporine on renal hemodynamics and blood pressure in healthy subjects. Transplantation 2002;73(5):732–6.

62. Watson WA, Litovitz TL, Rodgers GC Jr, et al. 2004 Annual report of the American Association of Poison Control Centers Toxic Exposure Surveillance System. Am J Emerg Med 2005;23(5):589–666.

63. Fagerholm U, Bjornsson MA. Clinical pharmacokinetics of the cyclooxygenase inhibiting nitric oxide donor (CINOD) AZD3582. J Pharm Pharmacol 2005;57(12):1539–54.

64. Schnitzer TJ, Kivitz AJ, Lipetz RS, et al. Comparison of the COX-inhibiting nitric oxide donor AZD3582 and rofecoxib in treating the signs and symptoms of osteoarthritis of the knee. Arthritis Rheum 2005;53(6):827–37.

65. Heyman SN, Kaminski N, Brezis M. Dopamine increases renal medullary blood flow without improving regional hypoxia. Exp Nephrol 1995;3(6):331–7.

66. Juillard L, Lerman LO, Kruger DG, et al. Blood oxygen level-dependent measurement of acute intra-renal ischemia. Kidney Int 2004;65(3):944–50.

67. Alford SK, Sadowski EA, Unal O, et al. Detection of acute renal ischemia in swine using blood oxygen level-dependent magnetic resonance imaging. J Magn Reson Imaging 2005;22(3):347–53.

68. Textor SC, Glockner JF, Lerman LO, et al. The use of magnetic resonance to evaluate tissue oxygenation in renal artery stenosis. J Am Soc Nephrol 2008;19(4):780–8.

69. Cheung CM, Shurrab AE, Buckley DL, et al. MR-derived renal morphology and renal function in patients with atherosclerotic renovascular disease. Kidney Int 2006;69(4):715–22.

70. Kurtkoti J, Snow T, Hiremagalur B. Gadolinium and nephrogenic systemic fibrosis: association or causation. Nephrology (Carlton) 2008;13(3):235–41.

71. Martin DR. Nephrogenic system fibrosis: a radiologist's practical perspective. Eur J Radiol 2008;66(2):220–4.

72. Penfield JG, Reilly RF Jr. What nephrologists need to know about gadolinium. Nat Clin Pract Nephrol 2007;3(12):654–68.

73. Todd DJ, Kagan A, Chibnik LB, et al. Cutaneous changes of nephrogenic systemic fibrosis: predictor of early mortality and association with gadolinium exposure. Arthritis Rheum 2007;56(10):3433–41.

74. Thoeny HC, Kessler TM, Simon-Zoula S, et al. Renal oxygenation changes during acute unilateral ureteral obstruction: assessment with blood oxygen level-dependent MR imaging—initial experience. Radiology 2008;247(3):754–61.

75. Knowles HC Jr. Magnitude of the renal failure problem in diabetic patients. Kidney Int Suppl 1974;1:2–7.

76. Palm F, Cederberg J, Hansell P, et al. Reactive oxygen species cause diabetes-induced decrease in renal oxygen tension. Diabetologia 2003;46(8):1153–60.

77. Ries M, Basseau F, Tyndal B, et al. Renal diffusion and BOLD MRI in experimental diabetic

nephropathy. Blood oxygen level-dependent. J Magn Reson Imaging 2003;17(1):104–13.

78. dos Santos EA, Li LP, Ji L, et al. Early changes with diabetes in renal medullary hemodynamics as evaluated by fiberoptic probes and BOLD magnetic resonance imaging. Invest Radiol 2007;42(3): 157–62.

79. Cowley AW, Roman RJ, Fenoy FJ, et al. Effect of renal medullary circulation on arterial pressure. J Hypertens Suppl 1992;10(7):S187–93.

80. Johnson RJ, Herrera-Acosta J, Schreiner GF, et al. Subtle acquired renal injury as a mechanism of salt-sensitive hypertension. N Engl J Med 2002; 346(12):913–23.

81. Cowley AW Jr, Mattson DL, Lu S, et al. The renal medulla and hypertension. Hypertension 1995; 25(4 Pt 2):663–73.

82. Mattson DL, Roman RJ, Cowley AW Jr. Role of nitric oxide in renal papillary blood flow and sodium excretion. Hypertension 1992;19(6 Pt 2):766–9.

83. Dananberg J, Sider RS, Grekin RJ. Sustained hypertension induced by orally administered nitro-L-arginine. Hypertension 1993;21(3):359–63.

84. Manning RD Jr, Hu L, Mizelle HL, et al. Cardiovascular responses to long-term blockade of nitric oxide synthesis. Hypertension 1993;22(1):40–8.

85. Majid DS, Williams A, Navar LG. Inhibition of nitric oxide synthesis attenuates pressure-induced natriuretic responses in anesthetized dogs. Am J Physiol 1993;264(1 Pt 2):F79–87.

86. Salazar FJ, Alberola A, Pinilla JM, et al. Salt-induced increase in arterial pressure during nitric oxide synthesis inhibition. Hypertension 1993; 22(1):49–55.

87. Nakanishi K, Mattson DL, Cowley AW Jr. Role of renal medullary blood flow in the development of L-NAME hypertension in rats. Am J Physiol 1995; 268(2 Pt 2):R317–23.

88. Mattson DL, Lu S, Nakanishi K, et al. Effect of chronic renal medullary nitric oxide inhibition on blood pressure. Am J Physiol 1994;266(5 Pt 2):H1918–26.

89. Panza JA, Casino PR, Kilcoyne CM, et al. Role of endothelium-derived nitric oxide in the abnormal endothelium-dependent vascular relaxation of patients with essential hypertension. Circulation 1993;87(5):1468–74.

90. Schnackenberg CG, Welch WJ, Wilcox CS. Normalization of blood pressure and renal vascular resistance in SHR with a membrane-permeable superoxide dismutase mimetic: role of nitric oxide. Hypertension 1998;32(1):59–64.

91. Schnackenberg CG, Wilcox CS. Two-week administration of tempol attenuates both hypertension and renal excretion of 8-Iso prostaglandin f2alpha. Hypertension 1999;33(1 Pt 2):424–8.

92. Feng MG, Dukacz SA, Kline RL. Selective effect of tempol on renal medullary hemodynamics in spontaneously hypertensive rats. Am J Physiol Regul Integr Comp Physiol 2001;281(5):R1420–5.

93. Fenoy FJ, Ferrer P, Carbonell L, et al. Role of nitric oxide on papillary blood flow and pressure natriuresis. Hypertension 1995;25(3):408–14.

94. Ojo AO, Wolfe RA, Held PJ, et al. Delayed graft function: risk factors and implications for renal allograft survival. Transplantation 1997;63(7):968–74.

95. Breza J, Navratil P. Renal transplantation in adults. BJU Int 1999;84(2):216–23.

96. Gainza FJ, Minguela I, Lopez-Vidaur I, et al. Evaluation of complications due to percutaneous renal biopsy in allografts and native kidneys with color-coded doppler sonography. Clin Nephrol 1995; 43(5):303–8.

97. Preda A, Van Dijk LC, Van Oostaijen JA, et al. Complication rate and diagnostic yield of 515 consecutive ultrasound-guided biopsies of renal allografts and native kidneys using a 14-gauge Biopty gun. Eur Radiol 2003;13(3):527–30.

98. Sadowski EA, Fain SB, Alford SK, et al. Assessment of acute renal transplant rejection with blood oxygen level-dependent MR imaging: initial experience. Radiology 2005;236(3):911–9.

99. Djamali A, Sadowski EA, Samaniego-Picota M, et al. Noninvasive assessment of early kidney allograft dysfunction by blood oxygen level-dependent magnetic resonance imaging. Transplantation 2006;82(5):621–8.

100. Colvin RB. Chronic allograft nephropathy. N Engl J Med 2003;349(24):2288–90.

101. Wu G, Luo F, Li Z, et al. Transient relationships among BOLD, CBV, and CBF changes in rat brain as detected by functional MRI. Magn Reson Med 2002;48(6):987–93.

102. Zhao JM, Clingman CS, Narvainen MJ, et al. Oxygenation and hematocrit dependence of transverse relaxation rates of blood at 3T. Magn Reson Med 2007;58(3):592–7.

103. Spees WM, Yablonskiy DA, Oswood MC, et al. Water proton MR properties of human blood at 1.5 Tesla: magnetic susceptibility, T(1), T(2), T*(2), and non-Lorentzian signal behavior. Magn Reson Med 2001;45(4):533–42.

104. Hess W. [Affinity of oxygen for hemoglobin—its significance under physiological and pathological conditions]. Anaesthesist 1987;36(9):455–67 [in German].

105. Grenier N, Basseau F, Ries M, et al. Functional MRI of the kidney. Abdom Imaging 2003;28(2):164–75.

106. Wang ZJ, Yeh BM. Is assessing renal oxygenation by using blood oxygen level-dependent MR imaging a clinical reality? Radiology 2008;247(3):595–6.

Molecular Magnetic Resonance Imaging of the Genitourinary Tract: Recent Results and Future Directions

Nicolas Grenier, MD[a,b],*, Olivier Hauger, MD, PhD[a,b], Omer Eker[b],
Christian Combe, MD, PhD[c], Frank Couillaud, PhD[a],
Chrit Moonen, PhD[a]

KEYWORDS
- Kidney diseases • MR imaging • Molecular imaging
- Macrophages • Stem cells • Gene expression

Specific diagnosis of most renal diseases still requires pathologic examination after percutaneous biopsy. Current renal imaging techniques, including ultrasound, computed tomography, and magnetic resonance (MR) imaging does not provide, up to now, detection of specific changes in the kidneys that could enable an accurate characterization of different types of kidney diseases, which could have a tremendous impact on patient management.

Molecular imaging techniques aim to identify and to characterize cellular and molecular processes in vivo. Using appropriate tracers, positon emission tomography (PET), optical imaging, and MR imaging techniques have demonstrated capabilities in imaging cellular and molecular targets. Renal PET has a great potential in that field.[1] Its high sensitivity to detect a signal from a tracer at a picomolar level is a serious advantage but it suffers from a low spatial resolution. Specific tracers have also to be developed and many applications are still at an experimental level. Optical techniques are very useful for proof of concepts of new molecular imaging approaches. However, it requires the development of specific tracers and, because of a high attenuation of the signal by tissues, clinical applications will be driven by the depth of the target organs: if kidneys are far too deep to expect potential renal applications, the prostate and the testis could benefit from these developments in the future.

The new developments of MR systems, providing higher signal-to-noise ratio and higher spatial and/or temporal resolution, and specific MR contrast agents, offer the opportunity to drive new challenges for obtaining functional and biological information on tissue characteristics relevant for diagnosis, prognosis, and treatment follow-up.

This article focuses on preclinical and early clinical applications of renal cell MR imaging, on new developments in MR control of intrarenal gene therapy, and finally, on several potential applications of molecular imaging techniques, mainly targeting cell receptors and enzyme activity, which

[a] UMR-CNRS 5231 Imagerie Moléculaire et Fonctionnelle, Université Victor Segalen-Bordeaux 2, 146 Rue Léo Saignat, 33076 Bordeaux-Cedex, France
[b] Service d'Imagerie Diagnostique et Thérapeutique de l'Adulte, Groupe Hospitalier Pellegrin, Place Amélie Raba-Léon, 33076 Bordeaux-Cedex, France
[c] Département de Néphrologie, Groupe Hospitalier Pellegrin, Place Amélie Raba-Léon, 33076 Bordeaux-Cedex, Bordeaux, France
* Corresponding author. Service d'Imagerie Diagnostique et Thérapeutique de l'Adulte, Groupe Hospitalier Pellegrin, Place Amélie Raba-Léon, 33076 Bordeaux-Cedex, France.
E-mail address: nicolas.grenier@chu-bordeaux.fr (N. Grenier).

Magn Reson Imaging Clin N Am 16 (2008) 627–641
doi:10.1016/j.mric.2008.07.004
1064-9689/08/$ – see front matter © 2008 Elsevier Inc. All rights reserved.

could find exciting applications within the genito-urinary tract.

MAGNETIC RESONANCE–GUIDED CELL TARGETING AND CELL TRACKING WITHIN THE KIDNEY
MR Imaging of Intrarenal Macrophage Activity

Whereas only a small number of interstitial leucocytes (predominantly monocytes and differential macrophages) are present in the normal kidney, their number can be considerably increased in specific nephropathies such as acute proliferative-types of human and experimental glomerulonephritides (GN),[2] renal graft dysfunctions (rejection and acute tubular necrosis),[3] and non-specific kidney diseases such as hydronephrosis.[4] This increase of the inflammatory cellular infiltration is a result of both a recruitment of circulating cells and a proliferation in situ. This macrophagic attraction is a dynamic process controlled by both chemotactic molecules (chemokines, Fc fragment of immunoglobulins, tumor necrosis factor [TNF]-α) and changes in expression level of leucocyte adhesion molecules. The degree of macrophagic infiltration and proliferation is correlated with the severity of renal disease, whereas it remains unclear if macrophages produce direct renal insults or if they are a consequence of the disease to regulate the inflammatory response. Their role is complex, contributing to glomerular and tubulointerstitial injury through the secretion of various cytokines and proteases that induce changes in extracellular matrix and progressive fibrotic changes (glomerulosclerosis, tubulointerstitial fibrosis).[5] The macrophagic activity may vary, depending on the type of kidney disease and its severity. It predominates within the glomeruli (ie, within the cortex) in glomerulonephritis, or within the interstitium (ie, diffuse, within all kidney compartments) in interstitial nephritis or in hydronephrosis.

In current clinical practice, the degree of inflammatory response in the kidney can be approached only by renal biopsy. Therefore, identification of intrarenal macrophage infiltration with a noninvasive technique has a great potential since it could help for the characterization of kidney disease, the evaluation of its level of inflammatory activity, and for monitoring response to treatment.

Intravenous injection of superparamagnetic particles of iron oxide (SPIO) has been proposed for targeting phagocytic cells in several inflammatory diseases such as multiple sclerosis and atherosclerosis. For this purpose, ultrasmall (U)SPIO are preferred because of a longer half-life in the blood stream (2 hours in rats) allowing a more effective capture by extrahepatic phagocytic cells including blood-circulating monocytes and resident macrophages already present in most of tissues.[6] The exact mechanism of particle capture is not perfectly known and may be cell specific. Two different mechanisms might be involved: first, and most likely, the particles could be taken up directly from the vascular space of the kidney by macrophages or mesangial cells gaining endocytic activity. This cellular uptake could be mediated by fluid-phase endocytosis. Another possibility could be a cellular uptake of the particles by circulating blood monocytes secondarily recruited into the kidney. Also, little is known about the fate of these macrophages, that is, whether they die in situ or emigrate and how long this takes. There is evidence suggesting migration of activated macrophages into the periglomerular interstitium.

Macrophage targeting in experimental models
Macrophage targeting within the kidney using USPIO was first proposed for a model of nephrotic syndrome, induced by intravenous injection of puromycin amino-nucleoside in rats.[7] This model induces both lesions of glomerular epithelial cells and a glomerular and tubulointerstitial infiltration by macrophages. It has been emphasized that accumulation of macrophages in the tubulointerstitium plays a role in renal injury and represents an important pathway of progressive renal functional impairment. After intravenous (IV) injection of 90 μmol Fe/kg (Sinerem, Guerbet Group, Aulnay-sous-Bois, France) on USPIO-enhanced MR images performed 24 hours after injection, our group demonstrated a diffuse decrease of signal intensity predominantly within the outer medulla. The degree of signal decrease was correlated with the number of macrophages within each renal compartment and to the amount of iron within the tissue measured with inductively coupled plasma emission spectroscopy. Normal rats did not show any decrease of intrarenal signal intensity after injection of USPIO (**Fig. 1**).

A diffuse interstitial macrophagic infiltration of renal parenchyma is a well-documented feature of chronic ureteral obstruction.[4] This cellular influx peaks the second day after the obstruction. Delayed USPIO-enhanced MR imaging demonstrated a diffuse but significant decrease of signal intensity in the three renal compartments, slightly more pronounced in the cortex (**Fig. 2**).[8]

In acute proliferative types of GN, such as Goodpasture syndrome or vascular nephritis, macrophages play also a role in the development of glomerular inflammation.[2] They accumulate in the Bowman space as a primary feature in the

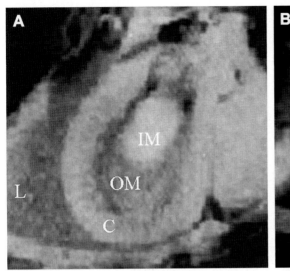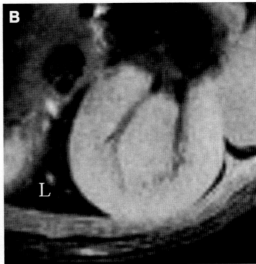

Fig. 1. T2*-weighted MR imaging of normal rat kidney at 4.7 T, before (*A*) and 24 hours after (*B*) intravenous infusion of USPIO. Iron oxide particles are captured by the liver (L) but not by kidney. C, cortex; OM, outer medulla; IM, inner medulla.

development of advanced cellular crescents, which is a known as a feature of rapidly progressive GN that is associated with a poor prognosis. A model of antiglomerular basal membrane (GBM) GN, comparable to Goodpasture syndrome in humans, was evaluated with MR imaging.[8] This model was induced in rats by IV injection of sheep anti-rat-GBM serum. In this model, kinetics of the immunologic response is characterized by two inflammatory phases (heterologous at day 2 involving neutrophils and autologous at day 14, involving macrophages), and a spontaneous resolution around day 21. The kinetics of signal intensity followed the biphasic evolution of the disease with a decrease of signal intensity within the cortex only at days 2 and 14 (**Fig. 3**A) and no change at day 21. This effect was a result of endocytosis of USPIO by macrophages at day 14 and by activated mesangial cells at both phases (see **Fig. 3**B). The degree of signal intensity decrease was strongly correlated with the degree of proteinuria (see **Fig. 3**C).

The mesangial cell is located in the glomerulus between the capillaries and plays a major role in the glomerular filtration by maintaining the capillary lumen open. Mesangial cell proliferation is a prominent feature of most human and experimental glomerular diseases: in various types of conditions, this cell can express phenotypic modifications and acquire myofibroblast cell characteristics such as proliferation, smooth muscle α-actin expression, increase synthesis of extracellular matrix components, and possibility of secondary renal impairment. These macrophagic-like

cells can potentially have deleterious effects by initializing the immune response, by producing mediators of inflammation, and by activating other mesangial cells with contractile phenotype. A noninvasive method for functional assessment of mesangial cells would therefore be crucial in the future. We demonstrated, using USPIOs, that the phagocytic phenotype of these cells could be assessed in an irreversible rat model of glomerulopathy, whereas no phagocytosis occurred in a reversible model.[9]

Intrinsic acute renal failure (ARF) is a multifactorial disease with concomitant ischemic, nephrotoxic, and septic components[10] and acute tubular necrosis (ATN) is its pathologic counterpart. Besides alterations in hemodynamics, tubule dynamics, tubule cell metabolism, and structure, the intrarenal inflammatory response plays a major role in the ischemic ARF. Neutrophils are the first leucocytes to accumulate in the postischemic kidney and macrophages are the next. Macrophages migrate into the outer medulla of rat kidneys and accumulate within peritubular capillaries, interstitial space, and even within tubules.[11,12] In an ischemia-reperfusion model in rats, USPIO-enhanced MR imaging demonstrated the same endocytosis pattern with a decrease of signal intensity within the outer medulla only from 24 to 120 hours after injection of particles (**Fig. 4**).[13] Signal intensity decrease was also correlated with level of renal function.

After renal transplantation, acute and chronic rejection episodes play a major role on long-term graft survival and involve T-cells and

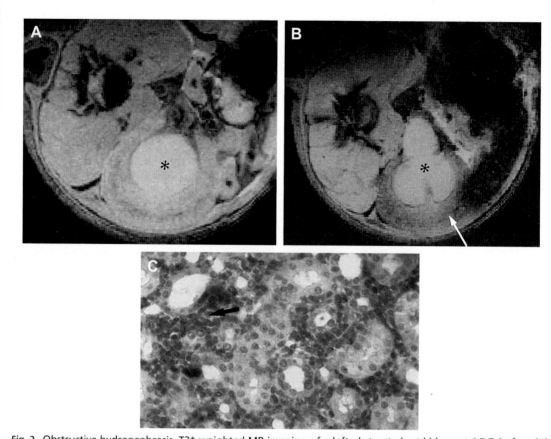

Fig. 2. Obstructive hydronephrosis. T2*-weighted MR imaging of a left obstructed rat kidney at 4.7 T, before (*A*) and 24 hours after (*B*) intravenous infusion of USPIO. There is a notable decrease in signal intensity in all kidney compartments after injection (*arrow* in *B*). Note the dilated renal collecting system (*). (*C*) Histologic section shows a diffuse infiltration of the interstitium by macrophages (original magnification ×40). (*From* Hauger O, Delelande C, Deminiere C, et al. Nephrotoxic nephritis and obstructive nephrology: evaluation with MR imaging enhanced with ultrasmall superparamagnetic iron oxide—preliminary findings in a rat model. Radiology 2000;217:819–26; with permission.)

macrophages. Two studies evaluated a rat model of acute rejection and showed a decrease of signal intensity within the cortex and medulla, increasing with iron dosage[14] and inhibited by immunosuppressive treatments.[15] Beckmann and colleagues[16] used SPIO to label macrophagic infiltration in a model of chronic rejection. They showed a dose-dependent decrease in cortical signal intensity in allografts between 8 and 16 weeks after transplantation (**Fig. 5**). The relative cortical signal intensity in the grafts was negatively correlated to the Banff score 6 weeks after transplantation and changes in creatinine clearance occurred only after 28 weeks. Groups treated with immunosuppressive and antiproliferative drugs showed lesser degree of signal intensity change.[17]

All these experimental results showed that USPIO-enhanced MR imaging could demonstrate intrarenal internalization of particles by macrophages or by glomerular cells gaining endocytic activity, ie, mesangial cells, and could localize precisely this endocytic activity in the different kidney compartments. Different types of experimental renal diseases showed different patterns of signal intensity changes but the degree of renal dysfunction appeared always correlated to the degree of endocytic activity, which may have significant implications in clinical practice.

Macrophage targeting in humans

These results led to the first pilot clinical study,[18] based on 12 patients exhibiting a dysfunction of either their native kidneys or of their transplant. As the blood half-life of USPIO is 36 hours in humans, MR imaging was performed 3 days after USPIO injection (Sinerem, Guerbet Group) to ensure avoiding signal changes from vascular blood

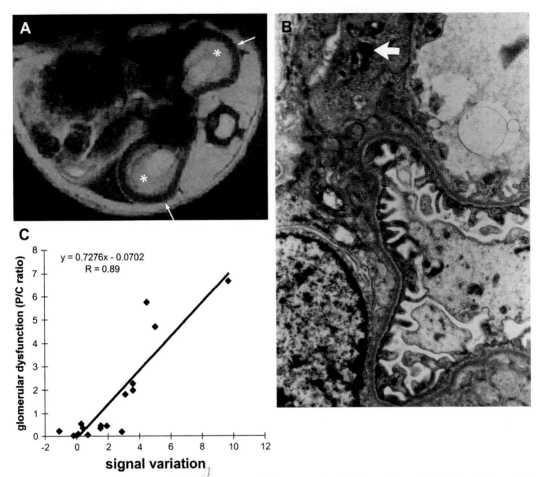

Fig. 3. Nephrotoxic anti-rat-GBM glomerulonephritis. (*A*) T2*-weighted MR imaging at 4.7 T, of rat kidneys in the day-2 pathologic group 24 hours after injection of USPIO. There is a notable decrease in signal intensity in the renal cortex (*arrows*) after injection, whereas no signal intensity change is observed in any portion of the medulla (***). (*B*) Electron microscopic image shows the presence of iron particles (*arrow*) in a lysosome of a mesangial cell. (*C*) A strong correlation between the degree of signal intensity variation (SI decrease?) and the estimate of glomerular damage is observed. P/C, protein-to-creatinine ratio. (*From* Hauger O, Delelande C, Deminiere C, et al. Nephrotoxic nephritis and obstructive nephrology: evaluation with MR imaging enhanced with ultrasmall superparamagnetic iron oxide—preliminary findings in a rat model. Radiology 2000;217:819–26; with permission.)

volume. Patients with chronic and fibrotic disease, without inflammatory component on biopsy did not show any significant change (**Fig. 6**A, B). Three patients with ATN (two transplanted kidneys and one native kidney) showed a significant decrease of signal intensity within the medulla only (see **Fig. 6**C, D). All patients but one with an inflammatory component on cortical biopsy showed a significant decrease of signal intensity after USPIO injection (see **Fig. 6**E, F). These preliminary clinical findings seem to corroborate experimental results, with the same topographic patterns, and call for larger multicenter clinical trials, and evaluation of imaging at 2 days after injection to reduce delay in the diagnosis.

MR Imaging and Intrarenal Stem Cell Therapy

Recovery of renal function after acute nephrotoxic or ischemic insult is dependent on the replacement of necrotic tubular cells by functional tubular epithelium.[19] This cellular regeneration may originate from renal resident cells or from extrarenal ones. Mesenchymal stem cells (MSC) have been shown to be able to repair damaged tissues, whether genetically modified or not.[20,21] They also have per se potential therapeutic effects such as with regard to the degradation of the extracellular matrix in experimental models of fibrosis[22] or the facilitation of the grafting of transplanted bone marrow progenitor cells by providing

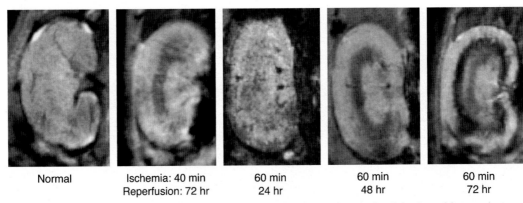

| Normal | Ischemia: 40 min
Reperfusion: 72 hr | 60 min
24 hr | 60 min
48 hr | 60 min
72 hr |

Fig. 4. Ischemia-reperfusion. T2*-weighted gradient-echo MR image 24 hours after injection of ferumodextran-10 USPIO particles. Rats were normal or subjected to 40 or 60 minutes of bilateral ischemia. A black band in the outer medulla is detected after 40 or 60 minutes of ischemia, at 48 to 120 hours after the beginning of reperfusion. (*From* Dagher PC, Herget-Rosenthal S, Ruehm SG, et al. Newly developed techniques to study and diagnose acute renal failure. J Am Soc Nephrol 2003;14:2188; with permission.)

a competent stroma.[23] They have a well-established ability to differentiate into the mesoderm lineage, which makes them potentially useful in strategies aiming at targeting the kidney mesangium for instance.

Recently, the possibility for bone marrow–derived MSC to differentiate into mesangial cells[24,25] and for hematopoietic stem cells into tubular cells was demonstrated in vivo,[26] bringing great therapeutic promise for the future. Noninvasive imaging techniques allowing in vivo assessment of the location of stem cells could be of great value for experimental studies in which these cells are transplanted. It provides a tool to verify immediately if the grafted cells have reached the target organ, to estimate the number of cells that were seeded, and to assess the permanence of these cells over time with sequential imaging. Using SPIO preparations to magnetically label the cells, several groups have demonstrated the feasibility of grafting and subsequent visualization of progenitor of different organs.[27–29] A strong relaxation rate effect was observed in vitro after MSC labeling for 48 hours with 50 μg Fe/mL and increased linearly with the iron dose.[30] Labeled cells were still able to differentiate into adipocytes (**Fig. 7**A) and osteocytes, but proliferation was limited with a 100 μg Fe/mL dose or greater. After intravascular administration, the renal distribution of SPIO-labeled MSC has been investigated recently. When administered into the renal artery of normal kidneys, labeled MSCs could be detected in vivo within the cortex as long as 7 days after injection at 1.5 T (see **Fig. 7**B, C) and iron-loaded cells

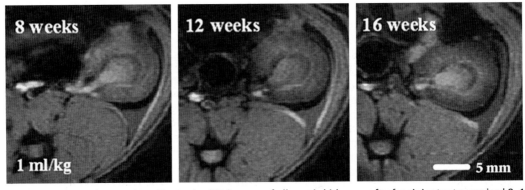

Fig. 5. SPIO-enhanced coronal gradient-echo MR images of allogenic kidney graft of recipient rats acquired 8, 12, and 16 weeks after transplantation. Imaging was performed 24 hours after injection of 1 mL/kg of SPIO. Darkening of the kidney cortex was apparent at different times after transplantation only in allogenic transplants, not in syngenic ones (not shown). (*Adapted from* Beckmann N, Cannet C, Zurbruegg S, et al. Macrophage infiltration detected at MR imaging in rat kidney allografts: early marker of chronic rejection? Radiology 2006;240:717; with permission.)

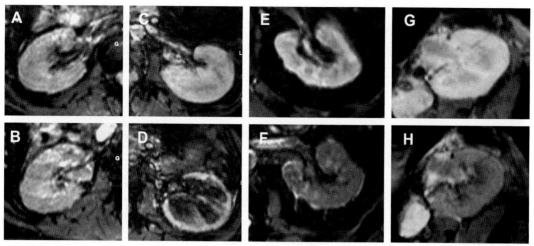

Fig. 6. USPIO-enhanced MR imaging in four patients with different patterns of signal intensity (SI) changes according to the type of disease. *A, C, E,* and *G* are T2*-weighted MR images before injection of USPIO. *B, D, F,* and *H* are T2*-weighted MR images 72 hours after injection of USPIO: (*A, B*) chronic glomerulohyalinosis and glomerulosclerosis with no SI change; (*C, D*) drug-induced acute renal failure with medullary SI drop; (*E, F*) extracapillary glomerulonephritis and (*G, H*) type Ia acute rejection, both with numerous interstitial macrophageson histology, and both showing diffuse SI drop after contrast. (*Adapted from* Hauger O, Grenier N, Deminere C, et al. USPIO-enhanced MR imaging of macrophage infiltration in native and transplanted kidneys: initial results in humans. Eur Radiol 2007;17:2898; with permission.)

were identified in renal glomeruli using histology.[30] The same experiment was repeated at 3 T[31] with similar results in normal kidneys. In kidneys with acute renal injury (40' ischemia-reperfusion), the improvement of renal function was accelerated in rats treated by cell graft: lower plasma creatinine levels at day 2 and day 3.[31] In a model of acute experimental glomerulopathy (Thy1+PAN), a homing effect was identified ex vivo, at 9.4 T, when the magnetically labeled MSCs were administered intravenously. A large proportion of cells was trapped within the liver, precluding their detection in the kidneys in vivo at 1.5 T. When comparing the enhancing renal segments in ex vivo images and pathologic lesions in histologic sections, the areas of low signal intensity correlated well with alpha-actin and Prussian blue stains, indicating that MSCs specifically homed to injured tissues (**Fig. 8**).[32]

MR IMAGING AND MONITORING OF GENE THERAPY

Up to now, MR imaging of transgene expression has been limited to demonstration of proof-of-principle experiments, using a change of signal intensity under the control of the expression of a reporter gene. As with PET, two approaches have been proposed with MR imaging using either an enzymatic pathway or a receptor pathway. The first method is based on the expression of a reporter gene (Lac-z) coding for an enzyme (β-galactosidase) that is able to activate a gadolinium (Gd)-chelate by giving access of water to the first coordination sphere of the Gd ions.[33] The second method is based on the targeting, with iron oxide particles, of cells overexpressing the transferrin receptors on their membrane.[34,35] None of these methods has been applied in the field of urogenital diseases.

MR imaging could also play a role in controlling gene expression in space and in time. The possibility to limit the effect of a therapeutic gene to a target diseased tissue and during a predefined time window is a key challenge for the future of gene therapy. For such a purpose, expression of a transgene can be controlled by a heat-sensitive promoter, such as promoter of the inducible heat shock protein systems, HSP70.[36] These promoters can activate gene expression several thousand-fold in response to hyperthermia.[37] Heating of deep parts of the body can be achieved with high-intensity focused ultrasound (HIFU). However, a precise control of the heating is absolutely necessary to reach the target temperature (around 42° to 43°) without any deleterious effect on the tissue. This temperature control is made possible by using temperature-sensitive MR sequences based on the proton resonance frequency (PRF) method[38] and by using an automatic monitoring of the acoustic power. The feasibility of such approach has been shown both in vitro and in vivo,[39,40] including the expression of suicide genes

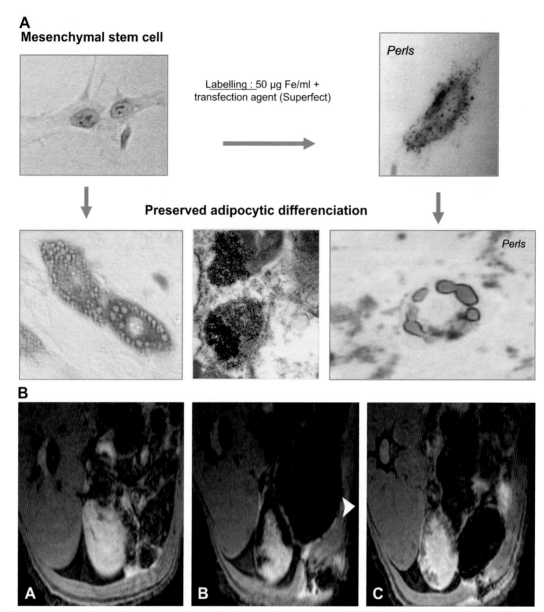

Fig. 7. Renal cell therapy by intraarterial graft of mesenchymal stem cells (MSC). (*A*) In vitro labeling of MSC with SPIO and a transfection agent. After labeling, cells keep their capacities of differentiation into adipocytes. (*B*) Transverse 3-dimensional T2*-weighted MR images of rat kidney obtained with water-selective excitation. Arrowhead indicates ventral side of animal. SPIO-labeled MSCs were injected into left renal artery. *A*, Image obtained before injection. *B*, Image obtained within 1 hour after injection: lower pole of kidney shows distinct cortical signal intensity decrease, which indicated presence of MSCs. *C*, Image obtained after 7 days. *(From Bos C, Delmas Y, Desmouliere A, et al. In vivo MR imaging of intravascularly injected magnetically labeled mesenchymal stem cells in rat kidney and liver. Radiology 2004;233:781; with permission.)*

in a transfected mammary cancer cell line.[41] The same approach was experimented within the prostate of three dogs, after direct injection in the gland of an adenoviral vector containing a transgene encoding firefly luciferase under the control of the hsp70B promoter. The prostate was heated using HIFU under MR imaging guidance. High levels of luciferase expression were demonstrated in vitro in prostate sections only in areas exposed to ultrasonic heating.[42]

Genetically modified stem and progenitor cells have been shown to be potentially useful vectors for cell therapy. They provide a way to express a transgene at the site where these cells are

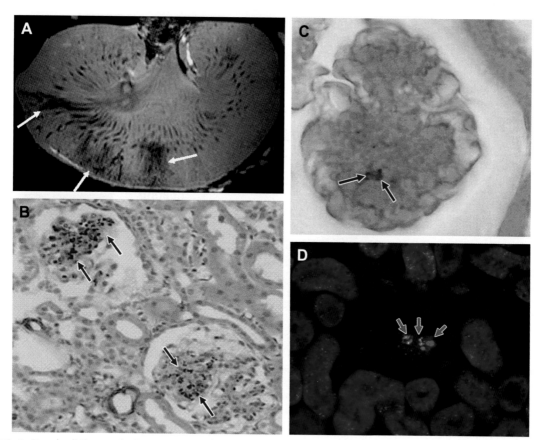

Fig. 8. Renal cell therapy by intravenous graft of mesenchymal stem cells (MSC). (*A*) Ex vivo sagittal 3-dimensional T2*-weighted 9.4-T MR images of pathologic kidney 6 days after intravenous injection of 10^7 labeled MSCs (the upper pole is oriented left). The corticomedullary differentiation is absent and distinct areas of cortical signal intensity decrease are present in the superior and superior midportion (*arrows*) poles. (*B*) Micrograph of a pathologic kidney portion shows grade 2–positive area for α-actin staining, with brown spots corresponding to activated mesangial cells (*arrows*). (*C, D*) These inflamed areas show a substantial number of Prussian blue– and DiI-positive glomeruli (*arrows*). Prussian blue– and DiI-positive spots correspond to labeled MSCs. (*From* Hauger O, Frost EE, Deminiere C, et al. MR evaluation of the glomerular homing of magnetically labeled mesenchymal stem cells in a rat model of nephropathy. Radiology 2006;238:200; with permission.)

grafted, either through direct administration within the tissue or intra-arterial injection. More importantly, because of their ability to differentiate in various cell lineages, they offer the additional potential of repairing and regenerating tissues in response to disease or injury.

This approach has been recently experimented in vivo within the rat kidney. First, modified MSC expressing the luciferase reporter gene under the control of the hsp70B promoter were administered through the left renal artery (**Fig. 9**). Luciferase expression in MR-guided HIFU heated regions was first demonstrated in vitro, using immunostaining.[43] More recently, using modified C6 cells with hsp70B-luc expression injected in the artery of superficialized rat kidneys, local luciferase expression was demonstrated for the first time in vivo, by using bioluminescence imaging (**Fig. 10**).[44] The

optimal heating protocol was found to be 43° during 5 minutes to get reproducible significant expression without parenchymal deleterious effect of heating. Application of this method in the kidney of large animals or humans will require the application of movement correction methods for an accurate temperature mapping.[45]

MR IMAGING OF CELL RECEPTORS

Molecular MR imaging of cell receptors is a growing field and requires development of specific contrast agents. The most developed strategy for targeting cells using MR imaging is to bind a contrast agent with a monoclonal antibody, an aptamer, or a peptide, able to recognize specifically a surface antigen expressed on the cell membrane surface. Up until now, main applications focused

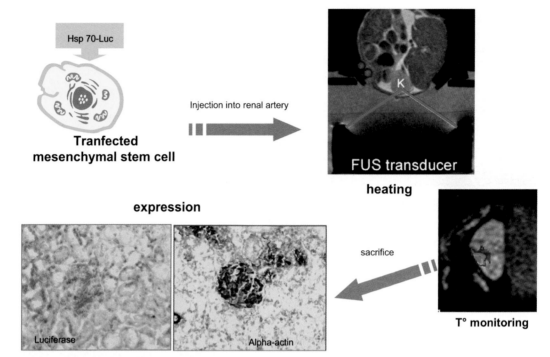

Fig. 9. Principle of ex vivo demonstration of intrarenal reporter gene expression under MR control. Genetically modified mesenchymal stem cells (MSC) with a luciferase reporter gene under control of the hsp70B promoter were injected into renal artery. Kidney was heated by focused ultrasound under control of MR thermometry. After sacrifice, histopathology revealed a positive alpha-actin immunostaining within glomeruli (brown) in heated rat kidneys compatible with MSCs and positive staining for luciferase activity (with luciferase antibody), not shown in kidneys injected and not heated.

on targeting inflammatory receptors, such as P-selectin,[46] E-selectin,[47] vascular cell adhesion molecule (VCAM),[48] intercellular adhesion molecule (ICAM),[49] or tumor-specific receptors, such as HER2/neu.[50] To our knowledge, targeting of the prostate-specific membrane antigen (PSMA) is the first application of these strategies involving the urinary system.

Dosage of prostate specific antigen (PSA) has transformed diagnosis of prostate cancer leading to downstaging of this tumor at diagnosis.[51] Patients with abnormal digital rectal examination or elevated PSA are referred to prostatic biopsies. However, about 28% of these patients show negative histologic results, leading to a second round of biopsies. In such cases, high-resolution MR imaging using endorectal coils, coupled with dynamic contrast-enhanced sequences and spectroscopic acquisitions are suggested to identify possible targets for subsequent biopsies. However, the provided findings are not specific for cancer tissue and a significant percentage of patients remain undiagnosed. Therefore, development of specific molecular probes for cancer targeting appears worthwhile.

PSMA, a type II transmembrane glycoprotein, is a potential cell surface antigen overexpressed in prostatic carcinomas.[52] PSMA also exhibits carboxypeptidase enzymatic activity. It is overexpressed in prostatic cancer, but also in the neovasculature of other cancers (breast, colon, neuroendocrine) and in duodenal epithelial cells and proximal tubule cells of the kidney. PSMA content has been shown to be correlated with both tumor grade and tumor progression. This antigen has been already targeted with radioactive antibodies (Prostascint)[53] but images are lacking spatial resolution for intraprostatic localization of missed tumors.

Recently, anti-PSMA antibodies conjugated with iron oxide nanoparticles, using a biotin-streptavidin linkage, were used to specifically image prostate cancer cells.[54] These authors showed that these particles targeted PSMA at the surface cells and are internalized by receptor-mediated endocytosis mechanism involving formation of clathrin-coated vesicles. Their accumulation on and within tumor cells enhanced in vitro T1 and T2 relaxation rates, leading to enhanced contrast in MR images. Besides the diagnostic potential of this agent in clinics, which remains to be

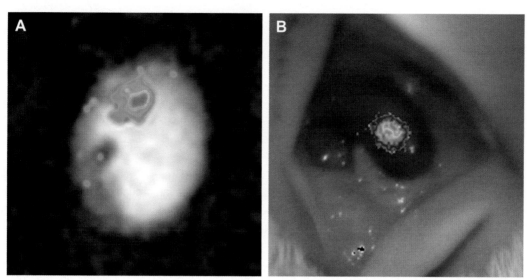

Fig. 10. In vivo demonstration of intrarenal reporter gene expression under MR control. Genetically modified C6-glioma cells, with a luciferase reporter gene under control of the hsp70B promoter, are injected into renal artery of rats and heated in vivo under control of MR thermometry (A). Optical imaging of the superficialized kidney shows an area of luminescence corresponding to the heated region (B).

demonstrated, a local intracellular delivery of therapeutics could also be suggested in the future, according to the authors.[52]

MR IMAGING OF APOPTOSIS

Apoptosis and its regulatory mechanisms contribute to cell number regulation in acute renal failure.[55] Tubular cell apoptosis is promoted by both exogenous factors such as nephrotoxic drugs and bacterial products, and endogenous factors such as lethal cytokines. Conversely to necrosis, which is a nonreversible process, apoptotic pathways are potentially accessible to therapeutic modulation.[56] Therefore, targeting apoptosis within the kidney would play a major role from a pathophysiological point of view and for the follow-up of acute ischemic disease under treatment.

There is actually a growing interest in using MR imaging for detection of apoptosis, mainly in the oncology field and in ischemic diseases. This approach requires labeling of apoptotic cells using USPIOs as a marker and phosphatidylserine as a target. This necessitates linking the superparamagnetic nanoparticle to annexin V or synaptotagmin I, which both bind to the phosphatidylserine present on the outer leaflet of the plasma membrane of apoptotic cells.[57] Several preclinical applications using MR imaging have been reported to target apoptotic cells within the heart[58] or within tumors during chemotherapy[59] but, to our knowledge, this approach has never been applied to an ischemic kidney model.

MR IMAGING OF ENZYME SYNTHESIS OR ACTIVITY

Whereas enzyme activity is highly involved in renal physiopathology of many renal parenchymal diseases and urinary cancers, nothing has been done in that field using MR imaging. We will focus here on potential applications of molecular imaging techniques that have been proposed for other organs.

MR Imaging of Matrix Metalloproteases

Matrix metalloproteases (MMPs) are zinc-containing endopeptidases that are involved in degradation and remodeling the extracellular matrix (ECM), crucial for tissue development and homeostasis.[60] They localize to the cell surface or extracellular compartments. Their spatial expression in the kidney is complex and has not been completely characterized. MMP activity is associated with tumor invasion and metastasis, justifying the development of MMP inhibitors as anticancer alternatives. Within the kidney, an aberrant MMP expression is related to a number of renal pathologies, both acute and chronic. In acute renal diseases, there is strong evidence that MMPs mediate acute kidney injury and are involved in changes in the vascular endothelium, glomeruli, and tubular epithelial cells. In the ischemia-reperfusion model, increased MMP-9 activity was associated with an increased vascular and tubular permeability, owing to degradation of cell adhesion molecules.[61] In chronic kidney diseases (CKD), a role for MMPs has been demonstrated in several experimental models. For example, decreased MMP-9 expression was correlated with the development of tubulointerstitial fibrosis and glomerulosclerosis in rats.[62] A number of studies have also demonstrated a link between aberrant MMP expression and the progression of diabetic nephropathy in animal models.[63] Overexpression of a single MMP may be a critical mediator of CKD. However, the relationship between MMP activity and inflammation remains an important component of CKD that remains to be addressed.

A Gd-chelate coupled with an MMP-inhibitor was recently developed for MR imaging of atherosclerotic plaques.[64] The affinity of this agent in vitro was broad toward MMP-1, 2, 3, 8, 9, and 13. In vivo, its affinity and specificity allowed accurate discrimination of MMP-poor and MMP-rich plaques. Another type of MR contrast agent, specific for MMPs, was proposed by Lepage and colleagues,[65] based on the concept of solubility switch, from hydrophilic to hydrophobic, modifying its pharmacokinetic properties. This agent, associating Gd-tetraazacyclododecanetetraacetic acid (Gd-DOTA) and a proteinase-sensitive peptide, was designed to display a reduced solubility after cleavage by MMP-7, responsible for an increased retention, making the detection of its activity possible. Applications of such agents in the nephro-urological sphere, as acute and chronic renal diseases and urological cancers, are really attractive but must still be developed.

MR Imaging of Myeloperoxidase

Myeloperoxidase (MPO) is one of the most abundant enzymes secreted by inflammatory mononuclear cells (neutrophils and macrophages), able to generate reactive oxygen species as hypochlorous acid/hypochlorite ($HOCl/OCl^-$) from hydrogen peroxide in the presence of chloride ions. Within the kidney, this reaction leads to a variety of chlorinated protein and lipid adducts that in turn may cause dysfunction of cells in different compartments of renal parenchyma.[66] MPO is an important pathogenic factor in glomerular and tubulointerstitial diseases: for example, MPO and HOCl-modified proteins can be seen in glomerular peripheral basement membranes and podocytes in human membranous glomerulonephritis; MPO antibody complexes induce and exacerbate the inflammation in necrotizing glomerulonephritis. Anti-neutrophil cytoplasm antibodies with anti-MPO specificity have a key role in the pathogenesis of microscopic polyangeitis, which may damage the kidneys and other organs.

An MPO-sensitive Gd-based MR contrast agent has been developed recently.[67] MPOs are able to activate this agent by inducing oligomerization and protein binding and, consequently, by increasing its relaxivity. Experiments have shown that this MPO activity could be targeted in vivo within reperfused ischemic myocardium[68] and within inflammatory demyelinating plaques in brain.[67,69] Applications of this technique within the kidney should be numerous in the future.

SUMMARY

Molecular MR imaging has already demonstrated its great potential in characterizing diseases because of the association of its high spatial resolution capabilities and the use of contrast agents specific for different kinds of cellular or molecular targets. The low MR sensitivity, when compared with PET, may be compensated by original methods of signal amplification. In the future, many parenchymal renal diseases could benefit from these new imaging techniques, which provide a better characterization of the diseases and offer noninvasive, objective prognostic criteria. Cellular targeting with superparamagnetic contrast agents have already found a broad range of applications in kidney diseases and potential clinical applications will emerge soon. Unfortunately, whereas the feasibility to image in vivo all the mentioned molecular processes using MR imaging was demonstrated in many preclinical experiments, little attention has been paid to validate them in the urinary tract. Therefore, in the future, much effort is required to extend such applications and turn this potential into use in clinical practice.

ACKNOWLEDGMENTS

Acknowledgments for collaborations in many experimental studies to: Clemens Bos, Jeff Bulte, Y. Delmas, Colette Deminière, Baudouin Denis de Senneville, Jean Ripoche.

REFERENCES

1. Szabo Z, Xia J, Mathews WB, et al. Future direction of renal positron emission tomography. Semin Nucl Med 2006;36(1):36–50.
2. Cattell V. Macrophages in acute glomerular inflammation. Kidney Int 1994;45(4):945–52.
3. Grau V, Herbst B, Steiniger B. Dynamics of monocytes/macrophages and T lymphocytes in acutely rejecting rat renal allografts. Cell Tissue Res 1998; 291(1):117–26.
4. Schreiner GF, Harris KP, Purkerson ML, et al. Immunological aspects of acute ureteral obstruction: immune cell infiltrate in the kidney. Kidney Int 1988;34(4): 487–93.

5. Erwig LP, Kluth DC, Rees AJ. Macrophages in renal inflammation. Curr Opin Nephrol Hypertens 2001; 10(3):341–7.

6. Modo M, Hoehn M, Bulte JW. Cellular MR imaging. Mol Imaging 2005;4(3):143–64.

7. Hauger O, Delalande C, Trillaud H, et al. MR imaging of intrarenal macrophage infiltration in an experimental model of nephrotic syndrome. Magn Reson Med 1999;41(1):156–62.

8. Hauger O, Delalande C, Deminiere C, et al. Nephrotoxic nephritis and obstructive nephropathy: evaluation with MR imaging enhanced with ultrasmall superparamagnetic iron oxide-preliminary findings in a rat model. Radiology 2000;217(3):819–26.

9. Hauger O, Delmas Y, Deminere C, et al. Assessment of phagocytic and nonphagocytic phenotypes of activated mesangial cells with experimental iron oxide-enhanced MR imaging. Presented at the International Society of Magnetic Resonance in Medicine, Honolulu, May 18–24, 2002.

10. Devarajan P. Update on mechanisms of ischemic acute kidney injury. J Am Soc Nephrol 2006;17(6): 1503–20.

11. Friedewald JJ, Rabb H. Inflammatory cells in ischemic acute renal failure. Kidney Int 2004;66(2):486–91.

12. Ysebaert DK, De Greef KE, Vercauteren SR, et al. Identification and kinetics of leukocytes after severe ischaemia/reperfusion renal injury. Nephrol Dial Transplant 2000;15(10):1562–74.

13. Jo SK, Hu X, Kobayashi H, et al. Detection of inflammation following renal ischemia by magnetic resonance imaging. Kidney Int 2003;64(1):43–51.

14. Ye Q, Yang D, Williams M, et al. In vivo detection of acute rat renal allograft rejection by MRI with USPIO particles. Kidney Int 2002;61(3):1124–35.

15. Zhang Y, Dodd SJ, Hendrich KS, et al. Magnetic resonance imaging detection of rat renal transplant rejection by monitoring macrophage infiltration. Kidney Int 2000;58(3):1300–10.

16. Beckmann N, Cannet C, Zurbruegg S, et al. Macrophage infiltration detected at MR imaging in rat kidney allografts: early marker of chronic rejection? Radiology 2006;240(3):717–24.

17. Beckmann N, Cannet C, Fringeli-Tanner M, et al. Macrophage labeling by SPIO as an early marker of allograft chronic rejection in a rat model of kidney transplantation. Magn Reson Med 2003;49(3): 459–67.

18. Hauger O, Grenier N, Deminere C, et al. USPIO-enhanced MR imaging of macrophage infiltration in native and transplanted kidneys: initial results in humans. Eur Radiol 2007;17(11):2898–907.

19. Gupta S, Verfaillie C, Chmielewski D, et al. A role for extrarenal cells in the regeneration following acute renal failure. Kidney Int 2002;62(4):1285–90.

20. Baksh D, Song L, Tuan RS. Adult mesenchymal stem cells: characterization, differentiation, and application in cell and gene therapy. J Cell Mol Med 2004;8(3):301–16.

21. Pittenger MF, Martin BJ. Mesenchymal stem cells and their potential as cardiac therapeutics. Circ Res 2004;95(1):9–20.

22. Fang B, Shi M, Liao L, et al. Systemic infusion of FLK1(+) mesenchymal stem cells ameliorate carbon tetrachloride-induced liver fibrosis in mice. Transplantation 2004;78(1):83–8.

23. Bacigalupo A. Mesenchymal stem cells and haematopoietic stem cell transplantation. Best Pract Res Clin Haematol 2004;17(3):387–99.

24. Imasawa T, Utsunomiya Y, Kawamura T, et al. The potential of bone marrow-derived cells to differentiate to glomerular mesangial cells. J Am Soc Nephrol 2001;12(7):1401–9.

25. Ito T, Suzuki A, Imai E, et al. Bone marrow is a reservoir of repopulating mesangial cells during glomerular remodeling. J Am Soc Nephrol 2001;12(12):2625–35.

26. Lin F, Cordes K, Li L, et al. Hematopoietic stem cells contribute to the regeneration of renal tubules after renal ischemia-reperfusion injury in mice. J Am Soc Nephrol 2003;14(5):1188–99.

27. Bulte JW, Zhang S, van Gelderen P, et al. Neurotransplantation of magnetically labeled oligodendrocyte progenitors: magnetic resonance tracking of cell migration and myelination. Proc Natl Acad Sci U S A 1999;96(26):15256–61.

28. Hoehn M, Kustermann E, Blunk J, et al. Monitoring of implanted stem cell migration in vivo: a highly resolved in vivo magnetic resonance imaging investigation of experimental stroke in rat. Proc Natl Acad Sci U S A 2002;99(25):16267–72.

29. Kraitchman DL, Heldman AW, Atalar E, et al. In vivo magnetic resonance imaging of mesenchymal stem cells in myocardial infarction. Circulation 2003; 107(18):2290–3.

30. Bos C, Delmas Y, Desmouliere A, et al. In vivo MR imaging of intravascularly injected magnetically labeled mesenchymal stem cells in rat kidney and liver. Radiology 2004;233(3):781–9.

31. Ittrich H, Lange C, Togel F, et al. In vivo magnetic resonance imaging of iron oxide-labeled, arterially-injected mesenchymal stem cells in kidneys of rats with acute ischemic kidney injury: detection and monitoring at 3T. J Magn Reson Imaging 2007; 25(6):1179–91.

32. Hauger O, Frost EE, Deminière C, et al. MR evaluation of the glomerular homing of magnetically labeled mesenchymal stem cells in a rat model of nephropathy. Radiology 2006;238(1):200–10.

33. Louie AY, Huber MM, Ahrens ET, et al. In vivo visualization of gene expression using magnetic resonance imaging. Nat Biotechnol 2000;18(3):321–5.

34. Moore A, Josephson L, Bhorade RM, et al. Human transferrin receptor gene as a marker gene for MR imaging. Radiology 2001;221(1):244–50.

35. Weissleder R, Mahmood U. Molecular imaging. Radiology 2001;219(2):316–33.

36. Rome C, Couillaud F, Moonen CT. Spatial and temporal control of expression of therapeutic genes using heat shock protein promoters. Methods 2005; 35(2):188–98.

37. Dreano M, Brochot J, Myers A, et al. High-level, heat-regulated synthesis of proteins in eukaryotic cells. Gene 1986;49(1):1–8.

38. Quesson B, de Zwart JA, Moonen CT. Magnetic resonance temperature imaging for guidance of thermotherapy. J Magn Reson Imaging 2000;12(4):525–33.

39. Huang Q, Hu JK, Lohr F, et al. Heat-induced gene expression as a novel targeted cancer gene therapy strategy. Cancer Res 2000;60(13):3435–9.

40. Smith RC, Machluf M, Bromley P, et al. Spatial and temporal control of transgene expression through ultrasound-mediated induction of the heat shock protein 70B promoter in vivo. Hum Gene Ther 2002; 13(6):697–706.

41. Braiden V, Ohtsuru A, Kawashita Y, et al. Eradication of breast cancer xenografts by hyperthermic suicide gene therapy under the control of the heat shock protein promoter. Hum Gene Ther 2000;11(18):2453–63.

42. Silcox CE, Smith RC, King R, et al. MRI-guided ultrasonic heating allows spatial control of exogenous luciferase in canine prostate. Ultrasound Med Biol 2005;31(7):965–70.

43. Letavernier B, Salomir R, Delmas Y, et al. Ultrasound induced expression of a heat-shock promoter-driven transgene delivered in the kidney by genetically modified mesenchymal stem cells. A feasibility study. In: Hynynen K, Jolesz F, editors. MR-guided focused ultrasound surgery. New-York: Taylor & Francis; 2007. p. 171–9.

44. Eker O, Quesson B, Frulio N, et al. In vivo visualization of an optical reporter gene expression transported by a cellular vector and locally activated by MRI-guided HIFU in rat kidney. Presented at the International Society of Magnetic Resonance in Medicine, Toronto, May 3–9, 2008.

45. de Senneville BD, Mougenot C, Quesson B, et al. MR thermometry for monitoring tumor ablation. Eur Radiol 2007;17(9):2401–10.

46. Chaubet F, Bertholon I, Serfaty JM, et al. A new macromolecular paramagnetic MR contrast agent binds to activated human platelets. Contrast Media Mol Imaging 2007;2(4):178–88.

47. Reynolds PR, Larkman DJ, Haskard DO, et al. Detection of vascular expression of E-selectin in vivo with MR imaging. Radiology 2006;241(2):469–76.

48. Nahrendorf M, Jaffer FA, Kelly KA, et al. Noninvasive vascular cell adhesion molecule-1 imaging identifies inflammatory activation of cells in atherosclerosis. Circulation 2006;114(14):1504–11.

49. Choi KS, Kim SH, Cai QY, et al. Inflammation-specific T1 imaging using anti-intercellular adhesion molecule 1 antibody-conjugated gadolinium diethylenetriaminepentaacetic acid. Mol Imaging 2007; 6(2):75–84.

50. Daldrup-Link HE, Meier R, Rudelius M, et al. In vivo tracking of genetically engineered, anti-HER2/neu directed natural killer cells to HER2/neu positive mammary tumors with magnetic resonance imaging. Eur Radiol 2005;15(1):4–13.

51. Hricak H, Choyke PL, Eberhardt SC, et al. Imaging prostate cancer: a multidisciplinary perspective. Radiology 2007;243(1):28–53.

52. Chang SS. Overview of prostate-specific membrane antigen. Rev Urol 2004;6(Suppl 10):S13–8.

53. Hinkle GH, Burgers JK, Neal CE, et al. Multicenter radioimmunoscintigraphic evaluation of patients with prostate carcinoma using indium-111 capromab pendetide. Cancer 1998;83(4):739–47.

54. Serda RE, Adolphi NL, Bisoffi M, et al. Targeting and cellular trafficking of magnetic nanoparticles for prostate cancer imaging. Mol Imaging 2007;6(4): 277–88.

55. Ortiz A, Justo P, Sanz A, et al. Targeting apoptosis in acute tubular injury. Biochem Pharmacol 2003;66(8): 1589–94.

56. Rana A, Sathyanarayana P, Lieberthal W. Role of apoptosis of renal tubular cells in acute renal failure: therapeutic implications. Apoptosis 2001;6(1-2): 83–102.

57. Hakumaki JM, Brindle KM. Techniques: visualizing apoptosis using nuclear magnetic resonance. Trends Pharmacol Sci 2003;24(3):146–9.

58. Hiller KH, Waller C, Nahrendorf M, et al. Assessment of cardiovascular apoptosis in the isolated rat heart by magnetic resonance molecular imaging. Mol Imaging 2006;5(2):115–21.

59. Zhao M, Beauregard DA, Loizou L, et al. Non-invasive detection of apoptosis using magnetic resonance imaging and a targeted contrast agent. Nat Med 2001;7(11):1241–4.

60. Catania JM, Chen G, Parrish AR. Role of matrix metalloproteinases in renal pathophysiologies. Am J Physiol Renal Physiol 2007;292(3):F905–11.

61. Caron A, Desrosiers RR, Beliveau R. Ischemia injury alters endothelial cell properties of kidney cortex: stimulation of MMP-9. Exp Cell Res 2005;310(1): 105–16.

62. Bolbrinker J, Markovic S, Wehland M, et al. Expression and response to angiotensin-converting enzyme inhibition of matrix metalloproteinases 2 and 9 in renal glomerular damage in young transgenic rats with renin-dependent hypertension. J Pharmacol Exp Ther 2006;316(1):8–16.

63. McLennan SV, Kelly DJ, Cox AJ, et al. Decreased matrix degradation in diabetic nephropathy: effects of ACE inhibition on the expression and activities of matrix metalloproteinases. Diabetologia 2002; 45(2):268–75.

64. Lancelot E, Amirbekian V, Brigger I, et al. Evaluation of matrix metalloproteinases in atherosclerosis using a novel noninvasive imaging approach. Arterioscler Thromb Vasc Biol 2008;28(3):425–32.

65. Lepage M, Dow WC, Melchior M, et al. Noninvasive detection of matrix metalloproteinase activity in vivo using a novel magnetic resonance imaging contrast agent with a solubility switch. Mol Imaging 2007;6(6):393–403.

66. Malle E, Buch T, Grone HJ. Myeloperoxidase in kidney disease. Kidney Int 2003;64(6):1956–67.

67. Chen JW, Querol Sans M, Bogdanov A Jr, et al. Imaging of myeloperoxidase in mice by using novel amplifiable paramagnetic substrates. Radiology 2006;240(2):473–81.

68. Nahrendorf M, Sosnovik D, Chen JW, et al. Activatable magnetic resonance imaging agent reports myeloperoxidase activity in healing infarcts and noninvasively detects the antiinflammatory effects of atorvastatin on ischemia-reperfusion injury. Circulation 2008;117(9):1153–60.

69. Chen JW, Breckwoldt MO, Aikawa E, et al. Myeloperoxidase-targeted imaging of active inflammatory lesions in murine experimental autoimmune encephalomyelitis. Brain 2008;131(Pt 4):1123–33.

MR Urography: Technique and Results for the Evaluation of Urinary Obstruction in the Pediatric Population

J. Damien Grattan-Smith, MBBS[a,b,*], Richard A. Jones, PhD[a,b]

KEYWORDS

- MR urography • Hydronephrosis
- Urinary tract obstruction
- Ureteropelvic junction obstruction

MR urography provides a comprehensive evaluation of the urinary tract in a single examination that does not use ionizing radiation and represents the next step in the evolution of uroradiology in children. Over the last few years, there has been rapid development and refinement of imaging protocols for evaluating the urinary tract in children using MR urography.[1–5] Several authors recognized early in its development the potential use of MR imaging in the evaluation of renal tract disease in children.[6–16] MR urography combines intrinsically high spatial and contrast resolution with rapid temporal resolution. In addition to high-resolution anatomic images of the entire urinary tract, functional information about the concentration and excretion of the individual kidneys can be obtained. By scanning dynamically after injection of contrast agents, the signal changes related to perfusion, concentration, and excretion of the contrast agent can be evaluated sequentially both in the renal cortex and medulla. Urinary tract anatomy is assessed using a combination of both T2-weighted and contrast-enhanced images. The functional information obtained routinely includes renal transit time (RTT) calculation, graphs of signal intensity versus time curves, differential renal function calculation, and estimation of individual kidney glomerular filtration rate (GFR) using a Patlak plot.

The improved anatomic and functional information obtained simultaneously with MR urography provides new insights into the underlying pathophysiology of urinary tract disorders. As a result, it is likely that MR urography will replace renal scintigraphy in the evaluation of renal tract disorders in children in the near future.

TECHNIQUE

The imaging protocols used for clinical studies consist of conventional T1-weighted, fast spin echo T2-weighted sequences before contrast administration, and dynamic three-dimensional gradient echo sequences after contrast administration and have been outlined in detail in earlier publications (**Figs. 1–3**).[1,2] There is a fundamentally complex relationship between signal intensity and gadolinium concentration, with T1 effects predominating at lower concentrations and T2* effects at higher concentrations, which may lead to signal loss. Phantom studies have shown that the relationship between signal intensity and

[a] Department of Radiology, Children's Healthcare of Atlanta, 1001 Johnson Ferry Road, Atlanta, GA 30342, USA
[b] Department of Radiology, Emory University School of Medicine, 1364 Clifton Road NE, Atlanta, GA 30322, USA
* Corresponding author. Department of Radiology, Children's Healthcare of Atlanta, 1001 Johnson Ferry Road, Atlanta, GA 30342, USA.
E-mail address: damien.grattan-smith@choa.org (J.D. Grattan-Smith).

Magn Reson Imaging Clin N Am 16 (2008) 643–660
doi:10.1016/j.mric.2008.07.003
1064-9689/08/$ – see front matter © 2008 Elsevier Inc. All rights reserved.

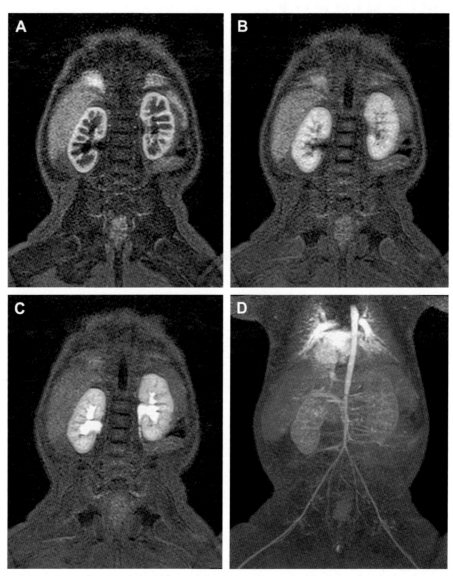

Fig. 1. Normal MR urogram in a 7-week-old boy with suspected antenatal hydronephrosis. (*A–C*) Same slice from each of three separate volume acquisitions. (*D–F*) Maximum intensity projection (MIP) projections derived from the same three separate time points. *A* and *D* show the cortical phase. *B* and *E* were acquired 60 seconds later and demonstrate enhancement of both the cortex and medulla with the signal intensity of the medulla exceeding the cortex. *C* and *F* were acquired 130 seconds after the vascular phase and show excretion into the calyces, renal pelvis, and ureters. Fetal folds are seen in the ureters bilaterally. The renal transit time was normal at 2 minutes and 20 seconds bilaterally (normal renal transit time is less than 240 seconds) and the volumetric differential renal function (DRF) was 51:49.

gadolinium concentration is relatively linear at low concentrations.[17] To stay within this linear portion of the curve, the authors keep the gadolinium concentration low by hydrating the patient, by giving furosemide 15 minutes before the contrast is administered, and by infusing the contrast agent slowly for the dynamic series.

For protocols, all children are hydrated before the study with an intravenous infusion of lactated Ringer's solution; for sedated children the volume infused is calculated to replace the NPO deficit, otherwise the volume is calculated using a guideline of 10 mL/kg. Typically, all children less than 7 years of age require sedation for the examination and the department's standard sedation procedures are followed. A bladder catheter is placed to eliminate the possibility of reflux and to ensure free drainage of the bladder. Once the patient is positioned in the scanner, scout images are acquired to determine both the positioning of the

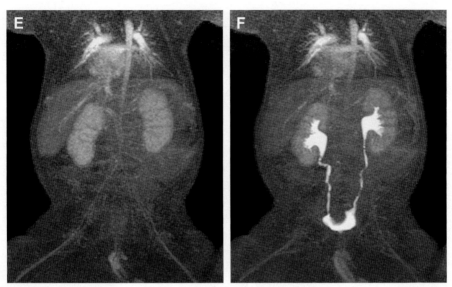

Fig. 1. (*continued*)

kidneys and bladder and the combination of spine coil elements required to optimize the signal-to-noise ratio for these anatomic structures. After the scout images were completed axial T2-weighted images through the kidneys are obtained. Furosemide (1 mg/kg, maximum 20 mg) is then administered intravenously. The authors administer furosemide 15 minutes before injecting contrast for three reasons: (1) the urinary tract is distended; (2) the gadolinium concentration is diluted, which reduces the susceptibility artifacts and helps maintain the contrast-induced signal changes to within the range where they are linearly related to contrast agent concentration;[17] and (3) the examination time is shortened. Coronal, two-dimensional, flow compensated T1- and T2-weighted series and a respiratory gated, heavily T2-weighted three-dimensional sequence are then acquired. The two-dimensional series served to provide detailed anatomic reference scans, whereas the heavily T2-weighted three-dimensional scan provided the basis for a precontrast maximum intensity projection (MIP) of the collecting system, ureters, and bladder. To create

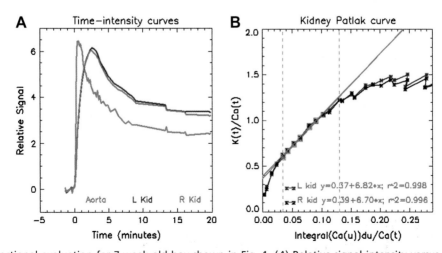

Fig. 2. Functional evaluation for 7-week-old boy shown in Fig. 1. (*A*) Relative signal intensity versus time curve showing curves for the aorta and both kidneys. Note the symmetric parenchymal curves with equivalent perfusion, concentration, and excretion of contrast agent. (*B*) The Patlak plot is used as an index of the individual kidney GFR. The slope of each plot reflects the GFR of each kidney (6.8 mL/min on left and 6.7 mL/min on right). The y intercept represents the fractional blood volume of each kidney. The body surface area corrected Patlak (BSA Patlak) is 92 mL/min. The Patlak DRF is calculated at 50:50.

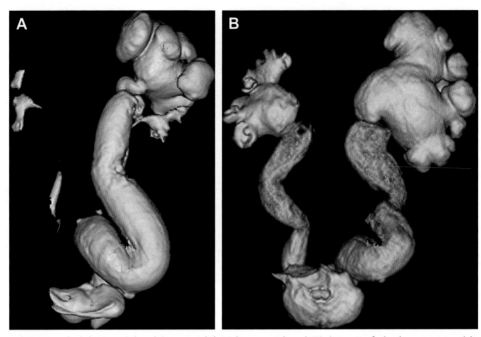

Fig. 3. Volume-rendered T2-weighted images. (*A*) Volume-rendered T2 image of duplex system with poorly functioning and obstructed upper pole moiety on the left. Despite minimal excretion of contrast agent, anatomic images of the duplex system can be obtained that show the anatomy of the upper pole moiety and the ureter. (*B*) Volume-rendered T2 image of bilateral hydroureteronephrosis in an infant. Underlying renal function was poor so that even after 20 minutes, little contrast was excreted into the collecting system. The anatomic analysis was based on the T2-weighted images.

the MIP other T2 structures with long T2 relaxation times, such as cerebrospinal fluid and the gallbladder, are manually edited out from the images. The T2-weighted images are particularly useful to define the anatomy of nonfunctioning or poorly functioning systems. These systems are generally associated with marked hydronephrosis or cystic changes and heavily T2-weighted images are able to delineate the anatomy even if little contrast excretion occurs (see **Fig. 3**).

Once these sequences are complete the acquisition of a three-dimensional, coronal, dynamic, gradient echo sequence orientated along the axis of the kidneys and including the bladder begins. The start of the dynamic series is approximately 15 minutes after the injection of furosemide, which coincides with the maximum effect of the furosemide.[18] There is significant diuretic effect from about 5 minutes to 30 minutes after injection, so there is considerable latitude in the timing of the furosemide administration. A dose of 0.1 mmol/kg Gd-DTPA (Magnevist; Bayer HealthCare Pharmaceuticals, Wayne, New Jersey) is slowly infused using a power injector (a minimum dose of 2 mL is used in smaller babies). Previously, the authors administered a compact bolus of contrast but this resulted in an aortic signal well above the

linear range of gadolinium concentration. They then instill the contrast typically at a rate of 0.25 mL/s so that the injection lasts 20 or more seconds. Each time point of the dynamic sequence consisted of 36 slices, with the outer two slices on each side being discarded to limit variations in the flip angle related to the slice profile, and also to limit wraparound artifacts. Parallel imaging with an acceleration factor of 2 is used to reduce the acquisition time per volume to 8 seconds. The scans are acquired contiguously for the first 3 minutes; subsequently intervals of progressively increasing duration are inserted between the scans until the scans are at 30-second intervals. For each volume acquisition, MIP of the whole volume is automatically generated.

After the completion of the dynamic series sagittal and coronal three-dimensional images with high spatial resolution are acquired for the purpose of reformatting and volume rendering on a three-dimensional workstation. Additional dynamic images are acquired between each of the three-dimensional volumes to allow the evaluation of the evolution of the time-intensity curves over a longer time period. These images from the high spatial resolution three-dimensional series provide exquisite anatomic evaluation of the kidneys and ureters. After the acquisition of the three-dimensional data sets is complete, if there is a significant amount of contrast in the renal pelvis (usually a clear "fluid level" can be seen because of gravity-dependent drainage) but where poor drainage from the renal pelvis means that no contrast is seen in the ureters, the patient may be turned prone to promote mixing of the contrast agent in the collecting system before the acquisition of additional high spatial resolution coronal and sagittal images. The total imaging time for nonobstructed patients is typically 45 minutes; for poorly draining kidneys the imaging time is closer to 1 hour. The MIP images from each volume acquisition are placed in a single cine sequence to provide a rapid overview of the transit of the contrast agent through the kidney. The delayed high-resolution anatomic images are particularly valuable in the evaluation of congenital malformations including ureteric strictures and ectopic ureteric insertion and complex postoperative anatomy (see **Fig. 3**).

POSTPROCESSING

Differential renal function (DRF) is among the most widely used measures of renal function. The DRF as measured by dynamic renal scintigraphy is based on the integration of the tracer curve over a range of time points at which the tracer is assumed to be located predominately in the parenchyma. Because of the limited spatial resolution of dynamic renal scintigraphy studies fixed time points are used because the exact location of the tracer cannot be confirmed by visual inspection of the images. Because dynamic renal scintigraphy measurements are based on projection images of the whole kidney they measure the activity in the whole kidney. Most techniques developed for measuring the DRF with MR imaging have attempted to duplicate this approach by combining the area under the time-intensity curve obtained from either a single slice, or a few slices, with a separate volume measurement.[19–22] The authors use a slightly different approach because the three-dimensional volumes used in this study cover the full extent of both kidneys and the uptake of the contrast in each kidney can be followed volumetrically. They make the assumption that voxels represent either functional or nonfunctional tissue and that by summing the voxels that show a significant uptake of contrast one can calculate the functional volume of each kidney and hence the split renal function. The dynamic series are visually inspected to determine the volumes in which contrast is first seen in the

collecting system of each kidney; the volume before this is then used for the calculation of the functional volume of each kidney (**Fig. 4**). In this way, possible differences between the two kidneys are taken into account and it is not necessary to assume a particular time point, or range of times, for the calculation. In previous studies, several authors have shown that the calculation of the DRF based on renal volume agrees well with the DRF calculated using nuclear medicine.[5,23,24] The volume of functioning tissue has also been shown to be well correlated with creatinine clearance rates.[25] For the dose of contrast and the pulse sequence parameters used in the studies, the segmentation of the kidneys at this homogeneous enhancement phase is straightforward and can be performed using semiautomatic segmentation. Although the renal volume can be estimated from T1- or T2-weighted images this is much more user intensive.[20,26] The methodology presented here makes a clear distinction between functioning and nonfunctioning tissue and accounts for the effects of cortical scarring or patchy enhancement, such as that seen in

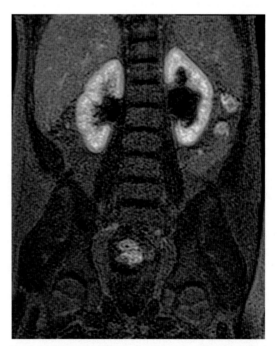

Fig. 4. Volumetric differential function. The time point for calculation of renal volumes is determined visually by defining the time when the kidneys have enhanced maximally and before contrast has been excreted into the collecting systems. At this time the kidneys are easily separated from background with semiautomated techniques that produce volume calculations for each kidney depending on a user-defined threshold.

uropathic or dysplastic kidneys. In the evaluation of duplex kidneys, MR urography can separate the boundaries between the upper and lower pole moieties by delineating the column of cortex separating the upper and lower poles so that the relative contributions of the upper and lower poles can be calculated.

Signal intensity versus time curves for each kidney is generated (**Fig. 2A**). Although it is possible to generate separate curves for the cortex and medulla, this is currently too time consuming for routine studies. The global curves for each kidney describe the perfusion, concentration, and excretion of the contrast agent over time. The two kidneys are easily compared and contrasted, which is especially helpful when one kidney is normal. The signal versus time curves are converted to relative signal versus time curves by calculating $(S_t-S_0)/S_0$, where S_0 is the mean precontrast signal, for each time point. The relative signal has a linear relationship with contrast agent concentration over a limited range of concentrations and compensates for spatial variations in the background signal, facilitating comparison of the two kidneys.[17]

The most widely used nonimaging clinical test of renal function is to measure the serum creatinine level. This test is a relatively insensitive measure of decreased GFR, however, and only measures the global, rather than single kidney, function. Although GFR can be accurately measured using such techniques as inulin clearance, such tests are invasive and are not feasible in a clinical setting. Several methods have been developed for estimating the GFR from dynamic nuclear medicine data but all of these are hampered by the poor counting statistics of such dynamic studies and the problem of accounting for the extrarenal component of the signal. More recently, several groups have applied the methods developed for nuclear medicine to dynamic MR imaging data acquired in conjunction with an injection of the contrast agent Gd-DTPA.[20,27] When applying these techniques to MR imaging data several issues have to be addressed.

First, whereas nuclear medicine directly measures the activity, and hence the concentration, of the contrast agent, the MR imaging contrast agents change signal by altering the relaxation times of the tissue and this produces a linear relationship with the concentration only over a limited range of concentrations. One either has to measure the relaxation rate or limit oneself to the range of concentrations where a linear relationship between signal and concentration exists. Second, the exact relationship between the signal and concentration depends on the flip angle used and, because the flip angle varies across the slice

in two-dimensional studies, time-consuming corrections are required for two-dimensional data, making these unsuitable for routine clinical applications. Third, to obtain adequate signal-to-noise it is generally necessary to use surface array coils for the reception of the signal, which in turn can lead to local variations in signal intensity, which complicate the analysis of the data. The authors' approach these problems by using a slow injection of contrast to limit the arterial concentration, by using a three-dimensional technique and discarding the outer slices to ensure a uniform flip angle, and by using the precontrast signal to correct for spatial variations in the signal intensity.

To estimate the GFR they use the Rutland-Patlak technique, which is based on a two-compartment model with unilateral flow of tracer from the first compartment (vasculature) into the second compartment (nephrons) (**Fig. 2B**).[28–30] The amount of contrast in any one kidney at a time point t, K(t), before the excretion of contrast can be expressed as the sum of the contrast in the vascular space and the contrast in the nephrons. Assuming that the plasma concentration of the contrast agent in the vascular space is proportional to that in the aorta, $c_a(t)$, then defining the constants k1 and k2 to represent the vascular volume within the kidney and the clearance of the contrast from the vascular space respectively, one can write

$$K(t) = k_1 c_a(t) + k_2 . \int_0^t c_a(u) \, du$$

where $t = 0$ is the time of arrival of the contrast. This can be rewritten in the form

$$\frac{K(t)}{c_a(t)} = k_1 + \frac{k_2 . \int_0^t c_a(u) \, du}{c_a(t)}$$

If one measures the average concentration of contrast within the kidney then k_2 represents the clearance per unit volume of tissue. A more conventional measurement of GFR can be obtained by multiplying k_2 by the renal volume. Alternatively, because K(t) represents the total amount of contrast in the kidney it can be replaced by $c_k(t).V_k$ where $c_k(t)$ is the mean tissue concentration of Gd-DTPA in the kidney and V_k is the volume of the kidney. The equation can now be written as

$$\frac{c_k(t)}{c_a(t)} = \frac{k_1}{V_k} + \frac{k_2 . \int_0^t c_a(u) \, du}{V_k . c_a(t)}$$

This can be plotted using an equation of the form $y = k_1 + k_2 . x$ (see **Fig. 2B**). The slope of the graph between the time points following uniform distribution of the contrast in the vasculature and before excretion of contrast into the collecting system is equal to the clearance of contrast from the vasculature (ie, the GFR). The x intercept (k_1) represents the fractional blood volume of the kidney. On the assumption of a linear relationship between the relative signal and the concentration of contrast agent the terms $c_a(t)$ and $c_k(t)$ can be replaced by the relative signal from the aorta and kidney. The relative signal versus time curves from the aorta and kidney can be used to generate a Patlak plot, and hence estimate the GFR. The precontrast relaxation times of, and the relaxivity of the contrast agent in, the blood and kidneys are different. Similarly, these quantities also differ between the subcompartments within each of these compartments (eg, plasma and red cells). When relative signal, as opposed to a measurement of the relaxation time, is used this may lead to errors in the Patlak analysis. A correction for the difference in relaxation rates can be estimated from phantom studies[31,32] or from mathematical simulations based on the measured signal but these do not accurately reflect the in vivo situation where exchange effects between different compartments (eg, plasma and red cells) contributes to the observed relaxivity.[33] For this reason the value derived from the slope of the Patlak plot is probably best regarded as a GFR index rather than an absolute measure of the GFR. When the Patlak DRF is calculated such effects are assumed to be common to both kidneys and can hence be ignored. Other possible sources of error in the Rutland-Patlak analysis include the fact that the interstitial space is neglected, that pulsation of the descending aorta may distort the measurement of the vascular signal, and the T2* shortening effects of the contrast agent may distort the relative signal measurements.

For each patient the key features derived from MR urography include calculation of DRF (both volume vDRF and Patlak pDRF); signal versus time curves for each kidney and the aorta; individual kidney GFR index of each kidney; concentration and excretion from each compartment; renal and calyceal transit times; and overall anatomic diagnosis. It is important to understand that there are two methods to determine the DRF: one based on volume and one based on the individual kidney GFR as determined by the Patlak plot. The vDRF is probably most analogous to the DRF obtained with DMSA renal scintigraphy because one is measuring the maximal amount of parenchyma that enhances. The pDRF is more analogous to the DRF obtained with DTPA renal scintigraphy in that one is measuring GFR and excretion. In

most cases these two parameters are symmetric; however, when there is a difference in these two measures of DRF it implies a change in renal hemodynamics, which may ultimately provide information about underlying renal pathophysiology.

Other approaches to measuring the GFR include fitting the signal from the renal cortex to a three-compartment model.[34,35] To achieve robust fitting for this model a higher temporal resolution is required, however, which means that the spatial resolution has to be significantly reduced. Annet and colleagues[34] found that the three-compartment model provided a better correlation with 51Cr-EDTA clearance measurements of GFR than the Patlak model, providing the measurements were confined to the renal cortex. Both MR imaging techniques yielded GFR values lower than the plasma clearance technique. Although Buckley and colleagues[35] were able to achieve a good fit to the time-intensity curves using the three-compartment model, the results of comparing the GFR calculated with their model with that measured using radioisotopes were no better than those obtained using the Patlak model.

EVALUATION OF HYDRONEPHROSIS

The most common indication for MR urography has been the evaluation of hydronephrosis, especially in infants and young children. Most experts currently advocate primary conservative management for infants with hydronephrosis with close follow-up and surgery only if there is evidence of decreased renal function or progressive hydronephrosis.[36–38] The definition of obstruction is difficult clinically and is usually defined in one of two ways: either as a restriction to urinary outflow that, when left untreated, causes progressive renal deterioration; or as a condition that hampers optimal renal development. Obstructive uropathy refers to obstruction of urine flow from the kidney to the bladder that results in renal damage.[39] In children, this is usually a result of chronic partial obstruction typically related to ureteropelvic junction (UPJ) obstruction or obstructive megaureter. The consequences of the obstruction depend not only on the degree of obstruction but occur secondarily to a complex syndrome resulting in alterations of both glomerular hemodynamics and tubular function caused by the interaction of a variety of vasoactive factors and cytokines.[40–42]

Two distinct populations of UPJ obstruction are seen: young infants diagnosed with antenatal hydronephrosis who are usually asymptomatic, and older children who present with symptoms related to abdominal pain or infection. The decision to operate is usually straightforward in the symptomatic population. The decision to operate in the antenatal and asymptomatic group is more difficult, with up to 50% of these children ultimately requiring surgical repair.[43]

Any attempt to separate obstructed from nonobstructed kidneys as distinct entities on the basis of renal drainage is artificial and unrealistic.[38,44] All hydronephrotic systems have some impairment of renal drainage and sensitive measures to predict early renal functional deterioration need to be developed. The ultimate goal of the management of obstruction is the preservation of renal function. Currently, there is no imaging modality that can accurately assess the degree of obstruction and hence identify which kidneys are at risk for progressive loss of renal function.

Initially, MR urography was used to evaluate hydronephrosis and obstruction by calculating the RTT, which is defined as the time it takes for the contrast agent to pass from the renal cortex to the ureter below the lower pole of the kidney.[23,44] If the transit time is less than 245 seconds, the system is considered nonobstructive. If the RTT is greater than 490 seconds, the system is probably obstructed. RTT times between 245 seconds and 490 seconds are considered equivocal and are managed conservatively with close follow-up to ensure that renal function is stable. Calculating the RTT from the images is relatively straightforward, because each individual volume acquisition is time-stamped: the time at which the cortex first enhances and the time when contrast is identified in the ureter are determined visually from the images. The RTT is simply the difference between these two time points. Experience with RTT has emphasized that obstruction represents a spectrum of impairment to urinary flow and is dependent on the anatomy of the UPJ and the rate at which urine is produced. Although it has been shown that RTT calculation is similar to dynamic renal scintigraphy for categorizing dilated systems, it still does not prospectively identify kidneys that lose function if left untreated. It has also become apparent from the high-resolution anatomic images that the RTT or renal drainage is dependent on the anatomy of the UPJ particularly the insertion of the ureter into the renal pelvis. For drainage to occur down the ureter, the contrast agent has to reach the orifice of the UPJ. In some children, the ureteric insertion is anteriorly located and in others posteriorly. Because the Gd-DTPA macromolecule is heavier than water, there is a tendency for the contrast agent to layer in the dependent portions of the renal pelvis. Knowing the position of the ureteric insertion into the UPJ helps in the interpretation of the RTT

and it is important to realize that the RTT is simply a measure of renal drainage and does not indicate which kidneys are likely to sustain progressive injury. Prolonged RTTs simply indicate poor drainage and stasis of urine is manifested by fluid levels (**Fig. 5**). When there has been significant loss of renal parenchyma and little urine is being produced, calculation of RTTs is of limited value in evaluating the presence of superimposed obstruction. The RTT is most useful when it is normal, indicating that there is no significant obstruction.

The calyceal transit time is the time it takes for the contrast to pass through the kidney (ie, from the initial enhancement of the cortex until it first appears as high signal intensity in the dependent calyces). The calyceal transit time is usually symmetric and is used as an indicator of hemodynamic and pathophysiologic changes in the renal parenchyma itself. The calyceal transit time is determined both by the GFR and the tubular reabsorption of urine. Delayed calyceal transit is usually seen in the setting of acute-on-chronic obstruction and occasionally with renal artery stenosis. Rapid calyceal transit times may be the result of glomerular hyperfiltration (pressure effect) or impaired concentration within the tubules (volume effect). The signal intensity and Patlak

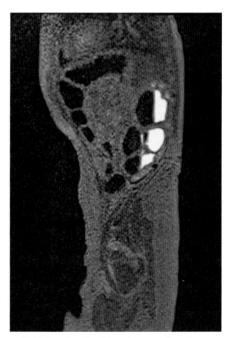

Fig. 5. Fluid levels. Fluid levels are often seen in the setting of marked hydronephrosis and are an indicator of stasis within the collecting system with the heavier contrast material layering along the dependent portions.

curves help to differentiate the level of the abnormality within the nephron.

Recently, the authors have begun to classify hydronephrotic systems as either compensated or decompensated based on the contrast dynamics within the renal parenchyma in response to the fluid and diuretic challenge (**Figs. 6 and 7**). It is more logical to focus on changes that occur to the kidney itself rather than relying on drainage patterns because progressive renal damage occurs as a consequence of vasoactive factors and cytokines that are released into the kidney parenchyma.[40–42]

In response to the fluid challenge created by the administration of intravenous fluids and furosemide, some kidneys develop signs of an acute-on-chronic obstruction with edema in the renal parenchyma seen as T2 hyperintensity. There may be a delay in excretion of contrast on the affected side with a delayed calyceal transit time. Additionally, the nephrogram becomes dense and persistent indicating ongoing tubular reabsorption of fluid. Functionally, there is a discrepancy between the pDRF and the vDRF and a difference of greater than 4% is classified as indicating a significant hemodynamic affect. The pDRF is typically decreased indicating a relative decrease in single kidney GFR presumably secondarily to an acute increase in the intrapelvic pressure. Similarly, analysis of signal intensity versus time curves shows persistent increase in signal intensity within the decompensated system. If a hydronephrotic system is "compensated" and able to accommodate the fluid challenge, there is symmetric calyceal transit time and symmetric nephrograms and signal intensity versus time curves. The pDRF and vDRF are within 4% points.

Following successful pyeloplasty there is typically rapid calyceal transit time, symmetric nephrograms, and signal intensity curves, and almost equivalent pDRF and vDRF (**Fig. 8**). The degree of hydronephrosis is typically improved, although dilation and calyceal clubbing persist. The RTT often remains prolonged indicating stasis and poor mechanical drainage.[45] Initial experience suggests that those children who have decompensated systems have significant improvement in renal function following pyeloplasty, whereas in those with compensated systems there is little change in renal function.[46]

An advantage of MR urography is the ability to identify ureters reliably in most children using the combination of T2 and postcontrast images. The ability to delineate the ureteric anatomy has allowed with confidence the diagnosis of midureteric strictures and persistent fetal folds (**Fig. 9**).[1] Fetal folds are typically seen in young infants being evaluated for antenatal hydronephrosis and are seen as a corkscrew appearance to the upper ureter. They are considered a normal variant in that the hydronephrosis tends to be mild and self-limited and there is no or only minimal impairment of renal function. The combination of transition in ureteric caliber and delayed excretion are the key features in the diagnosis of ureteric stricture. Although midureteric strictures have been considered a rare anomaly in children, it can be readily diagnosed by MR urography and this condition has probably been underdiagnosed by traditional modalities.[47]

The distal ureteric anatomy is also well demonstrated with MR urography.[48] Ectopic ureteric insertion either in single systems or in combination with duplex systems can usually be obtained on the delayed postcontrast images or on the T2-weighted images in markedly dilated or poorly functioning system (**Fig. 10**). The diagnosis of primary megaureter is made when the ureter measures more than 7 mm in diameter and the ureteric insertion into the bladder is normally located. The differentiation of obstructed from nonobstructed megaureter is arbitrarily made on the basis of RTTs because most cases are followed conservatively. Most cases of megaureter appear as compensated hydronephrosis and with follow-up studies there is elongation and lengthening of the ureter with improvement in RTT. MR urography can also demonstrate both simple and ectopic ureteroceles.

Another advantage of MR urography over other modalities is the ability to characterize the anatomy and morphology of the renal parenchyma itself. The diagnosis of obstructive uropathy is made after analysis of the high resolution T2-weighted images of the kidney and the quality of the nephrogram (**Fig. 11**). Signs of uropathy include small subcortical cysts, poor corticomedullary differentiation, decreased signal intensity in the cortex, and a poorly defined or patchy nephrogram indicating microvascular injury and impaired concentration by the renal parenchyma. These findings are similar to the pathologic changes described in the literature.[49–51] In these papers there is poor correlation between the pathologic changes and the renal functional studies. With MR urography, however, a kidney contributing 30% of total renal GFR may simply be a decompensated system with normal renal parenchyma or it may be severely uropathic with little chance for return of function. Identification of obstructive uropathy has prognostic implications in that these changes seem to be permanent and that functional improvement is unlikely if surgery is performed.

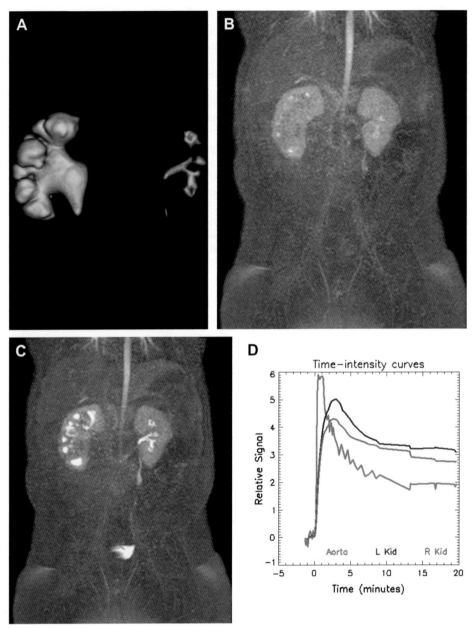

Fig. 6. A 3-month-old boy with compensated hydronephrosis. (*A*) Volume-rendered T2-weighted images demonstrate moderate hydronephrosis and caliectasis on the right with transition at the level of the UPJ. (*B*) Although the renal transit time on the right was delayed at 13 minutes, the caliceal transit time is symmetric. Contrast is excreted into the collecting systems simultaneously suggesting that there is no significant increase in pressure in the renal pelvis. (*C*) MIP image obtained 10 minutes after contrast injection shows normal ureteric excretion on the left with incomplete filling of the renal pelvis on the right. The density of the nephrograms is symmetric. (*D*) Signal intensity versus time curve demonstrating symmetric perfusion and excretion of the contrast agent in both kidneys. The peak signal intensity for the right kidney is lower than the left indicating an underlying concentrating defect presumably from medullary volume loss. The volumetric and Patlak differential functions were equivalent. All these parameters suggest that the hydronephrotic system can accommodate the fluid challenge with furosemide. It is categorized as a compensated system that is unlikely to deteriorate and can be followed conservatively.

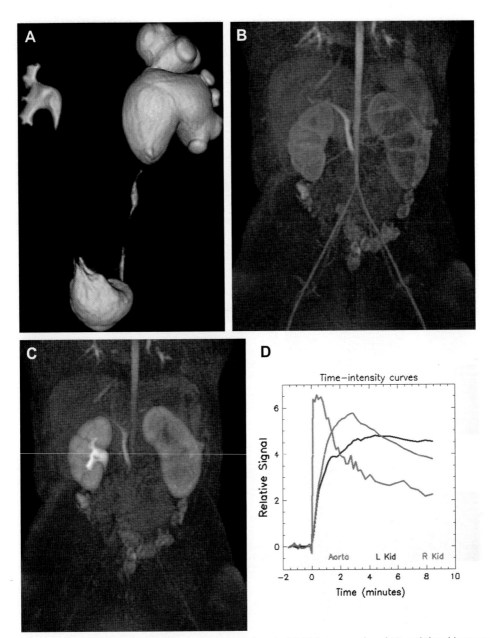

Fig. 7. A 9-month-old boy with decompensated hydronephrosis. (*A*) Volume-rendered T2-weighted images show-ing moderate hydronephrosis with "ballooning" of the pelvicaliceal system on the left. There is a kink at the level of the UPJ. (*B*) Coronal MIP from the dynamic series showing normal perfusion to both kidneys. The arterial phase shows no evidence of crossing vessel as an underlying cause for the UPJ. (*C*) The left kidney has a delayed dense nephrogram with delayed caliceal transit time. The renal transit time was greater than 15 minutes and catego-rized as obstructed. (*D*) Signal intensity versus time curves demonstrating asymmetric concentration and excre-tion of contrast agent. The curve for the right kidney is normal and on the left represents the dense delayed nephrogram. The volumetric differential renal function was 48% on the left and the Patlak differential renal function was 39% indicating a significant change in the GFR presumably related to acute increase in intratubular pressure secondary to the fluid challenge. As a result this is classified as a decompensated system and typically has improved function following pyeloplasty.

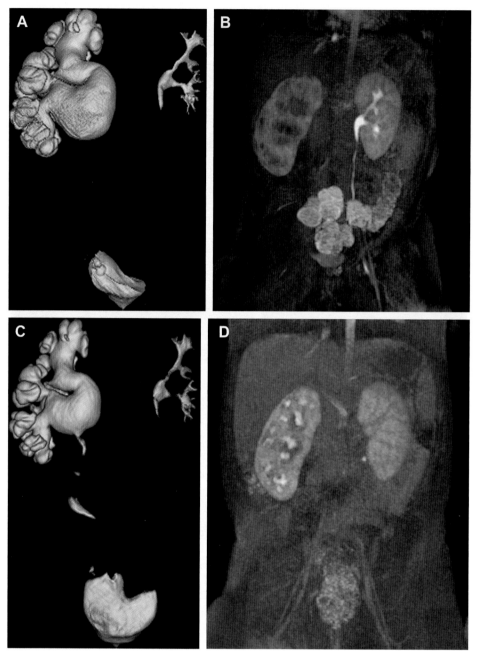

Fig. 8. Successful pyeloplasty in a 3-year-old boy. (A) Volume-rendered T2-weighted images showing typical morphology of UPJ obstruction on the right. (B) Coronal MIP from the dynamic series demonstrating delayed caliceal excretion on the right. For the right kidney, the volumetric differential renal function was 43% and the Patlak differential renal function was 35% (with a difference of 8% between the volumetric differential renal function and the Patlak differential renal function). The anatomic and functional features are typical for a decompensated hydronephrosis. (C) Following pyeloplasty, volume-rendered T2-weighted images showed decrease in the degree of hydronephrosis with postsurgical visualization of the UPJ and right ureter. (D) Coronal MIP from the dynamic series now demonstrates rapid excretion of contrast into the pelvicaliceal system. Postoperatively, functional analysis of the right kidney improved with volumetric differential renal function = 48% and Patlak differential renal function = 46%, so that the difference was lowered to 2%. In almost all successful pyeloplasties there is decrease in the degree of hydronephrosis and rapid caliceal transit on the operated side. If the caliceal transit is delayed, this is usually an early indicator of a failed pyeloplasty.

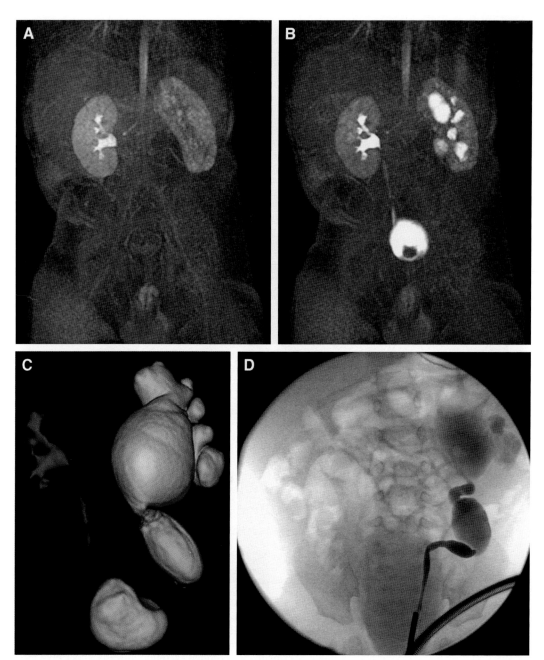

Fig. 9. A 2-month-old boy with left-sided antenatal hydronephrosis secondary to midureteric stricture. (*A*) Coronal MIP image from the dynamic series demonstrating a delayed dense nephrogram on the left. (*B*) Coronal MIP image 15 minutes after contrast injection shows incomplete filling of the pelvicaliceal system and moderate hydronephrosis. (*C*) Volume-rendered T2-weighted images demonstrated the hydroureteronephrosis extending to the level of the iliac vessels. The combination of T2 and contrast-enhanced imaging enables evaluation of ureteric anatomy in almost all cases. (*D*) Retrograde urogram showing confirming midureteric stricture.

FUTURE DIRECTIONS

This article concentrates on the use of exogenous contrast agents in the evaluation of renal function; however, endogenous contrast agents can also be used. The blood in large vessels can be used as a diffusible tracer and red blood cells can be used as a surrogate for blood oxygenation. Of these applications the use of blood as an endogenous tracer to measure tissue perfusion is probably the most promising clinical application. This

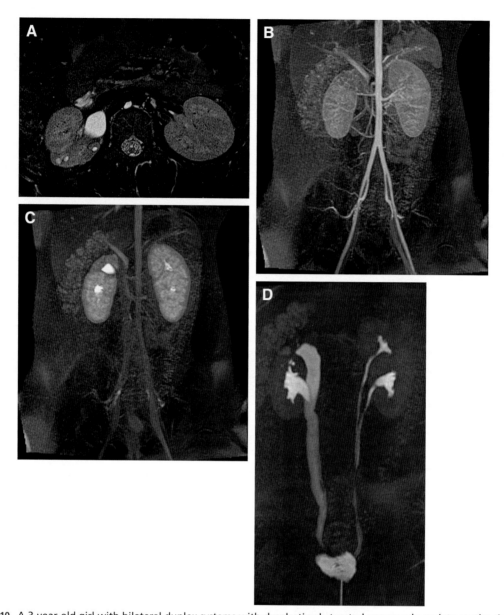

Fig. 10. A 3-year-old girl with bilateral duplex systems with dysplastic obstructed upper pole moiety on the right. (*A*) High-resolution axial T2-weighted image shows disorganized architecture and cyst formation of right upper pole. (*B*) Coronal MIP from vascular phase of dynamic series demonstrating poor perfusion to the upper pole on the right. (*C*) Coronal MIP from excretory phase of dynamic series shows excretion into the upper pole moiety with a diminished nephrogram. (*D*) Delayed coronal MIP image from dynamic series shows dilatation of the upper pole moiety to the level of the bladder.

application requires that the magnetization of the inflowing arterial blood be manipulated (labeled) in some way (ie, by inverting the magnetization of the blood in the descending aorta). After a delay a fraction of the blood has passed into kidneys. By acquiring images with and without this manipulation background effects can be removed and the remaining signal then reflects the tissue perfusion and delay time. The size of this effect is rather small, typically a few percent, and the lifetime of the labeling is determined by the T1 of the blood but by repeating the procedure a more reliable difference signal can be obtained. These techniques are generally referred to as "arterial spin labeling" techniques.[52–54] The reduced respiratory motion seen in young children and transplanted kidneys may make these categories most amenable to clinical implementations of this technique.

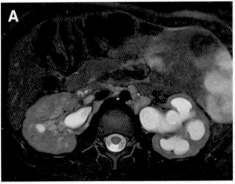
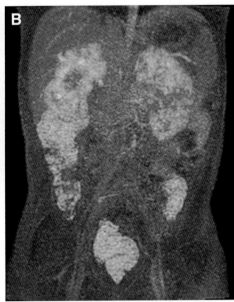

Fig. 11. Underlying uropathy in a 9-year-old girl with bilateral hydroureteronephrosis. (*A*) The axial T2-weighted image shows parenchymal loss with poor corticomedullary differentiation bilaterally. (*B*) Coronal MIP image from the dynamic series shows bilateral patchy and dim nephrograms indicating underlying microvascular damage.

Because of the small size of the labeling effect arterial spin labeling techniques are limited to lower spatial resolution than those using exogenous tracers. In addition, the low blood flow and longer transit time to the medulla probably means that this technique will be restricted to measuring the perfusion in the renal cortex.

The use of the blood oxygen level dependent technique is well established for functional MR imaging in the brain and a number of groups have applied this technique to study renal oxygenation. The technique relies on the fact that the magnetic properties of hemoglobin depend on whether it is oxygenated or deoxygenated, which in turn affects the transverse relaxation time (T2*) and hence the measured signal. By using a pulse sequence that is optimized for detecting this change, blood oxygen level dependent MR imaging can be used to measure changes in tissue Po_2.[52–54] In practice, the main problem with this technique is that it measures the change in T2* relaxation time and this parameter is affected by many other parameters and tissue oxygenation (homogeneity of the main magnetic field, presence of bowel gas, and so forth). To remove these other effects some sort of physiologic challenge is required so that baseline and postchallenge data sets can be compared. As yet there is no consensus on what challenges are both useful and practical in a clinical environment. The reduced motion, and a generally reduced level of field inhomogeneities, associated with transplanted kidneys may make these more amenable to the blood oxygenation level dependent technique.[55]

Water transport is the predominant phenomenon throughout the kidney because of its role in water reabsorption and concentration-dilution function. These movements are mainly within the tubular cells. Consequently, useful insights into the mechanisms of various renal diseases, such as chronic renal failure, renal artery stenosis, and ureteral obstruction, might be obtained by measuring the diffusion characteristics of the kidney. Diffusion MR imaging uses additional gradients to sensitize the pulse sequence to the microscopic motion of water within the tissue and is a well-established technique for evaluating cerebral ischemia (**Fig. 12**). Renal diffusion imaging is a challenging technique because of the extreme motion sensitivity of diffusion-weighted sequences, however, and in general has to be performed within one or more breathholds.[56,57] In the renal cortex the diffusion of the water is only slightly anisotropic, but the medulla is highly anisotropic.[58] The diffusion sequence has to measure rotationally invariant diffusion values, which tends to prolong the measurement time and complicates the use of diffusion imaging within a single breathhold. Similarly, the use of single-shot EPI restricts the spatial resolution such that only relatively large medullary compartments can be observed. To date, variation in the methodologies used for diffusion studies has made it difficult to compare the results, but it is hoped that the introduction of

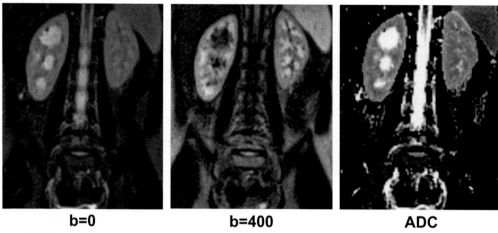

b=0   **b=400**   **ADC**

Fig. 12. Diffusion-weighted imaging. The images were acquired using a radial diffusion imaging sequence on a 1.5-T scanner. The diffusion weighting was applied along three separate axis to provide a direction independent measure of the diffusion. The images show an image with no diffusion weighting (b = 0 s/mm²); a diffusion-weighted image (b = 400 s/mm²); and a parametric map of the apparent diffusion coefficient. Because of the relatively long echo time required by this sequence the b = 0 and b = 400 images have substantial T2 weighting; the b = 400 image is a mixture of diffusion and T2 contrast. The diffusion weighting of b = 400 s/mm² is less than that used in the brain because of the higher rate of diffusion in the kidney. The apparent diffusion coefficient is calculated from the b = 0 and b = 400 images and shows a lower apparent diffusion coefficient in the medulla than in the cortex.

standardized procedures will improve this situation. Recently, radial diffusion sequences have also been shown to be useful for studying renal diffusion.[59]

SUMMARY

MR urography has the potential to revolutionize imaging of the urinary tract in both adults and children, providing an unprecedented level of anatomic information combined with quantitative functional evaluation of each kidney simultaneously. With attention to detail, specifically appropriate hydration and sedation, high-quality MR urograms can be obtained in almost every case. MR urography can now provide useful assessment of obstructive uropathy and may provide predictive information about which children benefit from surgery. It has the potential to identify parameters that indicate a significant obstruction as opposed to self-limited hydronephrosis. Further technical developments in the field, such as blood oxygenation level dependent and diffusion imaging, and molecular imaging with USPIO will produce greater insights into the pathophysiology of not only urologic disorders but also disorders of the kidney itself.

REFERENCES

1. Grattan-Smith JD, Jones RA. MR urography in children. Pediatr Radiol 2006;36:1119–32, quiz 1228–9.

2. Grattan-Smith JD, Little SB, Jones RA. MR urography in children: how we do it. Pediatr Radiol 2008; 38(Suppl 1):S3–17.

3. Grattan-Smith JD, Little SB, Jones RA. MR urography evaluation of obstructive uropathy. Pediatr Radiol 2008;38(Suppl 1):S49–69.

4. Grattan-Smith JD, Little SB, Jones RA. Evaluation of reflux nephropathy, pyelonephritis and renal dysplasia. Pediatr Radiol 2008;38(Suppl 1):S83–105.

5. Grattan-Smith JD, Perez-Bayfield MR, Jones RA, et al. MR imaging of kidneys: functional evaluation using F-15 perfusion imaging. Pediatr Radiol 2003; 33:293–304.

6. Avni EF, Bali MA, Regnault M, et al. MR urography in children. Eur J Radiol 2002;43:154–66.

7. Borthne A, Nordshus T, Reiseter T, et al. MR urography: the future gold standard in paediatric urogenital imaging? Pediatr Radiol 1999;29:694–701.

8. Borthne A, Pierre-Jerome C, Nordshus T, et al. MR urography in children: current status and future development. Eur Radiol 2000;10:503–11.

9. Nolte-Ernsting CC, Adam GB, Gunther RW. MR urography: examination techniques and clinical applications. Eur Radiol 2001;11:355–72.

10. Riccabona M. Pediatric MRU: its potential and its role in the diagnostic work-up of upper urinary tract dilatation in infants and children. World J Urol 2004;22:79–87.

11. Riccabona M, Riccabona M, Koen M, et al. Magnetic resonance urography: a new gold standard for the evaluation of solitary kidneys and renal buds? J Urol 2004;171:1642–6.

12. Riccabona M, Ruppert-Kohlmayr A, Ring E, et al. Potential impact of pediatric MR urography on the imaging algorithm in patients with a functional single kidney. AJR Am J Roentgenol 2004;183:795–800.

13. Rohrschneider WK, Becker K, Hoffend J, et al. Combined static-dynamic MR urography for the simultaneous evaluation of morphology and function in urinary tract obstruction. II. Findings in experimentally induced ureteric stenosis. Pediatr Radiol 2000;30:523–32.

14. Rohrschneider WK, Haufe S, Clorius JH, et al. MR to assess renal function in children. Eur Radiol 2003; 13:1033–45.

15. Rohrschneider WK, Haufe S, Wiesel M, et al. Functional and morphologic evaluation of congenital urinary tract dilatation by using combined static-dynamic MR urography: findings in kidneys with a single collecting system. Radiology 2002;224: 683–94.

16. Rohrschneider WK, Hoffend J, Becker K, et al. Combined static-dynamic MR urography for the simultaneous evaluation of morphology and function in urinary tract obstruction. I. Evaluation of the normal status in an animal model. Pediatr Radiol 2000;30:511–22.

17. Jones RA, Easley K, Little SB, et al. Dynamic contrast-enhanced MR urography in the evaluation of pediatric hydronephrosis. Part 1. Functional assessment. AJR Am J Roentgenol 2005;185: 1598–607.

18. Brown SC, Upsdell SM, O'Reilly PH. The importance of renal function in the interpretation of diuresis renography. Br J Urol 1992;69:121–5.

19. Huang AJ, Lee VS, Rusinek H. Functional renal MR imaging. Magn Reson Imaging Clin N Am 2004;12: 469–86, vi.

20. Lee VS, Rusinek H, Noz ME, et al. Dynamic three-dimensional MR renography for the measurement of single kidney function: initial experience. Radiology 2003;227:289–94.

21. Taylor J, Summers PE, Keevil SF, et al. Magnetic resonance renography: optimisation of pulse sequence parameters and Gd-DTPA dose, and comparison with radionuclide renography. Magn Reson Imaging 1997;15:637–49.

22. Teh HS, Ang ES, Wong WC, et al. MR renography using a dynamic gradient-echo sequence and low-dose gadopentetate dimeglumine as an alternative to radionuclide renography. AJR Am J Roentgenol 2003;181:441–50.

23. Perez-Brayfield MR, Kirsch AJ, Jones RA, et al. A prospective study comparing ultrasound, nuclear scintigraphy and dynamic contrast enhanced magnetic resonance imaging in the evaluation of hydronephrosis. J Urol 2003;170:1330–4.

24. Heuer R, Sommer G, Shortliffe LD. Evaluation of renal growth by magnetic resonance imaging and computerized tomography volumes. J Urol 2003; 170,1659–63 [discussion: 1663].

25. van den Dool SW, Wasser MN, de Fijter JW, et al. Functional renal volume: quantitative analysis at gadolinium-enhanced MR angiography–feasibility study in healthy potential kidney donors. Radiology 2005;236:189–95.

26. Bakker J, Olree M, Kaatee R, et al. Renal volume measurements: accuracy and repeatability of US compared with that of MR imaging. Radiology 1999;211:623–8.

27. Hackstein N, Heckrodt J, Rau WS. Measurement of single-kidney glomerular filtration rate using a contrast-enhanced dynamic gradient-echo sequence and the Rutland-Patlak plot technique. J Magn Reson Imaging 2003;18:714–25.

28. Rutland MD. A single injection technique for subtraction of blood background in 131I-hippuran renograms. Br J Radiol 1979;52:134–7.

29. Patlak CS, Blasberg RG, Fenstermacher JD. Graphical evaluation of blood-to-brain transfer constants from multiple-time uptake data. J Cereb Blood Flow Metab 1983;3:1–7.

30. Peters AM. Graphical analysis of dynamic data: the Patlak-Rutland plot. Nucl Med Commun 1994;15: 669–72.

31. Hackstein N, Kooijman H, Tomaselli S, et al. Glomerular filtration rate measured using the Patlak plot technique and contrast-enhanced dynamic MRI with different amounts of gadolinium-DTPA. J Magn Reson Imaging 2005;22:406–14.

32. Rusinek H, Lee VS, Johnson G. Optimal dose of Gd-DTPA in dynamic MR studies. Magn Reson Med 2001;46:312–6.

33. Pedersen M, Shi Y, Anderson P, et al. Quantitation of differential renal blood flow and renal function using dynamic contrast-enhanced MRI in rats. Magn Reson Med 2004;51:510–7.

34. Annet L, Hermoye L, Peeters F, et al. Glomerular filtration rate: assessment with dynamic contrast-enhanced MRI and a cortical-compartment model in the rabbit kidney. J Magn Reson Imaging 2004; 20:843–9.

35. Buckley DL, Shurrab AE, Cheung CM, et al. Measurement of single kidney function using dynamic contrast-enhanced MRI: comparison of two models in human subjects. J Magn Reson Imaging 2006; 24:1117–23.

36. Csaicsich D, Greenbaum LA, Aufricht C. Upper urinary tract: when is obstruction obstruction? Curr Opin Urol 2004;14:213–7.

37. Eskild-Jensen A, Gordon I, Piepsz A, et al. Congenital unilateral hydronephrosis: a review of the impact of diuretic renography on clinical treatment. J Urol 2005;173:1471–6.

38. Peters CA. Urinary tract obstruction in children. J Urol 1995;154:1874–83 [discussion:1883–4].

39. O'Reilly PH. Obstructive uropathy. Q J Nucl Med 2002;46:295–303.

40. Wen JG, Frokiaer J, Jorgensen TM, et al. Obstructive nephropathy: an update of the experimental research. Urol Res 1999;27:29–39.

41. Klahr S. Urinary tract obstruction. Semin Nephrol 2001;21:133–45.

42. Chevalier RL, Forbes MS. Generation and evolution of atubular glomeruli in the progression of renal disorders. J Am Soc Nephrol 2008;19:197–206.

43. Chertin B, Pollack A, Koulikov D, et al. Conservative treatment of ureteropelvic junction obstruction in children with antenatal diagnosis of hydronephrosis: lessons learned after 16 years of follow-up. Eur Urol 2006;49:734–8 [discussion: 739].

44. Jones RA, Perez-Brayfield MR, Kirsch AJ, et al. Renal transit time with MR urography in children. Radiology 2004;233:41–50.

45. Kirsch AJ, McMann LP, Jones RA, et al. Magnetic resonance urography for evaluating outcomes after pediatric pyeloplasty. J Urol 2006;176:1755–61.

46. Little SB, Jones RA, Grattan-Smith JD. Evaluation of UPJ obstruction before and after pyeloplasty using MR urography. Pediatr Radiol 2008;38(Suppl 1): S106–24.

47. Smith BG, Metwalli AR, Leach J, et al. Congenital midureteral stricture in children diagnosed with antenatal hydronephrosis. Urology 2004;64:1014–9.

48. Avni FE, Nicaise N, Hall M, et al. The role of MR imaging for the assessment of complicated duplex kidneys in children: preliminary report. Pediatr Radiol 2001;31:215–23.

49. Elder JS, Stansbrey R, Dahms BB, et al. Renal histological changes secondary to ureteropelvic junction obstruction. J Urol 1995;154:719–22.

50. Huang WY, Peters CA, Zurakowski D, et al. Renal biopsy in congenital ureteropelvic junction obstruction: evidence for parenchymal maldevelopment. Kidney Int 2006;69:137–43.

51. Pascual L, Oliva J, Vega- PJ, et al. Renal histology in ureteropelvic junction obstruction: are histological changes a consequence of hyperfiltration? J Urol 1998;160:976–9 [discussion: 994].

52. Detre JA, Leigh JS, Williams DS, et al. Perfusion imaging. Magn Reson Med 1992;23:37–45.

53. Fenchel M, Martirosian P, Langanke J, et al. Perfusion MR imaging with FAIR true FISP spin labeling in patients with and without renal artery stenosis: initial experience. Radiology 2006;238:1013–21.

54. Prasad PV, Edelman RR, Epstein FH. Noninvasive evaluation of intrarenal oxygenation with BOLD MRI. Circulation 1996;94:3271–5.

55. Sadowski EA, Fain SB, Alford SK, et al. Assessment of acute renal transplant rejection with blood oxygen level-dependent MR imaging: initial experience. Radiology 2005;236:911–9.

56. Muller MF, Prasad PV, Bimmler D, et al. Functional imaging of the kidney by means of measurement of the apparent diffusion coefficient. Radiology 1994;193:711–5.

57. Yamada I, Aung W, Himeno Y, et al. Diffusion coefficients in abdominal organs and hepatic lesions: evaluation with intravoxel incoherent motion echo-planar MR imaging. Radiology 1999;210:617–23.

58. Ries M, Jones RA, Basseau F, et al. Diffusion tensor MRI of the human kidney. J Magn Reson Imaging 2001;14:42–9.

59. Deng J, Omary RA, Larson AC. Multishot diffusion-weighted SPLICE PROPELLER MRI of the abdomen. Magn Reson Med 2008;59:947–53.

Dynamic Contrast-Enhanced MR Imaging of Ovarian Neoplasms: Current Status and Future Perspectives

Isabelle Thomassin-Naggara, MD[a,b,*],
Charles A. Cuenod, MD, PhD[b,c], Emile Darai, MD, PhD[d],
Claude Marsault, MD, PhD[a], Marc Bazot, MD[a]

KEYWORDS
- Perfusion • Ovarian tumor
- MR imaging • Angiogenesis • Neoplasm

Ovarian tumors are the leading indication for gynecologic surgery.[1] Imaging techniques can help identify patients in need of surgery and those qualifying for a wait-and-see approach.[2] Therapeutic management of epithelial ovarian tumors, which represent over two-thirds of ovarian tumors, depends mainly on whether the tumor is benign, borderline, or invasive. It is clinically important to distinguish borderline tumors from frankly invasive tumors preoperatively, as the former mainly occur in young women wishing to preserve their child-bearing potential and are associated with a low recurrence rate and good overall survival, warranting conservative laparoscopic surgery.[3–5] However, despite advances in imaging techniques, the diagnosis of borderline ovarian tumors remains difficult.

Ultrasonography is the first-line imaging technique for detecting and characterizing ovarian tumors.[6] In this specific setting, several investigators have proposed algorithms taking into account epidemiologic characteristics, serum tumor marker levels, and imaging features, including the presence of solid tissue.[7] However, ultrasound is operator-dependent, as shown in a prospective randomized trial.[8] Moreover, certain conditions that hinder accurate transvaginal examination, such as lesion complexity, large tumor size, obesity, and virginity, are indications for MR imaging, which is superior to CT for assessing complex and indeterminate ovarian tumors because of its better tissue contrast.[9,10] Finally, the accuracy of ultrasonography for the diagnosis of borderline ovarian tumors remains low (68.4%), with one-third of cases misdiagnosed as benign lesion because of the absence of typical features, such as unilocular cyst with a positive ovarian crescent sign and extensive papillary projections arising from the inner wall, or a cyst with a well-defined multilocular

[a] Division of Radiology, Hôpital Tenon-Assistance Publique des Hopitaux de Paris, 4 Rue de la Chine, 75020 Paris, France
[b] Laboratoire de Recherche en Imagerie LRI-EA 4062, Université Paris René Descartes, Paris, France
[c] Division of Radiology, Hopital Européen Georges Pompidou-Assistance Publique des Hopitaux de Paris, Paris, France
[d] Division of Gynecology and Obstetrics, Hôpital Tenon-Assistance Publique des Hopitaux de Paris, Paris, France
* Corresponding author. Service de Radiologie, Hôpital Tenon, 4 Rue de la Chine, 75020 Paris, France.
E-mail address: isabelle.thomassin@tnn.aphp.fr (I. Thomassin-Naggara).

Magn Reson Imaging Clin N Am 16 (2008) 661–672
doi:10.1016/j.mric.2008.07.012

nodule.[11,12] The morphologic criteria used to identify potentially malignant ovarian tumors on sonography and MR imaging are thickened irregular septations, vegetations, and solid portions.[13–16] A solid component with a high signal intensity on T2-weighted imaging is a further sign of malignancy.[14,17]

There are limited data on the use of dynamic contrast-enhanced (DCE) MR imaging for the characterization of ovarian tumors.[15,16,18,19] DCE MR imaging has proven useful for distinguishing malignant from benign tumors, and for characterizing gynecologic masses.[20,21] Applied to ovarian tumors, this technique might enable noninvasive in vivo assessment of angiogenesis.[22]

This article describes the DCE MR imaging technique, examines the relationship between estimated perfusion parameters obtained with DCE-MR imaging and histopathologic markers of angiogenesis in ovarian tumors, and suggests the potential applications of DCE MR imaging in patients with ovarian tumors.

CURRENT STATUS AND UNMET NEEDS OF IMAGING IN OVARIAN TUMORS

For unilocular ovarian simple cysts that are associated with a very low risk of malignancy (0.3% when <50 mm), ultrasonography is a sufficient technique to explore these masses.[23] However, in cysts with a diameter higher than 50 mm, papillary formations or solid parts may be missed by transvaginal ultrasonography, and yet increase the risk of malignancy by a factor of 3 to 6 relative to unilocular simple cysts.[23] Thus, MR imaging is useful in large cystic lesions or in cases of indeterminate ovarian masses by ultrasonography.[9] In the literature, the accuracy of MR imaging for distinguishing malignant from benign complex ovarian masses ranges from 83% to 93%,[14,15,24] compared with 63% with ultrasonography.[24]

The diagnostic criteria of conventional MR imaging may be classified into two features: those common to the different imaging modalities (ultrasonography, CT, MR imaging) and those that are specific to MR imaging, based on the signal contrast obtained on different sequences. In the first category, reported signs of malignancy include bilaterality, tumor diameter larger than 4 cm, predominantly solid mass, cystic tumor with vegetations, and secondary malignant features, such as ascites, peritoneal involvement, and enlarged lymph nodes.[14,15,24] However, bilaterality of ovarian lesions is not specific for malignancy, as the authors observed that 15% to 20% of dermoid cysts and up to 40% of endometriomas could be bilateral.[14,24,25] Likewise, lesion size is not

a specific predictor of malignancy because there is an overlap between benign and malignant tumors.[14] However, borderline tumors, especially those of the mucinous histologic subtype, are often larger than benign or frankly malignant tumors.[16] Sohaib and colleagues[15] consider that cystic ovarian tumors are usually benign, whereas mixed tumors (with solid and cystic components) have a high probability of malignancy. Umemoto and colleagues[26] reported that a solid component in an ovarian mass was the most statistically significant predictor of malignancy on MR imaging. In these studies, the overall accuracy of these criteria was low, because some benign tumors (such as ovarian fibromas, Brenner tumors, and cystadenofibromas) can display a solid fibrous component. Thus, a solid component lacks specificity, especially when it is the only sign of malignancy. Papillary projections (vegetations) are characteristic of some surface epithelial-stromal tumors of the ovary. Vegetations can be exocystic but are more commonly intracystic. Histopathologic studies show that these vegetations are present in 20% to 26% of benign tumors, 62% to 78% of borderline tumors, and 59% to 92% of ovarian cancers.[16,27] Likewise, MR imaging displays vegetations in respectively 13% to 22%, 61% to 62%, and 38% to 48% of benign, borderline, and invasive ovarian tumors.[16]

There are three important reasons for identifying vegetations on MR images. First, vegetations in an ovarian mass show that the mass is an ovarian epithelial tumor.[27] Second, recent reports suggest that the presence of vegetations within a cystic mass is the most significant predictor of malignancy[14,15]—with low accuracy (66%), however—in keeping with the authors' experience.[16] In the authors' series of 168 ovarian masses, intracystic vegetations were present in 37.5% of benign epithelial tumors. Thus, vegetations alone had poor sensitivity (52.2%) and acceptable specificity (77.8%) for malignancy on MR imaging. Finally, the size and extent of papillary projections may correlate with tumor aggressiveness.[28] Enhancing mural nodules (which are not different from vegetation, but the term of "vegetation" is reserved for epithelial ovarian tumors) have also been reported to be characteristic of malignancy in patients with endometriosis.[19] In clinical practice, however, enhancement of mural nodules is often difficult to evaluate on conventional T1-weighted images and can be confused with blood clots. In their preliminary study, Tanaka and colleagues[19] found that dynamic subtraction imaging easily depicted the enhancement of mural nodules in atypical endometriomas (unilateral, and without T2 shading).

In summary, the signs of malignancy described above could be diagnosed on any imaging technique and lack specificity.

The second category of criteria for diagnosis of malignancy includes those that are specific to MR imaging and are based on the T1 and T2 contrast. The low signal of solid components on T2-weighted imaging is suggestive of benign fibrous tissue (observed in cystadenofibromas, ovarian fibromas, and Brenner tumors)[17,29,30] and improves the characterization of solid components, with an overall accuracy of about 68% according to Sohaib and colleagues.[15] High signal intensity on T1-weighted images is highly suggestive of benign disease; this may correspond to fat (highly specific for benign teratomas)[31] or blood products. Non fat-suppressed and fat-suppressed T1-weighted sequences and in- and out-of-phase imaging[32] are used to differentiate fat from blood products.[33,34] Hemorrhagic lesions may exhibit low signal intensity on T2-weighted images ("shading"), which is highly suggestive of old hemorrhagic products consistent with endometrial cysts.[35,36]

RATIONALE FOR THE USE OF DCE MR IMAGING IN OVARIAN TUMORS

The diagnostic values of the different MR criteria are reported in **Table 1**. When comparing the value of different conventional MR criteria for distinguishing benign from malignant ovarian masses, the accuracy associated with the presence of fat or an endometriotic component is high (> 92%) and, in the

authors' opinion, DCE-MR imaging is not useful for characterizing these lesions. However, the accuracy of all the other features is below 75%. When a complex ovarian mass is detected, surgical treatment is usually the gold standard. Improving characterization of ovarian masses would result in avoiding surgery for benign tumors and avoiding aggressive surgery for borderline tumors. Thus, using additional sequence, such as DCE MR imaging, could improve preoperative characterization of ovarian lesions to better select treatment options.

TECHNIQUE AND PROCESSING OF DCE-MR IMAGING OF THE PELVIS
Image Acquisition

For the pelvic DCE-MR imaging protocol, the authors use a 1.5T system with high performance gradients and a six-element phased-array coil. All sequences are acquired with anterior and posterior saturation bands to eliminate high signal from subcutaneous fat. Patients are asked to fast for 3 hours, and they receive an antispasmodic drug intravenously (10-mg of tiemonium methylsulfate) immediately before the MR imaging to reduce bowel peristalsis.

Our protocol includes the following conventional sequences:

Sagittal T2-weighted fast spin-echo (repetition time or TR/echo time or TE, 5050/ 121; echo-train length, 15; slice thickness, 5 mm; gap, 1 mm; field of view,

Table 1
Value of conventional morphologic MR imaging findings for distinguishing benign from malignant ovarian tumors and the potential added value of DCE MR imaging to conventional MR imaging protocol

—	Accuracy (%)	Value of DCE MR Imaging
Signs of malignancy		
Bilaterality	55%	+
Predominantly solid mass	49%	+
Thickened irregular septa	67%	±
Papillary projections	54%–66%	+
Solid portion	56%–62%	+
Adenopathy	70%	+
Ascites or peritoneal implants	67%–72%	+
Signs of benignity		
T2 shading	96%	−
Presence of fat	92%–95%	−
Low T2 signal of solid component	72%	+

Data from Refs.[15,16,33,36,39,62]

280 mm × 225 mm; excitations, 2; and matrix, 512 × 245).

Axial T2-weighted fast spin-echo from the renal hilum to the symphysis pubis (TR/TE, 6790/89; echo-train length, 15; slice thickness, 5 mm; gap, 1 mm; field of view, 370 mm × 275 mm; excitations, 2; and matrix, 512 × 187).

Axial T1-weighted gradient-echo images with breath hold (TR/TE, 170/4.8; flip angle, 70°; excitation, 1; slice thickness, 5 mm; gap, 1 mm; field of view, 370 mm to 275 mm; excitations, 2; and interpolated matrix, 256 × 145). This sequence is performed with and without fat suppression.

Delayed postcontrast axial and sagittal T1-weighted gradient-echo images with breath-hold are acquired 6 minutes after the gadolinium injection (after the DCE-MR imaging acquisition).

For DCE-MR imaging the authors use a free-breathing axial dynamic contrast-enhanced non fat-suppressed T1-weighted gradient-echo sequence (two-demensional fast low angle shot) acquired through the solid components (including solid portion, papillary projections, or thickened irregular septa, detected on precontrast T2-weighted images and confirmed on delayed postcontrast T1-weighted images) of the ovarian tumor and through the uterus with the following parameters: TR/TE, 27/2.24; flip angle, 80°; slice thickness, 5 mm; number of slices, 3; excitation, 1; field of view, 400 mm to 200 mm; interpolated matrix 256 × 134; bandwidth 300. Superior and inferior saturation bands (90-mm wide) are added to avoid the inflow effect and venous artefacts respectively. A dose of 0.1-mmol/kg^{-1} body weight of gadolinium contrast is given intravenously via a power injector at a rate of 2 mL/s^{-1}, followed by 20 mL of normal saline to flush the tubing. Images are obtained at 2.4-second intervals, beginning 10 seconds after the bolus injection and continuing for 320 seconds after the injection (130 time frames).

Image Analysis

Regions of interest (ROIs) are placed within solid tissue selected on precontrast MR images and on normal outer myometrium to measure signal intensity versus time (**Fig. 1**). Normal myometrium is used as an internal reference tissue.[17] Myometrial time intensity curve has a sigmoid pattern, which is in the same signal intensity range than those of ovarian tumors and thus is useful for tumor characterization. Time-intensity curves (over all 130 frames) are determined for semiquantitative or pharmacokinetic perfusion analysis. Because tumors are often heterogeneous, several ROIs are drawn, and only the maximum enhancement parameters are taken into account for analysis.

RESULTS OF DCE MR IMAGING FOR CHARACTERIZATION OF OVARIAN TUMORS AND CORRELATION WITH HISTOPATHOLOGIC MARKERS OF ANGIOGENESIS
Usefulness of DCE MR Imaging for Characterizing Ovarian Masses

Several studies have suggested that contrast-enhanced MR imaging is superior to noncontrast MR imaging for ovarian tumor characterization.[14,15,37] The overall accuracy of contrast-enhanced MR sequences for distinguishing benign from malignant ovarian lesions reaches 90% in some series.[14,38] In a recent study, Sohaib and

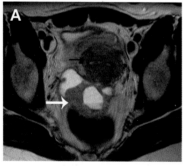
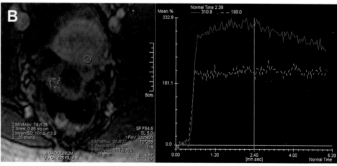

Fig. 1. A 43-year-old woman with ovarian serous cystadenocarcinoma. The figure shows the placement of ROIs in the tumor (*white arrow*) and normal myometrium (*black arrow*). (*A*) Axial fast spin-echo T2-weighted image shows a right cystic ovarian tumor containing solid component (*white arrow*), which display slightly higher signal intensity compared with the normal myometrium (*black arrow*). (*B*) DCE T1-weighted image shows ROI placement in the outer myometrium (*red line*) and the solid component of the ovarian tumor (*yellow line*). Ovarian tumor displays moderate enhancement not steeper than myometrium with a plateau (time intensity curve type 2).

colleagues[15] confirmed that malignant tumors exhibited stronger early enhancement (< 60 seconds) than benign tumors. However, borderline ovarian tumors were grouped among malignant tumors in their study. DCE-MR imaging could be especially useful for characterizing borderline ovarian tumors. In a small series of 11 tumors, Van Vierzen and colleagues[18] found that early enhancement might be a better diagnostic criterion for borderline tumors than the CA 125 level and ultrasonographic findings. The authors recently defined three patterns of enhancement of ovarian epithelial tumors, using myometrial enhancement as the internal reference[39] as for nonovarian gynecologic tumors.[20,40–42] This classification of the time-intensity curves of tumor enhancement correlated with histopathologic findings (**Fig. 2**): Type 1 is a curve showing a gradual increase in the signal of solid tissue, without a well-defined shoulder. Type 2 is a curve with moderate initial rise in the signal of solid tissue relative to that of myometrium, followed by a plateau. Type 3 is a curve with intense initial rise in the signal of solid tissue steeper than that of myometrium (see **Fig. 2**). In the authors' experience[39] on a population of 37 epithelial ovarian tumors proven by histopathology (10 benign, 11 borderline, and 16 malignant tumors), it was demonstrated that only invasive tumors displayed time intensity curve type 3 (specificity 100%) (**Fig. 3**). Enhancement curve types 1 and 2 corresponded to benign (**Fig. 4**) and borderline ovarian tumors, respectively,

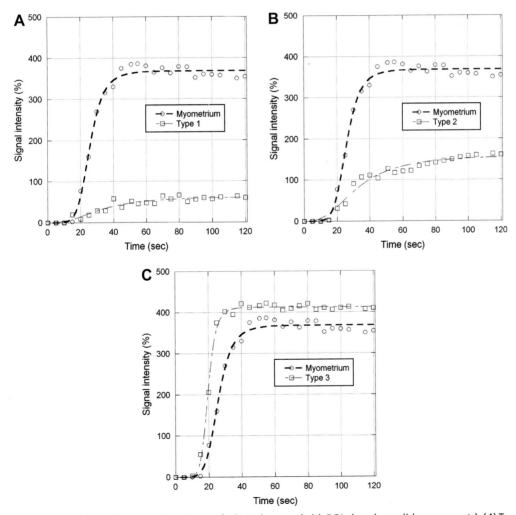

Fig. 2. DCE MR imaging enhancement patterns of adnexal masses (with ROI placed on solid components). (*A*) Type 1: gradual increase in the signal of solid tissue, without a well-defined shoulder. (*B*) Type 2: moderate initial rise in the signal of solid tissue relative to that of myometrium, followed by a plateau. (*C*) Type 3: initial rise in the signal of solid tissue, steeper than that of myometrium. Signal intensity (SI) is normalized to baseline as SI = (SI(t)-SI(0))/SI(0) and expressed as a percentage.

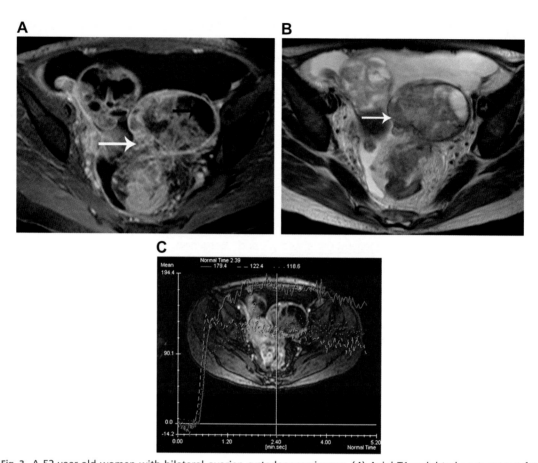

Fig. 3. A 52-year-old woman with bilateral ovarian cystadenocarcinoma. (*A*) Axial T1-weighted postcontrast fat suppressed image shows bilateral complex adnexal masses, with enhancing solid components (*white arrow*) and cystic components (*black arrow*). (*B*) Axial fast spin-echo T2-weighted image shows intermediate T2 signal of solid component (*white arrow*). (*C*) DCE T1-weighted image shows intense enhancement of these tumors (*yellow and green lines*) compared with the myometrium (*red line*) (curve type 3).

however, with a significant overlap. In addition, semiquantitative parameters, such as the enhancement amplitude, time of half rising, and the maximal slope were found to be useful for the characterization of ovarian epithelial tumors. The maximal slope was the best criterion for distinguishing invasive from noninvasive tumors. A cutoff of 3.9% per second distinguished between invasive and benign or borderline tumors with a sensitivity of 100% and a specificity of 92%.[43] Using the myometrium as the internal reference, the maximum slope ratios (tumor maximal slope divided by myometrial maximal slope) and the initial area under the curve (IAUC) 60 seconds after injection or IAUC60ratio (IAUC60 tumor divided by myometrial IAUC60) were combined to generate a decision tree demonstrating an 81% accuracy.[39] Using cutoff values of 0.366 for maximum slope ratio and 0.25 for the IAUC60ratio, only one invasive (6%), two (20%) benign, and four (36%) borderline tumors were misclassified.

DCE-MR imaging has also been proved to be useful for distinguishing solid pelvic masses, and especially ovarian fibromas and uterine leiomyomas.[44] Although Troiano and colleagues[45] found that low T2-weighted signal was highly suggestive of ovarian fibromas, subserosal pedunculated leiomyomas can mimic ovarian tumors, especially in premenopausal or menopausal women in whom normal ovaries are atrophic and sometimes not detectable. In the authors' experience, morphologic criteria (such as size, homogeneity, T1- or T2-weighted signal, cystic portion, ovarian tissue, pelvic fluid) are inadequate for distinguishing between subserosal uterine leiomyomas and ovarian fibromas. In a retrospective study comparing 15 leiomyomas and 15 ovarian fibromas, the authors found that DCE-MR imaging accurately distinguished uterine fibroids from ovarian fibromas.[44] With normal myometrium used as the reference, enhancement of ovarian fibromas was weaker and slower than

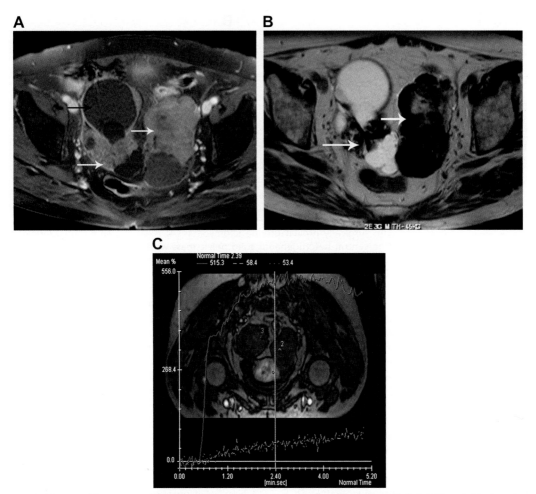

Fig. 4. A 48-year-old woman with bilateral benign ovarian cystadenofibromas. (A) Axial T1-weighted postcontrast fat-suppressed T1-weighted images show bilateral adnexal masses with enhancing solid components (*white arrows*) and cystic components (*black arrow*). (B) Axial non fat-suppressed T2-weighted image shows low T2-signal of the solid component (*white arrows*). (C) DCE T1-weighted image shows weak enhancement of the solid components of the tumors (*yellow and green lines*) compared with the myometrium (*red line*) (curve type 1).

that of uterine leiomyomas (**Figs. 5** and **6**), as shown with dynamic CT features.[46] Moreover, in the authors' study, cellular ovarian fibromas were able to be distinguished from classical ovarian fibromas. This form is defined by a degree of mitotic activity, which is intermediate between classical ovarian fibroma (lower than three mitotic figures per high 10 fields) and fibrosarcoma (higher than three mitotic figures per high 10 fields).[47] Cellular ovarian fibromas have a high rate of recurrence compared with classical ovarian fibromas. These tumors are hyperintense on T2-weighted images and displayed stronger and with earlier contrast uptake than ovarian fibromas, but weaker and with later uptake than uterine leiomyomas.[44]

Correlation of DCE MR Imaging with Angiogenesis Biomarkers

The mechanisms explaining the different enhancement curves after intravenous injection of gadolinium chelates are complex and depend on tissue-specific factors, such as the number and maturity of microvessels, interstitial space, and the interstitial pressure.[48] Malignant tumors are characterized by poorly formed and fragile neoangiogenic vessels. In addition, microvessels in malignant tumors lack a muscular coat and are highly permeable.[49] One way to assess the muscular coat of microvessels is to determine the pericyte coverage index (PCI). The density of smooth muscle cells within microvessels, based on the PCI, is significantly lower in malignant

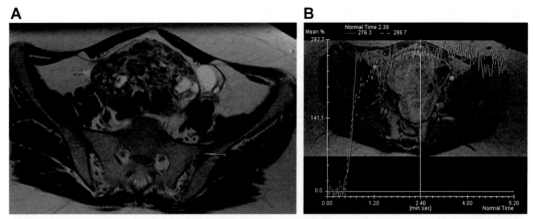

Fig. 5. A 46-year-old woman with surgically proven uterine leiomyoma. (*A*) Axial fast spin-echo T2-weighted image shows a well-defined large central heterogeneous solid pelvic mass with an intermediate T2-weighted signal. (*B*) DCE T1-weighted image shows intense and early enhancement of the tumor (*yellow line*), similar to myometrial enhancement (*red line*).

ovarian tumors than in benign tumors.[43,50] Another major determinant of microvascular permeability is vascular endothelial growth factor (VEGF) expression. Vascular endothelial growth factor receptor 2 (VEGFR-2) is an endothelial VEGF receptor specifically involved in ovarian tumor metastasis,[51] expressed both by tumor cells and by endothelial cells of blood vessels in the stroma adjacent to tumor nests. Overexpression of VEGF and VEGFR-1 and -2 has been observed in malignant ovarian tumors when compared with benign tumors.[43,52–54]

In the authors' experience, there was no observable correlation between semi-quantitative DCE MR imaging parameters and tumor microvascular density in a population of patients (*n* = 41) with ovarian tumors,[43] as opposed to prior studies involving different tumor tissues (breast and cervical tumors).[55–57] However, a correlation between DCE

MR imaging parameters and histopathologic markers of vascular maturity was observed. Enhancement amplitude correlated with VEGFR-2 expression on endothelial and epithelial cells, and maximal slope was associated with low smooth muscle actin expression and high VEGFR-2 expression on endothelial and epithelial cells (**Fig. 7**). The results confirmed that VEGF-2 influences MR signal enhancement, as reported Knopp and colleagues[58] in a study of breast tumors.

LIMITATIONS OF DCE MR IMAGING

A significant amount of solid tissue is needed to generate a time-intensity curve. In this specific setting, time-intensity curves obtained with small solid-tissue components can be limited by partial volume effect of adjacent structures. In the authors' study, benign and borderline mucinous tumors with

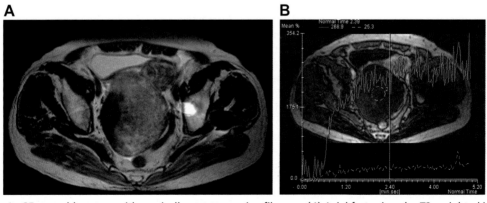

Fig. 6. An 85-year-old woman with surgically proven ovarian fibroma. (*A*) Axial fast spin-echo T2-weighted image shows a central heterogeneous solid pelvic mass with an intermediate T2-weighted signal similar to the one above (shown in **Fig. 5**). (*B*) DCE T1-weighted image shows weak enhancement of the tumor (*yellow line*) compared with the myometrium (*red line*).

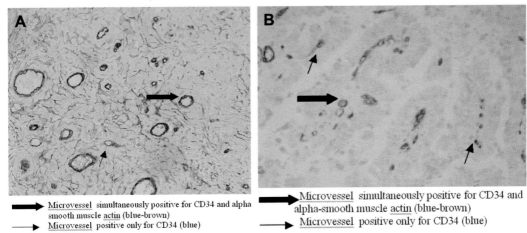

Fig. 7. Correlation between DCE MR parameters and histopathologic markers of angiogenesis. (A) Benign ovarian tumor. High pericyte coverage index: more than two-thirds of the number of cells simultaneously positive for CD34 and alpha-smooth muscle actin (*blue-brown, thick arrow*) compared with the number of cells positive for CD34 (*blue, thin arrow*). This tumor displayed a time intensity curve type 1 (not shown). (B) Malignant ovarian tumor. Low pericyte coverage index: ratio of number of cells simultaneously positive for CD34 and alpha-smooth muscle actin (*blue-brown, thick arrow*)/total number of cells positive for CD34 (*blue, thin arrows*) is less than one in three. This tumor displayed a time intensity curve type 3 (not shown).

small solid-tissue components (thickened irregular septa or small papillary projections) were the most commonly misclassified ovarian tumors.

The authors used descriptive and semiquantitative parameters that translate enhancement behavior without taking into account the arterial input function. This approach has the advantage of being efficient and straightforward, but it cannot be simply extrapolated to different platforms because of the use of different acquisition parameters. The latter must be optimized to extract quantitative parameters, such as perfusion, blood volume, and the capillary permeability product, using a MR pharmacokinetic compartmental model.

FUTURE PROSPECTS

Pharmacodynamic models allow the evaluation of microvascular parameters of tissue blood flow, tissue blood volume, tissue interstitial volume, mean transit time, and permeability.[58,59] Tissue enhancement depends on arterial input function, kinetic distribution of blood into the capillary bed, leakage across the capillary walls, and volume of the interstitial space. Hemodynamic characteristics of immature neovessels can be noninvasively assessed by DCE MR imaging, which has been shown to correlate with conventional outcome methods, such as histopathologic studies. The process of tumor neoangiogenesis plays a central role in the growth and spread of tumors. Evaluation of angiogenesis can be used as a prognostic

marker to evaluate the aggressiveness of tumor and as a potential predictive marker of antiangiogenic treatment response.[58] The authors have recently shown that MR kinetic parameters are highly correlated with VEGFR-2 expression in tumors,[43] which reflects the aggressiveness of ovarian carcinoma and has is also a prognostic marker in patients with ovarian carcinoma.[60] Many new drugs targeting the tumor neoangiogenic process are under development, especially for advanced ovarian tumors using an intraperitoneal technique. Thus, DCE MR imaging would be useful for patients with stage IV epithelial ovarian cancer receiving intraperitoneal chemotherapy, to predict the tumor response to therapy. MR kinetic parameters should be new predictors of overall survival and be integrated in clinical prognostic scores.[61] Moreover, multiparametric imaging combining DCE MR imaging, and other functional MR techniques such as diffusion-weighted imaging and MR spectroscopy, may further improve preoperative tissue characterization.

SUMMARY

DCE MR imaging is a promising emerging technique for characterizing ovarian masses based on semiquantitative perfusion parameters. Quantitative DCE MR parameters should be developed in future studies to obtain more reproducible kinetic parameters, potentially useful for better tumor characterization and to predict tumor aggressiveness.

REFERENCES

1. Curtin JP. Management of the adnexal mass. Gynecol Oncol 1994;55(3 Pt 2):S42–6.
2. Fauvet R, Boccara J, Dufournet C, et al. Restaging surgery for women with borderline ovarian tumors: results of a French multicenter study. Cancer 2004; 100(6):1145–51.
3. Fauvet R, Boccara J, Dufournet C, et al. Laparoscopic management of borderline ovarian tumors: results of a French multicenter study. Ann Oncol 2005;16(3):403–10.
4. Darai E, Tulpin L, Prugnolle H, et al. Laparoscopic restaging of borderline ovarian tumors. Surg Endosc May 2007;21(11):2039–43.
5. Morice P. Borderline tumours of the ovary and fertility. Eur J Cancer 2006;42(2):149–58.
6. Gynecologic sonography. Report of the ultrasonography task force. Council on Scientific Affairs, American Medical Association. JAMA 1991;265(21): 2851–5.
7. Timmerman D, Testa AC, Bourne T, et al. Logistic regression model to distinguish between the benign and malignant adnexal mass before surgery: a multicenter study by the International Ovarian Tumor Analysis Group. J Clin Oncol 2005;23(34): 8794–801.
8. Yazbek J, Raju SK, Ben-Nagi J, et al. Effect of quality of gynaecological ultrasonography on management of patients with suspected ovarian cancer: a randomised controlled trial. Lancet Oncol 2008;9(2):124–31.
9. Kinkel K, Lu Y, Mehdizade A, et al. Indeterminate ovarian mass at US: incremental value of second imaging test for characterization—meta-analysis and Bayesian analysis. Radiology 2005;236(1): 85–94.
10. Tsili AC, Tsampoulas C, Argyropoulou M, et al. Comparative evaluation of multidetector CT and MR imaging in the differentiation of adnexal masses. Eur Radiol 2008;18(5):1049–57.
11. Yazbek J, Aslam N, Tailor A, et al. A comparative study of the risk of malignancy index and the ovarian crescent sign for the diagnosis of invasive ovarian cancer. Ultrasound Obstet Gynecol 2006;28(3): 320–4.
12. Yazbek J, Raju KS, Ben-Nagi J, et al. Accuracy of ultrasound subjective "pattern recognition" for the diagnosis of borderline ovarian tumors. Ultrasound Obstet Gynecol 2007;29(5):489–95.
13. Brown DL, Doubilet PM, Miller FH, et al. Benign and malignant ovarian masses: selection of the most discriminating gray-scale and Doppler sonographic features. Radiology 1998;208(1):103–10.
14. Hricak H, Chen M, Coakley FV, et al. Complex adnexal masses: detection and characterization with MR imaging—multivariate analysis. Radiology 2000;214(1):39–46.
15. Sohaib SA, Sahdev A, Van Trappen P, et al. Characterization of adnexal mass lesions on MR imaging. AJR Am J Roentgenol 2003;180(5):1297–304.
16. Bazot M, Nassar-Slaba J, Thomassin-Naggara I, et al. MR imaging compared with intraoperative frozen-section examination for the diagnosis of adnexal tumors; correlation with final histology. Eur Radiol 2006;16:2687–99.
17. Siegelman ES, Outwater EK. Tissue characterization in the female pelvis by means of MR imaging. Radiology 1999;212(1):5–18.
18. Van Vierzen PB, Massuger LF, Ruys SH, et al. Borderline ovarian malignancy: ultrasound and fast dynamic MR findings. Eur J Radiol 1998;28(2):136–42.
19. Tanaka YO, Yoshizako T, Nishida M, et al. Ovarian carcinoma in patients with endometriosis: MR imaging findings. AJR Am J Roentgenol 2000;175(5): 1423–30.
20. Park BK, Kim B, Park JM, et al. Differentiation of the various lesions causing an abnormality of the endometrial cavity using MR imaging: emphasis on enhancement patterns on dynamic studies and late contrast-enhanced T1-weighted images. Eur Radiol 2006;16(7):1591–8.
21. Boss EA, Massuger LF, Pop LA, et al. Post-radiotherapy contrast enhancement changes in fast dynamic MRI of cervical carcinoma. J Magn Reson Imaging 2001;13(4):600–6.
22. Folkman J. Successful treatment of an angiogenic disease. N Engl J Med 1989;320(18):1211–2.
23. Ekerhovd E, Wienerroith H, Staudach A, et al. Preoperative assessment of unilocular adnexal cysts by transvaginal ultrasonography: a comparison between ultrasonographic morphologic imaging and histopathologic diagnosis. Am J Obstet Gynecol 2001;184(2):48–54.
24. Rieber A, Nussle K, Stohr I, et al. Preoperative diagnosis of ovarian tumors with MR imaging: comparison with transvaginal sonography, positron emission tomography, and histologic findings. AJR Am J Roentgenol 2001;177(1):123–9.
25. Kinkel K, Frei KA, Balleyguier C, et al. Diagnosis of endometriosis with imaging: a review. Eur Radiol 2006;16(2):285–98.
26. Umemoto M, Shiota M, Shimono T, et al. Preoperative diagnosis of ovarian tumors, focusing on the solid area based on diagnostic imaging. J Obstet Gynaecol Res 2006;32(2):195–201.
27. Scully E, Young J, Clement PB. Common "epithelial" tumors. In: Rosai J, editor, Tumors of the ovary and maldeveloped gonads, fallopian tube, and broad ligament, vol 23. Washington, DC: Armed Forces Institute of Pathology; 1998. p. 53–151.

28. Outwater EK, Huang AB, Dunton CJ, et al. Papillary projections in ovarian neoplasms: appearance on MRI. J Magn Reson Imaging 1997;7(4):689–95.

29. Outwater EK, Siegelman ES, Talerman A, et al. Ovarian fibromas and cystadenofibromas: MRI features of the fibrous component. J Magn Reson Imaging 1997;7(3):465–71.

30. Outwater EK, Siegelman ES, Kim B, et al. Ovarian Brenner tumors: MR imaging characteristics. Magn Reson Imaging 1998;16(10):1147–53.

31. Jung SE, Lee JM, Rha SE, et al. CT and MR imaging of ovarian tumors with emphasis on differential diagnosis. Radiographics 2002;22(6):1305–25.

32. Togashi K, Nishimura K, Itoh K, et al. Ovarian cystic teratomas: MR imaging. Radiology 1987;162(3):669–73.

33. Bazot M, Boudghene F, Billieres P, et al. Value of fat-suppression gradient-echo MR imaging in the diagnosis of ovarian cystic teratomas. Clin Imaging 2000;24(3):146–53.

34. Yamashita Y, Torashima M, Hatanaka Y, et al. Value of phase-shift gradient-echo MR imaging in the differentiation of pelvic lesions with high signal intensity at T1-weighted imaging. Radiology 1994;191(3):759–64.

35. Togashi K, Nishimura K, Kimura I, et al. Endometrial cysts: diagnosis with MR imaging. Radiology 1991;180(1):73–8.

36. Outwater E, Schiebler ML, Owen RS, et al. Characterization of hemorrhagic adnexal lesions with MR imaging: blinded reader study. Radiology 1993;186(2):489–94.

37. Stevens SK, Hricak H, Stern JL. Ovarian lesions: detection and characterization with gadolinium-enhanced MR imaging at 1.5 T. Radiology 1991;181(2):481–8.

38. Sohaib SA, Mills TD, Sahdev A, et al. The role of magnetic resonance imaging and ultrasound in patients with adnexal masses. Clin Radiol 2005;60(3):340–8.

39. Thomassin-Naggara I, Darai E, Cuenod CA, et al. Dynamic contrast-enhanced magnetic resonance imaging: a useful tool for characterizing ovarian epithelial tumors. JMRI 2008;28(1):111–20.

40. Yamashita Y, Baba T, Baba Y, et al. Dynamic contrast-enhanced MR imaging of uterine cervical cancer: pharmacokinetic analysis with histopathologic correlation and its importance in predicting the outcome of radiation therapy. Radiology 2000;216(3):803–9.

41. Manfredi R, Mirk P, Maresca G, et al. Local-regional staging of endometrial carcinoma: role of MR imaging in surgical planning. Radiology 2004;231(2):372–8.

42. Koyama T, Togashi K. Functional MR imaging of the female pelvis. J Magn Reson Imaging 2007;25(6):1101–12.

43. Thomassin-Naggara I, Bazot M, Darai E, et al. Epithelial ovarian tumors: value of dynamic contrast-enhanced MR Imaging and correlation with tumor angiogenesis. Radiology 2008;248(1):148–59.

44. Thomassin-Naggara I, Darai E, Nassar-Slaba J, et al. Value of dynamic enhanced magnetic resonance imaging for distinguishing between ovarian fibroma and subserous uterine leiomyoma. J Comput Assist Tomogr 2007;31(2):236–42.

45. Troiano RN, McCarthy S. Magnetic resonance imaging evaluation of adnexal masses. Semin Ultrasound CT MR 1994;15(1):38–48.

46. Bazot M, Ghossain MA, Buy JN, et al. Fibrothecomas of the ovary: CT and US findings. J Comput Assist Tomogr 1993;17(5):754–9.

47. Prat J, Scully E. Cellular fibromas and fibrosarcomas of the ovary: a comparative clinicopathologic analysis of seventeen cases. Cancer 1981;47:2663–70.

48. Jain RK. Determinants of tumor blood flow: a review. Cancer Res 1988;48(10):2641–58.

49. Fleischer AC, Rodgers WH, Kepple DM, et al. Color Doppler sonography of ovarian masses: a multiparameter analysis. J Ultrasound Med 1993;12(1):41–8.

50. Emoto M, Iwasaki H, Mimura K, et al. Differences in the angiogenesis of benign and malignant ovarian tumors, demonstrated by analyses of color Doppler ultrasound, immunohistochemistry, and microvessel density. Cancer 1997;80(5):899–907.

51. So J, Wang FQ, Navari J, et al. LPA-induced epithelial ovarian cancer (EOC) in vitro invasion and migration are mediated by VEGF receptor-2 (VEGF-R2). Gynecol Oncol 2005;97(3):870–8.

52. Abu-Jawdeh GM, Faix JD, Niloff J, et al. Strong expression of vascular permeability factor (vascular endothelial growth factor) and its receptors in ovarian borderline and malignant neoplasms. Lab Invest 1996;74(6):1105–15.

53. Yamamoto S, Konishi I, Mandai M, et al. Expression of vascular endothelial growth factor (VEGF) in epithelial ovarian neoplasms: correlation with clinicopathology and patient survival, and analysis of serum VEGF levels. Br J Cancer 1997;76(9):1221–7.

54. Chen H, Ye D, Xie X, et al. VEGFRs expressions and activated STATs in ovarian epithelial carcinoma. Gynecol Oncol 2004;94(3):630–5.

55. Hulka JF, Hulka CA. Preoperative sonographic evaluation and laparoscopic management of persistent adnexal masses: a 1994 review. J Am Assoc Gynecol Laparosc 1994;1(3):197–205.

56. Su MY, Cheung YC, Fruehauf JP, et al. Correlation of dynamic contrast enhancement MRI parameters with microvessel density and VEGF for assessment of angiogenesis in breast cancer. J Magn Reson Imaging 2003;18(4):467–77.

57. Cooper RA, Carrington BM, Loncaster JA, et al. Tumour oxygenation levels correlate with dynamic contrast-enhanced magnetic resonance imaging parameters in carcinoma of the cervix. Radiother Oncol 2000;57(1):53–9.

58. Knopp MV, Weiss E, Sinn HP, et al. Pathophysiologic basis of contrast enhancement in breast tumors. J Magn Reson Imaging 1999;10(3):260–6.

59. Cuenod CA, Fournier L, Balvay D, et al. Tumor angiogenesis: pathophysiology and implications for contrast-enhanced MRI and CT assessment. Abdom Imaging 2006;31(2):188–93.

60. Nishida N, Yano H, Komai K, et al. Vascular endothelial growth factor C and vascular endothelial growth factor receptor 2 are related closely to the prognosis of patients with ovarian carcinoma. Cancer 2004; 101(6):1364–74.

61. Sharma R, Hook J, Kumar M, et al. Evaluation of an inflammation-based prognostic score in patients with advanced ovarian cancer. Eur J Cancer 2008; 44(2):251–6.

62. Guinet C, Ghossain MA, Buy JN, et al. Mature cystic teratomas of the ovary: CT and MR findings. Eur J Radiol 1995;20(2):137–43.

Functional MR Imaging of the Uterus

Asako Nakai, MD, PhD*, Takashi Koyama, MD, PhD,
Koji Fujimoto, MD, Kaori Togashi, MD, PhD

KEYWORDS

- Uterus • Function • Cine MR imaging
- Diffusion-weighted MR imaging
- Dynamic contrast-enhanced MR imaging

MR imaging is an established method for the evaluation of a variety of gynecologic conditions and diseases. It is established as a problem-solving modality when ultrasound evaluation is equivocal, because of its excellent tissue contrast reflecting pathology compared with CT. MR imaging has additional advantages because it is noninvasive and more importantly free from ionizing radiation, being especially beneficial to evaluate reproductive-aged women. The standard technique involves the acquisition of spin-echo T1- and T2-weighted sequences. On T2-weighted images, the uterus in reproductive-aged women demonstrates distinct anatomic zonal differentiation (**Fig. 1**). The combination of these two types of sequences with different contrasts provides information on tissue contents so that a specific diagnosis is often reached.

Recent developments in MR techniques have enabled the functional assessment of the uterus. Cine MR imaging using rapid T2 sequences is used to evaluate the kinematic function of the uterus by demonstrating temporal morphologic changes. Diffusion-weighted imaging (DWI) provides tissue contrast based on molecular diffusion phenomenon. Finally, dynamic contrast-enhanced (DCE) MR imaging is a promising tool for evaluating vascular dynamics. Although most of these techniques are still in the experimental stage, they may provide functional information when used in combination with standard imaging methods.

UTERINE CONTRACTIONS ON CINE MR IMAGING
Technique

Recent developments in ultrafast MR imaging techniques have enabled the acquisition of serial images with few seconds between each acquisition, although spatial and contrast resolutions are worse than those of conventional imaging. Under quiet respiration, 60 serial rapid T2-weighted images in the midsagittal plane of the uterus can be obtained repeatedly within 2 to 3 minutes. T2-weighted half-Fourier rapid acquisition with the relaxation enhancement technique provides sufficient contrast between three layers of the uterus with an acquisition time of less than a second. Of great importance is the display of images in the cine mode at a faster speed than real time to enhance slow and subtle movements of uterine peristalsis. Assessment of uterine peristalsis can be performed visually or semiautomatically by using software with an automated contour-tracing method.[1]

Results

In nongravid myometrium, at least two patterns of myometrial contractions are known. One involves sustained contraction and the other consists of uterine peristalsis. Sustained contraction is mainly characterized by focal and sporadic myometrial contractility, which frequently involves the entire layer of the myometrium; this type of contraction may be sustained for several minutes.[2,3] On static

Department of Diagnostic Radiology, Kyoto University Hospital, 54 Kawahara-cho Shogoin Sakyo-ku, Kyoto 606-8507, Japan
* Corresponding author.
E-mail address: asanakai@kuhp.kyoto-u.ac.jp (A. Nakai).

Magn Reson Imaging Clin N Am 16 (2008) 673–684
doi:10.1016/j.mric.2008.07.010

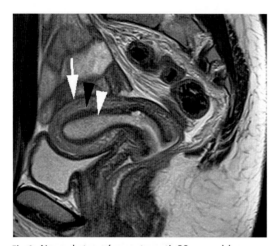

Fig. 1. Normal uterus (asymptomatic 28-year-old woman during periovulatory phase). Sagittal fast spin echo (FSE) T2-weighted image (TR/TE = 3800/105). The endometrium demonstrates high signal intensity (*white arrowhead*); the inner myometrium demonstrates low signal intensity also known as the "junctional zone" (*black arrowhead*); and the myometrium shows relatively high signal intensity (*arrow*).

T2-weighted images, sustained uterine contractions are seen as transient focal masses of low signal intensity, which bulge into the endometrium.[2] These focal contractions are known as "pseudolesions," which can mimic disease processes, such as leiomyomas and adenomyosis (**Fig. 2**).[2,3]

Uterine peristalsis is identifiable on ultrasound as rhythmic and subtle wave-like endometrial movements associated with contractions of the subendometrial myometrium.[4–6] The frequency, height, and direction of the peristaltic waves have been reported to vary throughout the phases of the menstrual cycle.[4,5] It has been postulated that uterine peristalsis occurs for such activities as sperm transport, discharge of menstrual blood, and conservation of the gestational sac during the early stages of pregnancy.[4,5] Uterine peristalsis has not been identified on conventional T2-weighted images, however, because of insufficient temporal resolution. On cine MR imaging, uterine peristalsis can be depicted as the conduction of low-intensity areas in the subendometrial myometrium, usually associated with a stripping movement of the endometrium (**Fig. 3**).[7,8] The conduction of low-intensity areas seems directly to display subtle and rhythmic contractions of the subendometrial myometrium.

Cine MR imaging allows the observation of both sustained contractions and peristalsis, and is used for investigating the changes and impairment in uterine function in a variety of conditions and gynecologic disorders.

Uterine Peristalsis in Healthy Nongravid Women

Cine MR imaging demonstrates drastic changes in uterine peristalsis through the phases of the menstrual cycle. Peristaltic waves predominantly travel in a cervicofundal direction during the proliferative and periovulatory phases, and in a fundocervical direction during menstruation.[1,7–9] On cine MR imaging, it was observed that uterine peristalsis was most active during the periovulatory phase (91.7% positive) and most subdued during the luteal phase (27.1% positive). The average frequencies of the conduction waves are 4.5, 0.9, and 1.3 per 2 minutes for the periovulatory phase, luteal

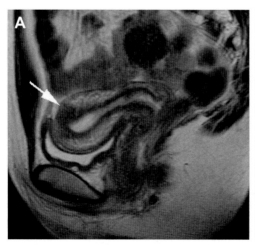
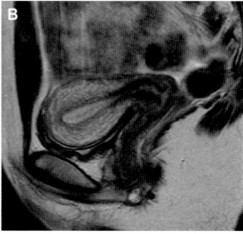

Fig. 2. Sustained contraction (asymptomatic 27-year-old woman). Sagittal FSE T2-weighted images (TR/TE = 4000/120). Ill-defined focal area with low signal intensity in the myometrium (*arrow* in A) disappears during repeated scans 12 days later (B). This pseudolesion can mimic adenomyosis.

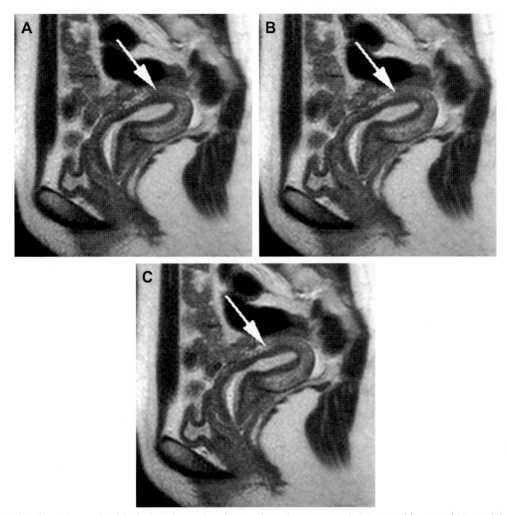

Fig. 3. (*A–C*) Uterine peristalsis during the periovulatory phase (asymptomatic 25-year-old woman). On serial sagittal half-Fourier rapid acquisition with the relaxation enhancement images (TR/TE = 3000/81) obtained every 3 seconds, uterine peristalsis appears as the conduction of low signal intensity areas (*arrows*) in the subendometrial myometrium, associated with a stripping movement of the endometrium.

phase, and menstrual phase, respectively.[1,9] A recent cine MR imaging study showed that there is no diurnal variation in uterine peristalsis.[9]

Uterine Contractions in Various Physiologic and Pathologic Conditions

Uterine contractions including uterine peristalsis, which might play important roles in uterine functions, may be affected by various physiologic and pathologic conditions. Dysmenorrhea is a condition that is thought to correlate with uterine contractility, affecting a large number of women. Infertility has recently become a more common concern because more women tend to delay childbearing. Moreover, contraception is also an important issue for some women. Various gynecologic benign conditions, such as endometriosis or

leiomyomas, are believed to be the causes of unfavorable symptoms related to the menstrual cycle. Disturbed uterine peristalsis might be a key factor for such symptoms, and cine MR imaging is a potential tool to evaluate dysfunctional uterine peristalsis with benign gynecologic conditions.

Dysmenorrhea
Primary dysmenorrhea that occurs in the absence of pelvic pathology is one of the most common gynecologic problems among young women. Around 10% of women are reported to have severe menstrual pain that limits work or daily activities. Several studies on intrauterine pressure have shown that dysmenorrhea is associated with higher tone and higher amplitude of uterine contraction. Such studies have been conducted rather

invasively, however, and they might have caused artifactual contractility. Because of these limitations and the difficulty of assessing subjective pain, the literature on dysmenorrhea is extremely limited. The evaluation of uterine contraction on MR imaging may provide a potential tool objectively to evaluate dysmenorrhea. On MR imaging, the volume of the myometrium is smaller when the subjects have maximum pain compared with those without pain.[10] Remarkable changes were noted on uterine cine MR imaging in early cycle with severe pain and on a different cycle date without pain (**Fig. 4**).[10] Increased pain is related to a thicker junctional zone, the presence of focal contractions, or endometrial distortion, all of these characteristics representing stronger uterine contractility.[10]

Cine MR imaging is also useful for the evaluation of treatment effects. During menstruation, women taking oral contraceptives (OC) for contraception or dysmenorrhea show less prominent endometrial distortion and a thinner subendometrial low-intensity area[11] compared with healthy women. There was a slight tendency for a larger myometrial area in women taking OCs, indicating less myometrial contractility, which might be one of the reasons for reduced menstrual pain.[11]

Effects of contraceptives

Intrauterine devices are very effective ways of contraception worldwide. Two major mechanisms are considered to be involved in this method of contraception: the interrupted implantation of the fertilized ovum, and a spermicidal effect by the inhibition of sperm transport.[12,13] The exact mechanisms, however, remain controversial.[12,13] In a previous study using cine MR imaging, dominant fundocervical directed peristaltic waves were demonstrated in as many as 4 of 11 intrauterine

device–bearing subjects during their periovulatory phase, whereas cervicofundal-directed peristalsis was dominant in healthy control women.[14] Such fundocervical waves spread through more than half of the thickness of the myometrium, and might serve for expelling intrauterine devices from the uterine cavity rather than supporting sperm transport. Furthermore, the peristaltic frequency in intrauterine device users (five per 3 minutes) was less than that of the control group (6.5 per 3 minutes).[14] Uncoordinated contractions on cine MR imaging and a significantly thick junctional zone on static images were also observed, which might be closely related to each other (**Fig. 5**).[14]

OCs are the most widely used and effective method of contraception, and are commonly used to minimize dysmenorrhea. Preliminary data show that uterine peristalsis was hardly discernable even at the midcycle in OC users on cine MR imaging.[15] Sporadic contractions were less frequent, and endometrial distortion was much less identified in the OC group. On static T2-weighted images, OC users showed a thin endometrium and junctional zone (**Fig. 6**).[15] The uterine myometrial area was larger in the OC group (19.8 cm^2) than in the control group (16.4 cm^2).[15] All these observations suggest that uterine contractility is suppressed in OC users. It is still unclear, however, how these facts affect the mechanisms of contraception and reduction of dysmenorrhea.

Infertility with endometriosis or leiomyoma

Infertility is associated with a wide variety of pathologic conditions, and much of the etiology of infertility remains unresolved. Endometriosis represents one of the most important factors of infertility, and 30% to 50% of women with endometriosis are infertile.[16] Preliminary results showed that uterine peristalsis was suppressed and identifiable in less

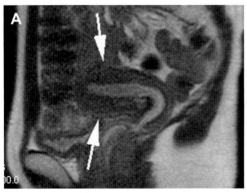
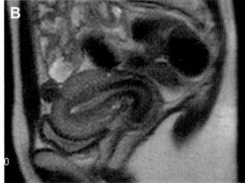

Fig. 4. Dysmenorrhea during menstruation (30-year-old woman). Sagittal RARE images (TR/TE = 2000/81) on cycle date 1 (A) and day 3 (B). The uterine myometrium on cycle date 1 with severe pain is smaller and exhibits lower signal intensity (*arrows* in A) compared with that on cycle date 3 without pain (B).

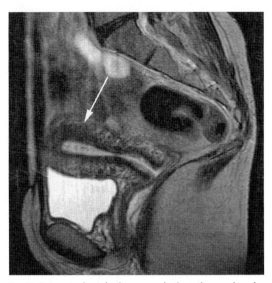

Fig. 5. Intrauterine device user during the periovulatory phase (34-year-old woman). On a sagittal FSE T2-weighted image (TR/TE = 5470/122), a thick junctional zone more than half of the myometrium is noted (*arrow*). This finding suggests the presence of strong myometrial contractility, which might serve for expelling the intrauterine device from the uterine cavity rather than supporting sperm transport. Intrauterine device is seen as dotted low-intensity areas lined at the center of the endometrium.

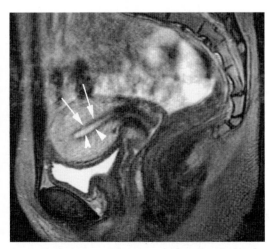

Fig. 6. Oral contraceptive user during the periovulatory phase (22-year-old woman). On a sagittal FSE T2-weighted image (TR/TE 5470/122), both the endometrium (*arrowheads*) and the junctional zone (*arrows*) are thin. On cine MR imaging (not shown), uterine peristalsis is not observed in this thin junctional zone even in the periovulatory phase, when normally frequent and strong uterine peristalsis is observed, suggesting sperm transport is not supported by the uterine motion.

than half of the patients with endometrioma even in the periovulatory phase when nearly 100% of healthy women demonstrated uterine peristalsis.[17] The frequency of peristalsis in the endometriosis group was also less than that in the control group. Decreased peristalsis in patients with endometriosis could be a possible cause of infertility, by adversely affecting sperm transport. Sporadic contractions were more frequently observed in the endometriosis group than in healthy controls, although this observation was not statistically significant.

Submucosal leiomyoma is a well-known uterine factor for miscarriage or infertility.[18] The role of submucosal leiomyoma in miscarriage or infertility has not been elucidated, although the mechanical prevention of sperm transportation and nidation, and hypercontractility, have been postulated as possible causes. Preliminary investigations using cine MR imaging demonstrated focal and irregular myometrial contractions that were different from peristalsis around submucosal leiomyomas in 55% of patients with submucosal leiomyomas.[19] The conduction of the peristaltic movements became indistinct at the site of submucosal leiomyomas.[19] These observations indicate that the obliteration of regular peristalsis or dysfunctional myometrial movements caused by submucosal leiomyomas may be one of the causative factors in pregnancy loss or infertility.

DIFFUSION-WEIGHTED IMAGING

DWI is a recently introduced technique that allows the observation of differences in molecular diffusion caused by the random and microscopic motion of molecules, also known as "brownian motion."[20] One of the attractive benefits of DWI is that it provides tissue contrast based on molecular diffusion, which differs from conventional T1- and T2-weighted images. The use of this technique has been initially established in the central nervous system, mainly for the diagnosis of acute stroke. This technique has now become available for the abdomen and pelvis. DWI can delineate malignant lesions displaying hyperintense signal because water diffusion is restricted in tissues of high cellularity.[21,22] Recent developments in parallel imaging techniques have improved the quality of abdominal DWI by reducing the acquisition time, and by minimizing the echoplanar imaging–related susceptibility artifacts. DWI also allows the quantitative measurement of the apparent diffusion coefficient (ADC) value. Decreased ADC values of malignant tumors compared with those of normal tissues or benign lesions have been previously reported in various organs.

Technique

DWI measures the loss of signal after a series of two symmetric gradient pulses called "motion-probing gradient" pulses, which are added to both sides of a 180 refocusing radiofrequency pulse to enhance the difference of molecular diffusion phenomena between tissues. Motion-probing gradient pulses are commonly applied in three directions on a X-Y-Z axis. DWI with single-shot echo-planar imaging can provide excellent contrast-to-noise ratio because the signals of most organs are very low, whereas the lesion signals remain high.[23,24] The intensity of motion-probing gradient pulses is represented by the b-value, which affects the signal intensity on DWI. On DWI with an intermediate b-value (eg, 500 s/mm^2), urine or ascites appear as comparatively high-signal intensity according to T2 contamination.[25] This T2 contamination is successfully excluded by looking at ADC maps. On DWI with a higher b-value (eg, 800 or 1000 s/mm^2), malignant tumors and lymph nodes are more conspicuous compared with images with lower b-value because most of the normal pelvic tissue is strongly suppressed, although anatomic detailed information is lost.

In body regions, short TI inversion recovery fat suppression may provide more homogeneous fat suppression compared with the chemical shift-selective method; the latter method has better signal-to-noise ratio.[22]

The authors' standard protocols for pelvic DWI are performed with a 1.5-T magnet unit, a multi-channel body phased-array coil, and a single-shot echo-planar imaging sequence under free breathing in the sagittal plane (**Table 1**).

Diffusion-Weighted Imaging Assessment

There are two methods for assessment: visual assessment and quantitative assessment of ADC values. The latter gives more specific information on molecular diffusion.

Visual assessment

A three-dimensional display of images acquired in two dimension with a reversed grayscale can produce positron emission tomography–like images because of a strong suppression of background signal. It may be difficult, however, to define the anatomic locations.[22] Recently fusion software, which overlays DWI onto conventional MR images, has become available.[26]

Assessment of apparent diffusion coefficient values

The ADC value describes microscopic water diffusivity, and decreases in the presence of factors

Table 1
Suggested parameters for acquisition of single shot echo planar diffusion imaging of the pelvis in the sagittal plane

TR (ms)	TE (ms)	Field of View (mm)	Thickness (mm)	Interslice Gap (mm)	Number of Slices	Acquisition Matrix	Bandwidth (Hz/Pixel)	Parallel Imaging Factor	NEX	Total Acquisition Time (min:s)	bValue (s/mm2)
2300–2600	75–79	260–300	5	1.5	19	128 × 61	1446	2	5	1:34	0, 500, 1000

that restrict water diffusion, such as cell membranes and the viscosity of the fluid. The ADC value can be obtained on a voxel-by-voxel basis, and depicted on an ADC map, allowing the measurement of a target tissue ADC value using regions of interest. In solid tumors, the ADC values are considered to be influenced by changes in the balance between extracellular and intracellular water molecules, and changes in cytologic morphology including the nuclear-to-cytoplasm ratio and cellular density.

Clinical Application

In the female pelvis, the expected clinical applications of DWI include tumor detection and differentiation between malignant and benign lesions. The latter role of DWI may be limited, however, because a variety of benign tumors can show restricted diffusion. Accordingly, it is important to refer to conventional MR images when interpreting DW images.

Endometrial cancer

To evaluate endometrial cancer, visual assessment of DWI is not useful because both endometrial cancerous tissues and the normal endometrium can appear hyperintense on diffusion images. Along with the calculation of the ADC values, however, DWI has the potential to demonstrate uterine endometrial cancer, and differentiate between normal and cancerous tissues of the endometrium. The ADC value of endometrial cancer is prominently lower than that of the normal endometrium (**Fig. 7**).[27] The ADC map image can be used for detecting endometrial cancer lesions. In addition, the ADC values of endometrial cancers of higher grade tend to decrease compared with those of lower grade, although there is considerable overlap.[27]

Cervical cancer

DWI has been shown to be useful in cervical cancer to detect tumor location and the extensions of tumor and the normal uterine cervical tissues, which have similar signal intensities on T2-weighted images. The ADC value of cervical cancer lesions has been reported to be lower than that of normal cervical tissues, and the ADC increase after chemotherapy or irradiation.[28]

Uterine sarcoma and leiomyoma

Uterine myometrial lesions with high signal intensity on T2-weighted images raise concerns if they are malignant. For such lesions, DWI is helpful in differentiating uterine sarcomas from leiomyomas, by showing restricted diffusion in the former, whereas ordinary leiomyomas (including degenerated leiomyomas, which demonstrate high intensity on T2-weighted images) do not display restricted

diffusion.[29] Cellular leiomyoma, however, which is a specific subtype of leiomyoma characterized by hypercellularity, also exhibits restricted diffusion; it is difficult to differentiate uterine sarcomas from cellular leiomyomas on DWI.[29,30] ADC values of sarcomas also overlap with those of cellular leiomyomas. Accordingly, conventional MR images should be meticulously observed to differentiate uterine sarcomas better from leiomyomas, although currently differentiation is limited. DWI cannot tell the difference between cellular leiomyomas and sarcomas but ordinary leiomyomas including degenerated leiomyomas.

For uterine leiomyomas, DWI and ADC maps may serve for assessing treatment response after uterine artery embolization by providing functional information at a cellular level. The ADC values of leiomyomas have been reported to decrease significantly after uterine artery embolization[31] or focused ultrasound ablation.[32] For the confirmation of the therapeutic effect, contrast-enhanced MR imaging is the standard technique recommended because it adds direct information on the lesion's vascularity.

DYNAMIC CONTRAST-ENHANCED MR IMAGING

DCE MR imaging is becoming a promising tool for assessment of cancer, and for monitoring tumor treatment response.[33,34] Malignant tumors tend to have increased vessel density and vascular permeability, with subsequent increased enhancement in the early phase of DCE MR imaging compared with normal tissues.[35] DCE MR imaging can quantify tumor perfusion and permeability, and potentially could be used as a noninvasive marker of angiogenesis, by showing correlation with histopathologic markers of angiogenesis (eg, microvessel density), which are performed on tissue samples and are not always easily available. Assessments of tumor perfusion and permeability with DCE MR imaging can be used for monitoring treatment response, for prediction of treatment response, and to predict clinical outcome.[35–37] Recent developments in anticancer drugs have been directed from cytotoxic therapies to more selective therapies that target the oncogenic abnormalities underlying the tumors. Novel therapies including antiangiogenic drugs and vascular targeting drugs are expected to improve the efficacy and tolerance of anticancer treatments.[36–38] In gauging the therapeutic effects of these treatments, there is a growing need to evaluate drug efficacy based on such factors as hypoxia and tumor blood supply.

Technique

DCE MR imaging is usually performed with the use of low-molecular-weight contrast media, such as

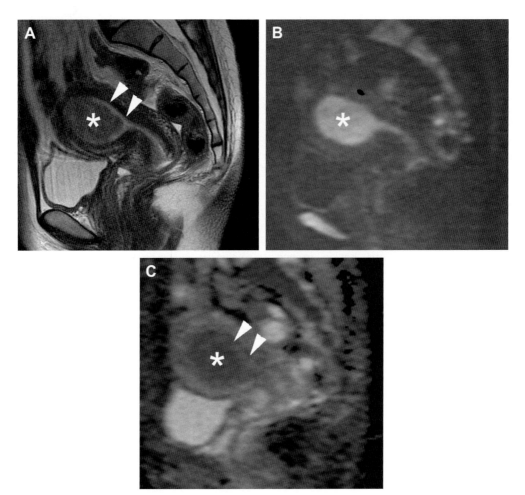

Fig. 7. Endometrial cancer, stage T1b, grade 2 (34-year-old woman). (*A*) On a sagittal T2-weighted image, endometrial cancer (*asterisk*) appears lower signal intensity compared with normal endometrium, which shows high intensity (*arrowheads*). (*B*) On single-shot echo-planar imaging diffusion-weighted image (using b = 1000), both the endometrial cancer (*asterisk*) and the normal endometrium appear hyperintense. (*C*) On the apparent diffusion coefficient map, however, the endometrial cancer (*asterisk*) displays lower apparent diffusion coefficient compared with normal endometrium (*arrowheads*).

gadopentetate dimeglumine. DCE MR imaging commonly uses T1-weighted gradient-echo pulse sequences. Standard gradient-echo sequences include spoiled gradient-echo (eg, fast low-angle shot) and magnetization-prepared gradient-echo (eg, turbo fast low-angle shot). The latter may be a preferable sequence for assessing T1-weighted perfusion because of excellent temporal resolution, although its decreased flip angle may result in a decreased contrast-to-noise ratio and impaired image quality. Compared with standard gradient-echo sequences, three-dimensional gradient-echo sequences have the potential to provide higher signal-to-noise ratio and contrast-to-noise ratio, and fewer partial-volume effects. The application of parallel imaging can improve the temporal resolution.

Assessment of Dynamic Enhancement

Tissue perfusion can be assessed in two ways: a semiquantitative method analyzing the changes in signal intensity, and a quantitative method using a pharmacokinetic model.

Semiquantitative assessment

The semiquantitative method analyzes the changes in signal intensity. This method is simple and commonly used in the clinical setting with a dynamic enhancement curve. Parameters include the onset time of enhancement, initial and mean gradients of the enhancement curves, maximum signal intensity, and washout gradient. Although this method has the advantage of relatively simplified calculations, it is difficult to

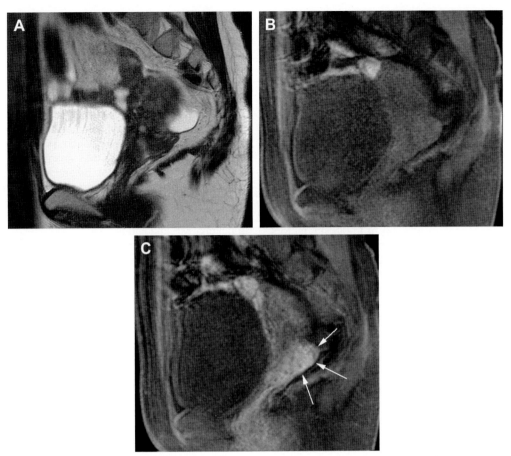

Fig. 8. Cervical cancer, stage T1b (38-year-old woman). (*A*) Sagittal FSE T2-weighted image. (*B*) Dynamic contrast sagittal T1-weighted images: precontrast and postcontrast 20 seconds after the intravenous injection of gadopentetate dimeglumine. Tumor detection is difficult on the T2-weighted image because of poor tumor contrast against normal cervical stromal tissue. (*C*) On an early postcontrast image, cervical cancer is more conspicuous because of strong enhancement (*arrows*).

compare data among patients and systems because the parameters provided by the signal intensity are relative values and are influenced by the cardiac output of the patients, sequence parameters, and machines used. Such a semiquantitative method still provides valuable information, however, to clinical management.

Quantitative assessment

The quantitative method uses pharmacokinetic modeling and provides details of several parameters including (1) the volume transfer constant K^{trans} (min^{-1}), which expresses blood flow and permeability; (2) the volume of extravascular-extracellular space per unit volume of tissue v_e ($0 < v_e < 1$); and (3) the flux rate constant between extravascular-extracellular space and plasma k_{ep}.[39] These three parameters are linked as follows: $k_{ep} = K^{trans} / v_e$. When a bolus of a paramagnetic contrast agent passes through a capillary bed, the contrast agent

rapidly passes into the extravascular-extracellular space at K^{trans}. Recently, K^{trans} has been chosen as the primary end point in antivascular clinical trials because it reflects contrast agent delivery (perfusion) and transport across the vascular endothelium (permeability).[36] If the contrast-agent concentration is properly measured, the pharmacokinetic parameters can be readily compared with the data obtained at different times in a given patient, in different patients, or with different systems. There are several limitations, however, with this technique: difficulties in data acquisition, need of an arterial input function, postprocessing, and image display using software.[39]

Clinical Applications for Uterine Cancers

DCE MR imaging is a technique used for assessing uterine pathologic conditions. It is especially useful for tumor detection and staging in malignant tumors by adding different contrast between the uterine layers (ie, strong contrast against normal uterine tissues). In addition, parametric assessment allows the quantitative evaluation of vascularity of tumor.

Cervical cancer

Although DCE MR imaging does not significantly improve staging accuracy compared with standard T2-weighted images, it may be additionally applied for detection of early stage cervical cancer (**Fig. 8**).[40] Furthermore, the functional assessment of the microcirculation using DCE MR imaging has been suggested to predict therapy outcome in cervical cancer, in addition to traditional factors, such as stage, extent of disease, histologic type, lymphatic spread, and vascular invasion. Oxygenation and perfusion (microcirculation) are believed to be important factors affecting the outcomes of the cytotoxic therapies.[41] In a preradiation therapy study, a favorable outcome was present in patients with strong tumor enhancement, suggesting good oxygenation. Tumors with baseline higher permeability (K^{trans}) tend to show a better response to radiotherapy.[40,41] After radiotherapy, the onset time of tumor enhancement has been delayed compared with that before therapy.[42] It is believed that local recurrence arises from radioresistant hypoxic tumor regions represented by the low-perfusion proportion of the pixel distribution.[41] A tendency of poorer prognosis has also been reported, however, in tumors with a fast initial rate of enhancement or vascular permeability.[43]

Endometrial cancer

When evaluating the local staging of endometrial cancers, early enhancement of the normal innermost muscle layer on DCE MR imaging is the first evident characteristic against the presence of myometrial invasion, and is considered to be relevant to the junctional zone on T2-weighted images.[44,45] This finding on DCE MR imaging for assessing myometrial invasion is valuable when the junctional zone on T2-weighted images is indistinct as in postmenopausal women.

Leiomyoma

DCE MR imaging is also useful for assessing benign myometrial lesions to select effective therapy. The extent of enhancement and the degree of hyaline degeneration seem to be related in leiomyomas.[46] Increased vascularity may be helpful in predicting the therapeutic effects of either uterine artery embolization or gonadotropin-releasing hormone analogue therapy.[47,48]

SUMMARY

Cine MR imaging is a useful tool for evaluating uterine kinematic functions derived from myometrial contractility, and for investigating the alteration of uterine contractility in a variety of conditions and gynecologic disorders. DWI can demonstrate abnormal signal in pathologic foci based on differences in molecular diffusion, and could provide useful information in evaluating malignant conditions. DCE MR imaging has the potential to improve tumor detection and local staging, and quantitative information may be useful for both monitoring therapeutic effects and predicting outcome. The use of these state-of-the-art functional MR imaging techniques is beneficial for elucidating various uterine conditions when used appropriately, and the findings provide the basis of future MR imaging investigations.

REFERENCES

1. Kido A, Nishiura M, Togashi K, et al. A semiautomated technique for evaluation of uterine peristalsis. J Magn Reson Imaging 2005;21:249–57.
2. Togashi K, Kawakami S, Kimura I, et al. Sustained uterine contractions: a cause of hypointense myometrial bulging. Radiology 1993;187:707–10.
3. Masui T, Katayama M, Kobayashi S, et al. Pseudolesions related to uterine contraction: characterization with multiphase-multisection T2-weighted MR imaging. Radiology 2003;227:345–52.
4. Lyons EA, Taylor PJ, Zheng XH, et al. Characterization of subendometrial myometrial contractions throughout the menstrual cycle in normal fertile women. Fertil Steril 1991;55:771–4.
5. de Vries K, Lyons EA, Ballard G, et al. Contractions of the inner third of the myometrium. Am J Obstet Gynecol 1990;162:679–82.
6. Chalubinski K, Deutinger J, Bernaschek G. Vaginosonography for recording of cycle-related myometrial contractions. Fertil Steril 1993;59:225–8.
7. Nakai A, Togashi K, Yamaoka T, et al. Uterine peristalsis shown on cine MR imaging using ultrafast sequence. J Magn Reson Imaging 2003;18:726–33.
8. Nakai A, Togashi K, Kosaka K, et al. Uterine peristalsis: comparison of transvaginal ultrasound and two different sequences of cine MR imaging. J Magn Reson Imaging 2004;20:463–9.
9. Kido A, Togashi K, Nakai A, et al. Investigation of uterine peristalsis diurnal variation. Magn Reson Imaging 2006;24:1149–55.
10. Kataoka M, Togashi K, Kido A, et al. Dysmenorrhea: evaluation with cine-mode-display MR imaging–initial experience. Radiology 2005;235:124–31.
11. Kido A, Togashi K, Kataoka M, et al. The effect of oral contraceptives on uterine contractility and

menstrual pain: an assessment with cine MR imaging. Hum Reprod 2007;22:2066–71.

12. Stanford JB, Mikolajczyk RT. Mechanisms of action of intrauterine devices: update and estimation of postfertilization effects. Am J Obstet Gynecol 2002;187:1699–708.

13. Kadanali S, Varoglu E, Komec D, et al. Evaluation of active and passive transport mechanisms in genital tracts of IUD-bearing women with radionuclide hysterosalpingoscintigraphy. Contraception 2001;63:41–5.

14. Kido A, Togashi K, Kataoka ML, et al. Intrauterine devices and uterine peristalsis: evaluation with MRI. Magn Reson Imaging 2008;26:54–8.

15. Kido A, Togashi K, Nakai A, et al. Oral contraceptives and uterine peristalsis: evaluation with MRI. J Magn Reson Imaging 2005;22:265–70.

16. Schenken RS, Guzick DS. Revised endometriosis classification: 1996. Fertil Steril 1997;67:815–6.

17. Kido A, Togashi K, Nishino M, et al. Cine MR imaging of uterine peristalsis in patients with endometriosis. Eur Radiol 2007;17:1813–9.

18. Donnez J, Jadoul P. What are the implications of myomas on fertility? A need for a debate? Hum Reprod 2002;17:1424–30.

19. Nishino M, Togashi K, Nakai A, et al. Uterine contractions evaluated on cine MR imaging in patients with uterine leiomyomas. Eur J Radiol 2005;53:142–6.

20. Le Bihan D, Breton E, Lallemand D, et al. MR imaging of intravoxel incoherent motions: application to diffusion and perfusion in neurologic disorders. Radiology 1986;161:401–7.

21. Nasu K, Kuroki Y, Nawano S, et al. Hepatic metastases: diffusion-weighted sensitivity-encoding versus SPIO-enhanced MR imaging. Radiology 2006;239:122–30.

22. Takahara T, Imai Y, Yamashita T, et al. Diffusion weighted whole body imaging with background body signal suppression (DWIBS): technical improvement using free breathing, STIR and high resolution 3D display. Radiat Med 2004;22:275–82.

23. Li TQ, Takahashi AM, Hindmarsh T, et al. ADC mapping by means of a single-shot spiral MRI technique with application in acute cerebral ischemia. Magn Reson Med 1999;41:143–7.

24. Edelman RR, Wielopolski P, Schmitt F. Echo-planar MR imaging. Radiology 1994;192:600–12.

25. Provenzale JM, Engelter ST, Petrella JR, et al. Use of MR exponential diffusion-weighted images to eradicate T2 shine-through effect. AJR Am J Roentgenol 1999;172:537–9.

26. Koyama T, Umeoka S, Kataoka M, et al. Utility of diffusion-weighted MR imaging in evaluation of esophageal cancers. Presented at the Proceedings of the 13th Annual Meeting of ISMRM. Miami Beach, Florida, May 7–13, 2005 [abstract 2820].

27. Tamai K, Koyama T, Saga T, et al. Diffusion-weighted MR imaging of uterine endometrial cancer. J Magn Reson Imaging 2007;26:682–7.

28. Naganawa S, Sato C, Kumada H, et al. Apparent diffusion coefficient in cervical cancer of the uterus: comparison with the normal uterine cervix. Eur Radiol 2005;15:71–8.

29. Tamai K, Koyama T, Saga T, et al. The utility of diffusion-weighted MR imaging for differentiating uterine sarcomas from benign leiomyomas. Eur Radiol 2008;18:723–30.

30. Burns B, Curry RH, Bell ME. Morphologic features of prognostic significance in uterine smooth muscle tumors: a review of eighty-four cases. Am J Obstet Gynecol 1979;135:109–14.

31. Liapi E, Kamel IR, Bluemke DA, et al. Assessment of response of uterine fibroids and myometrium to embolization using diffusion-weighted echoplanar MR imaging. J Comput Assist Tomogr 2005;29:83–6.

32. Jacobs MA, Herskovits EH, Kim HS. Uterine fibroids: diffusion-weighted MR imaging for monitoring therapy with focused ultrasound surgery—preliminary study. Radiology 2005;236:196–203.

33. Hayes C, Padhani AR, Leach MO. Assessing changes in tumour vascular function using dynamic contrast-enhanced magnetic resonance imaging. NMR Biomed 2002;15:154–63.

34. Ross BD, Chenevert TL, Rehemtulla A. Magnetic resonance imaging in cancer research. Eur J Cancer 2002;38:2147–56.

35. Padhani AR, Leach MO. Antivascular cancer treatments: functional assessments by dynamic contrast-enhanced magnetic resonance imaging. Abdom Imaging 2005;30:324–41.

36. Leach MO, Brindle KM, Evelhoch JL, et al. Pharmacodynamic/Pharmacokinetic Technologies Advisory Committee, Drug Development Office, Cancer Research UK. The assessment of antiangiogenic and antivascular therapies in early-stage clinical trials using magnetic resonance imaging: issues and recommendations. Br J Cancer 2005;92:1599–610.

37. Padhani AR, Hayes C, Assersohn L, et al. Prediction of clinicopathologic response of breast cancer to primary chemotherapy at contrast-enhanced MR imaging: initial clinical results. Radiology 2006;239:361–74.

38. Morgan B, Thomas AL, Drevs J, et al. Dynamic contrast-enhanced magnetic resonance imaging as a biomarker for the pharmacological response of PTK787/ZK 222584, an inhibitor of the vascular endothelial growth factor receptor tyrosine kinases, in patients with advanced colorectal cancer and liver metastases: results from two phase I studies. J Clin Oncol 2003;21:3955–64.

39. Tofts PS, Brix G, Buckley DL, et al. Estimating kinetic parameters from dynamic contrast-enhanced T(1)-weighted MRI of a diffusable tracer: standardized

quantities and symbols. J Magn Reson Imaging 1999;10:223–32.

40. Yamashita Y, Takahashi M, Sawada T, et al. Carcinoma of the cervix: dynamic MR imaging. Radiology 1992; 182:643–8.

41. Mayr NA, Hawighorst H, Yuh WT, et al. MR microcirculation assessment in cervical cancer: correlations with histomorphological tumor markers and clinical outcome. J Magn Reson Imaging 1999;10:267–76.

42. Boss EA, Massuger LF, Pop LA, et al. Post-radiotherapy contrast enhancement changes in fast dynamic MRI of cervical carcinoma. J Magn Reson Imaging 2001;13: 600–6.

43. Hawighorst H, Knapstein PG, Knopp MV, et al. Uterine cervical carcinoma: comparison of standard and pharmacokinetic analysis of time-intensity curves for assessment of tumor angiogenesis and patient survival. Cancer Res 1998;58:3598–602.

44. Yamashita Y, Harada M, Sawada T, et al. Normal uterus and FIGO stage I endometrial carcinoma: dynamic gadolinium-enhanced MR imaging. Radiology 1993; 186:495–501.

45. Ito K, Matsumoto T, Nakada T, et al. Assessing myometrial invasion by endometrial carcinoma with dynamic MRI. J Comput Assist Tomogr 1994;18: 77–86.

46. Shimada K, Ohashi I, Kasahara I, et al. Triple-phase dynamic MRI of intratumoral vessel density and hyalinization grade in uterine leiomyomas. AJR Am J Roentgenol 2004;182:1043–50.

47. Li W, Brophy DP, Chen Q, et al. Semiquantitative assessment of uterine perfusion using first pass dynamic contrast-enhanced MR imaging for patients treated with uterine fibroid embolization. J Magn Reson Imaging 2000;12:1004–8.

48. Yamashita Y, Torashima M, Takahashi M, et al. Hyperintense uterine leiomyoma at T2-weighted MR imaging: differentiation with dynamic enhanced MR imaging and clinical implications. Radiology 1993; 189:721–5.

Diffusion and Perfusion MR Imaging of the Prostate

Diederik M. Somford, MD[a], Jurgen J. Fütterer, MD, PhD[b,c],*,
Thomas Hambrock, MD[b], Jelle O. Barentsz, MD, PhD[b]

KEYWORDS

- Prostate cancer
- Magnetic resonance • Diffusion • Perfusion

MR imaging plays an important role in the initial detection, localization, and staging of prostate cancer and the assessment of posttreatment changes in prostate cancer. In the near future, more image-guided techniques will become available, permitting precise biopsies and targeted focal treatment. Accurate and detailed information on tumor localization and size is needed to perform these image-guided interventions and therapies optimally. This article focuses on the role of diffusion-weighted MR imaging (DWI) and dynamic contrast-enhanced (DCE) MR imaging (or perfusion-weighted MR imaging) of the prostate. Background aspects and the clinical usefulness of DWI and DCE MR imaging for assessment of prostate cancer are reviewed.

DIFFUSION WEIGHTED IMAGING
Diffusion and Prostate Cancer

Water molecules exhibit random motion in tissue, related to temperature (Brownian effect).[1] DWI can quantify this water motion in an indirect manner.[2,3] The DWI pulse sequence labels hydrogen nuclei in space, of which most is water molecules at any moment, and determines the length of the path that water molecules travel over a short period of time. DWI estimates the mean distance traveled by all hydrogen nuclei in every voxel of imaged tissue. The greater this mean distance the more self-diffusion of water molecules has occurred in a certain time interval.[4] The degree of restriction to water diffusion in biologic tissue is inversely correlated to tissue cellularity and the integrity of cell membranes. Free motion of water molecules is more restricted in tissues with a high cellular density. The sensitivity of the DWI sequence to water motion can be varied by changing the gradient amplitude, expressed as the b-value. By performing DWI using different b-values, quantitative analysis can be made to determine the apparent diffusion coefficient (ADC).

In a volume of pure water this self-diffusion is equal in all directions, hence isotropic, and not restricted by any barrier. Because diffusion in tissue is limited by cellular structures, to establish a reliable estimate of this mean distance traveled by hydrogen nuclei, DWI is acquired in at least three different orthogonal directions for each b-value.[4,5] This phenomenon of varying restriction of self-diffusion along different axes is called "anisotropy" and can also be used for tissue characterization. As in linear aligned tissue this anisotropy is more pronounced because there is one direction that contributes most to the DWI. Diffusion tensor imaging is a specific technique that

[a] Department of Urology, Radboud University, Nijmegan Medical Centre, Geert Grooteplein Zuid 10, NL 6500 HB, Nijmegen, The Netherlands
[b] Department of Radiology, Radboud University, Nijmegan Medical Centre, Geert Grooteplein Zuid 10, NL 6500 HB, Nijmegen, The Netherlands
[c] Department of Interventional Radiology, Radboud University, Nijmegan Medical Centre, Geert Grooteplein Zuid 10, NL 6500 HB, Nijmegen, The Netherlands
* Corresponding author. Department of Radiology, University Medical Center Nijmegen, Geert Grooteplein Zuid 10, NL 6500 HB, Nijmegen, The Netherlands.
E-mail address: j.futterer@rad.umcn.nl (J.J. Fütterer).

Magn Reson Imaging Clin N Am 16 (2008) 685–695
doi:10.1016/j.mric.2008.07.002

quantifies the level of anisotropy in tissue, expressed in a fractional anisotropy value. This is low in imaged tissue without substantial anisotropy and is higher in imaged tissue in which the larger part of diffusion takes place in one direction.[5,6] Diffusion tensor imaging can be used in addition to DWI to determine the structural organization of tissue along which diffusion takes place.

DWI typically has T2- and diffusion-weighted characteristics. The intensity of the signal on the diffusion-weighted image represents a combination of signal from the T2 relaxation and the dephasing caused by water motion in the presence of the diffusion gradients. At low b-values there is greater contribution from the T2 signal, and at higher b-values contrast is determined more by relative diffusion.[7] When a diffusion image is bright because of high T2 signal rather than restricted diffusion, it is known as "T2 shine-through" effect. ADC maps should be obtained with at least two b-values to correct for the T2 shine-through effect, typically a low b-value, between 0 and 50 s/mm^2, and a high b-value. Tissue microperfusion can contaminate the signal attenuation in DWI acquisition, which could be decreased by using an additional low b-value greater than 0 (eg, b = 50 s/mm^2) and a high b-value.

To minimize the influence of bulk motion as a distorting factor and minimizing T2 shine-through, typically a TE as short as possible is chosen. Typical sequence parameters for the prostate (as used in the authors' institution) include TR 2600 milliseconds; TE 91 milliseconds; and b-values of 0, 50, 500, 800 s/mm^2 in three orthogonal directions with parallel imaging (**Table 1**).

Diffusion-Weighted MR Imaging Characteristics of Prostate Tissue

DWI was initially used for the early detection of cerebral ischemia.[8] The evolution of DWI characteristics in cerebral ischemia over time has classically been attributed to the extracellular to intracellular distribution of hydrogen nuclei caused by different types of edema.[9] It has been postulated that extracellular water molecules have a far higher range of self-diffusion because they are not bound within membranes or by other cellular structures.[10,11] When this is translated to prostate tissue, which is predominantly glandular tissue, the predominant contribution of the extracellular component is from tubular structures and their fluid content, whereas the intracellular component is determined by the epithelial and stromal cells. Fractional anisotropy is determined along the axis of the tubular structures of normal prostate tissue. A prerequisite for the correct interpretation of diffusion and ADC images relies on good knowledge of the diffusion characteristics of the different anatomic zones of the prostate and of benign prostatic conditions compared with prostate cancer.[12]

The normal prostatic gland is rich in tubular structures. This allows for abundant self-diffusion of water molecules within their contents and provides high ADC values. In most cases, the peripheral zone can be easily discriminated from the central gland on DWI, because it displays relative higher ADC values.[13–15] The exact background of this phenomenon remains unclear, because the exact ratio of extracellular to intracellular components for the different anatomic zones of the prostate has not yet been described. The central gland by observation consists of more compact smooth muscle and sparser glandular elements than the peripheral zone, however, leading to lower extracellular to intracellular fluid ratio.[16] Furthermore, an age-related increase of T2 signal intensity of the peripheral zone compared with the central gland has been observed,[17] and an age-related increase in ADC values in both central gland and peripheral zone has been observed,[15] which are most likely caused by atrophy in the prostate leading to reduced cell volume and enlarged glandular ducts.

Benign prostatic hyperplasia (BPH) gives rise to nodular adenomas in the transition zone and with time these compress the central zone to form a pseudocapsule, occupying the complete central gland. The peripheral zone is usually not affected by BPH and retains its own histologic characteristics. BPH is defined by hyperplasia of all cells that constitute the central gland, with glandular, muscular, and fibrous compartments more or less evenly involved. This nodular hyperplasia gives rise to inhomogeneous diffusion patterns and because tubular structures often remain in place, the increased cellular density of hyperplasia, which is far less predominant than in prostate carcinoma, might explain the observed reduction in ADC levels of the central gland on DWI, because of decreased ratio of extracellular to intracellular volume. Because BPH has inhomogeneous diffusion characteristics, however, an increase in ADC also has been observed.[18]

Prostatitis almost uniquely originates in the peripheral zone. With respect to MR imaging, chronic prostatitis is of far more importance than the acute prostatitis counterpart because it is asymptomatic in many cases or its symptoms might mimic BPH, often associated with elevated prostate-specific antigen levels, raising the suspicion of prostate cancer. Histologically, chronic prostatitis is characterized by extracellular edema surrounding the involved prostatic cells with concomitant

Table 1
Diffusion-weighted and dynamic contrast-enhanced MR imaging parameters at 3 T with combination of endorectal and surface coils

	Diffusion-Weighted MR Imaging	Dynamic Contrast-Enhanced MR Imaging[a]
TR (ms)	2600	38
TE (ms)	91	1.35
Flip angle (degrees)	90	14
Slice thickness (mm)	3	3
b-values (s/mm²)	0, 50, 500, 800	NA
Matrix	128 × 128	128 × 128
Field of view (mm)	192	220
Temporal resolution (seconds)	NA	3[b]
Number of averages	8	1
Acquisition time (minutes)	3:40	3:00

[a] Three-dimensional gradient echo sequence.
[b] During at least 4 minutes.

aggregation of lymphocytes, plasma cells, macrophages, and neutrophils in the prostatic stroma. This abundance in cells as compared with normal prostatic tissue may lead to an ADC decrease because of decreased extracellular to intracellular fluid volume ratio. To the authors' knowledge, no reports are available on the DWI characteristics of chronic prostatitis.

Prostate carcinoma is histologically characterized by a higher cellular density than normal prostate tissue, with replacement of the normal glandular tissue. This leads to a decrease in ADC values, compared with normal prostate gland (**Fig. 1**).[12,19] Concomitantly with destruction of tubular structures in prostate carcinoma, fractional anisotropy is also reduced.[20,21] Interestingly, whereas well-differentiated prostate carcinomas display some tubular formation, with worsening differentiation the tubular structures become less predominant, and the cellular component of the cancer increases.

Diffusion-Weighted MR Imaging in Addition to T1- and T2-Weighted MR Imaging

One of the main drawbacks of DWI of the prostate is its suboptimal spatial resolution, even with currently widely available 3-T MR imaging scanners, combining pelvic phased array surface coil in combination with an endorectal coil for signal reception. T1-weighted imaging has a very limited role for the zonal delineation of the prostate and for tumor detection. The main usefulness of T1-weighted imaging is for the detection of

postbiopsy hemorrhage, which can cause restricted diffusion, a possible confounding factor for both T2-weighted images and DWI.[22]

T2-weighted imaging is currently the most widely used sequence for localization and staging of prostate carcinoma because it depicts anatomic details exceptionally well with high resolution.[23] T2-weighted imaging is also helpful for zonal delineation between the peripheral zone (high T2 signal) and the central gland (intermediate and inhomogeneous T2). In addition, T2-weighted imaging is necessary for a correct interpretation of ADC mapping. The typical nodular appearance of BPH on T2-weighted imaging helps in discriminating BPH from prostate carcinoma on DWI, which both can present with decreased ADC. For localization of prostate carcinoma T2-weighted MR imaging reaches fair sensitivity levels between 54% and 81%, with lower specificity levels, ranging from 46% to 61%, depending on the series.[24,25] When used as a staging tool, T2-weighted imaging has a lower performance. The addition of MR spectroscopy and DCE MR imaging may improve the staging performance[26,27], mostly because of the improved localization, and thereby better evaluation of the prostatic capsule on T2-weighted images.

Clinical Applications of Diffusion-Weighted MR Imaging for Prostate Carcinoma

Recently, several reports on the use of DWI in patients with prostate cancer, using endorectal or phased array coils have been published, with

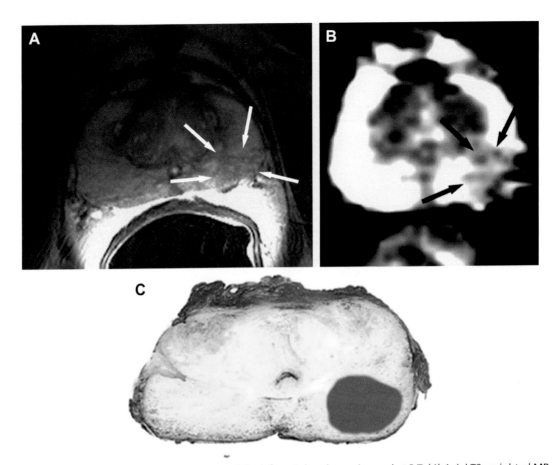

Fig.1. A 52-year-old man with prostate cancer of the left peripheral zone imaged at 3 T. (*A*) Axial T2-weighted MR image showing the presence of a low signal intensity area (*arrows*) in the left peripheral zone. (*B*) ADC map at the same level as in **Fig. 2**A shows decreased ADC compared with the normal peripheral zone. Whole-mount section histopathology (*C*) confirmed the findings and showed a tumor with Gleason Score of 3+3 = 6.

recent reports on the use of 3-T systems, proving that the clinical use of DWI is possible. The described diffusion acquisition parameters differ, however, mostly regarding the use of different b-values. This makes comparison between different reports difficult, but a clear identifiable trend in performance is present.

Several small studies have shown that prostate carcinoma displays significantly lower ADC values compared with benign prostatic tissue,[19,21,28,29] making it a potential useful measure for the localization of prostate carcinoma. In various reports, mean ADC values range between 1.30 and 1.35 $\times$ 10^{-3} mm^2/s for malignant prostate tissue and 1.60 and 1.96 $\times$ 10^{-3} mm^2/s for benign tissue, including peripheral zone and central gland.[14,21,28] DWI seems to perform better in localization of prostate carcinoma compared with T2-weighted imaging.[13,30] At 1.5 T, T2-weighted imaging yielded sensitivities of 50% to 73%, whereas DWI yielded sensitivities of 73% to 84%, with only slightly reduced or comparable specificity. These results

suggest a potential role of DWI in localization of prostate carcinoma, especially in combination with T2-weighted imaging.[14,25,31,32] Because of the higher baseline ADC of the peripheral zone, DWI performs best in differentiation of prostate cancer from normal peripheral zone in which more than 70% of the tumors originate. Compared with normal central gland ADC levels, prostate cancer ADC levels are significantly lower.[14,18]

Because of lack of spatial resolution, DWI alone is not very useful in staging of prostate carcinoma and lags behind conventional T2-weighted imaging. Like other advanced MR imaging techniques, however, such as DCE MR imaging and MR spectroscopy, DWI draws attention to suspicious lesions and this may help the radiologist in identifying regions of interest for local staging. Even with increasing spatial resolution caused by improved acquisition techniques the value of DWI alone in staging of prostate carcinoma remains limited, but improves localization of lesions in combined reading with conventional and other functional

MR imaging sequences. To the authors' knowledge, no reports have yet been published on this subject.

DWI might have potential for grading of prostate carcinoma. The histopathologic Gleason score remains one of the most important prognostic factors for progression-free and disease-specific survival in prostate cancer.[33–37] It is known that Gleason score obtained with transrectal ultrasound–guided biopsy can underestimate the final Gleason score obtained at prostatectomy in a substantial number of patients.[38–40] With evolving therapeutic options to consider in patients with localized prostate carcinoma, accurate pretreatment grading for clinical decision making is of paramount importance. These therapies range from active surveillance to minimally invasive therapies, such as cryotherapy and high-intensity focused ultrasound, to radical therapies, such as radical prostatectomy in all its forms, brachytherapy, and external beam radiation therapy. Wang and colleagues[41] investigated the ability of MR imaging to grade prostate cancer. They found that higher Gleason grades were associated with lower tumor-muscle signal intensity ratios on T2-weighted imaging. Hypothetically, DWI has far more potential than any other MR imaging sequence in grading of prostate carcinoma, because increased cellular density and loss of tubular structures implicate a higher Gleason score and also seriously hamper self-diffusion in the involved tissue leading to lower ADC levels on DWI.[12]

Few reports have been published on the detection of metastasis of prostate carcinoma using DWI and currently this technique is not used for this purpose. One report by Nakanishi and colleagues[42] did not show convincing superiority of DWI over skeletal scintigraphy for detection of osseous metastasis in a heterogeneous group of malignancies, 9 out of 30 being prostate cancer patients. Skeletal scintigraphy still remains the gold standard for detection of osseous metastasis in prostate cancer. This is supported by a recent report on patients who underwent cerebral MR imaging including DWI, in which DWI proved insensitive to skull metastasis of prostate carcinoma when compared with skeletal scintigraphy.[43] No significant reports on the detection of lymph node metastasis in prostate cancer have been reported to the authors' knowledge.

Technical Considerations in 3-T Diffusion-Weighted MR Imaging of the Prostate

3-T systems, which are increasingly available, provide improved signal-to-noise ratios, with improved spatial and temporal resolution compared with 1.5-T systems.[44] Functional MR imaging methods, such as MR spectroscopy, DCE MR imaging, and DWI, will likely benefit from 3-T systems, because those have so far been hampered by limited resolution.[45] T2-weighted imaging, which has been performed at 1.5 T for years with fair results, also has been proved to benefit; however, the window of improvement, as far as signal-to-noise ratio and spatial resolution is concerned, is much smaller. The authors' experience is that improved spatial resolution with the use of DWI at 3 T improves zonal and tumor delineation and allows improved ability to compare ADC mapping with whole-mount sectioned prostatectomy specimens for research purposes. It has been shown that use of an endorectal coil significantly improves imaging quality in T2-weighted imaging. Rectal gas in the absence of an endorectal coil may lead to susceptibility artifacts.[46] The endorectal coil enables better staging performance and improves sensitivity for the localization of prostate carcinoma with conventional MR imaging.[47,48] In the authors' experience, the use of an endorectal coil in conjunction with surface coils and parallel imaging improves image quality of DWI. This may result in improved overall performance of DWI in the localization, characterization, and delineation of prostate carcinoma.

Limitations of DWI in prostate carcinoma remain its low spatial resolution, which can be overcome by using this technique in combination with conventional T2 MR imaging at 3 T by projecting the ADC maps as color overlay images on T2 images. Furthermore, DWI is very susceptible to motion artifact, but when using a combination of surface and endorectal coil, these facilitate shortened imaging time and the use of a lower TE, while concomitantly improving image quality by diminishing susceptibility artifact from gas in the rectum.

DYNAMIC CONTRAST-ENHANCED MR IMAGING
Angiogenesis and Prostate Cancer

For a tumor, one critical factor that affects development, growth, invasiveness, and progression into the metastatic form is the ability of the tumor to generate new blood vessels. Angiogenesis, the sprouting of new capillaries from existing blood vessels, and vasculogenesis, the de novo generation of new blood vessels, are the two primary methods of vascular expansion by which nutrient supply to tumor tissue is adjusted to match physiologic needs.[49] Tumor growth beyond 1 to 2 mm in solid tissues cannot occur without vascular support.[50] The importance of angiogenesis in prostate cancer is well established. The angiogenic process is a complex multistep sequence involving many growth factors and interactions between varieties of cell types.[51] Circulating endothelial progenitor cells derived from bone marrow are recruited to sites of active angiogenesis by tumor-derived growth factors, such as vascular endothelial growth factor.[52] The angiogenic process in prostate cancer is highly dependent on vascular endothelial growth factor. Concomitantly, Jackson and colleagues[53] detected vascular endothelial growth factor in tumor cells and peritumoral stromal cells of prostate cancer specimens and in nonmalignant glandular epithelial cells and interglandular stromal cells in BPH specimens. With respect to the vasculature, it is clear that vascular endothelial growth factor is required for vascular homeostasis in BPH, and the overproduction of vascular endothelial growth factor maintains a high fraction of immature vessels (those without investigating pericytes or smooth muscle cells) in prostate cancer.[51,53,54]

A number of features are characteristic of malignant vasculature, many of which are amenable to study by DCE MR imaging and DWI techniques. These include (1) spatial heterogeneity and chaotic structure; (2) poorly formed fragile vessels with high permeability to macromolecules because of the presence of large endothelial cell gaps, incomplete basement membrane, and relative lack of pericytes or smooth muscle association with endothelial cells; (3) arteriovenous shunting; (4) intermittent or unstable blood flow; and (5) extreme heterogeneity of vascular density, with areas of low vascular density mixed with regions of high angiogenic activity.[51]

These tumor-induced vascular and structural abnormalities result in functional impairments that are important to DCE MR imaging observations. These include (1) increased interstitial pressure as a result of increased vascular permeability and poor lymphatic drainage, resulting in an enlarged interstitial space; (2) the transcapillary permeability is increased, allowing a more rapid exchange of low-molecular-weight contrast agents; and (3) the total vascular cross-sectional area may increase and can be combined with arteriovenous shunts. This gives rise to increased blood flow overall. The global increase in flow in cancers causes the bolus of contrast agent to arrive just a little earlier than it does in surrounding normal tissue. In the prostate, differences in arrival time between normal and abnormal tissues are short.[51]

Dynamic Contrast-Enhanced MR Imaging of the Prostate

DCE MR imaging is a noninvasive method to probe tumor angiogenesis. DCE MR imaging following the administration of low-molecular-weight contrast media (<1 kd) is the most common imaging method for evaluating human tumor vascular function in vivo.[55] Insights into these physiologic processes are obtained qualitatively by characterizing kinetic enhancement curves or quantitatively by applying complex compartmental modeling techniques.[56] Data reflecting the tissue perfusion (blood flow, blood volume, and mean transit time), the microvessel permeability, and the extracellular leakage space can be obtained.

MR imaging sequences can be designed to be sensitive to the vascular phase of contrast medium delivery, so-called "susceptibility-weighted (T2*-weighted) DCE MR imaging," which reflects tissue perfusion and blood volume; or to the presence of contrast agent, so-called T1-weighted DCE MR imaging, which reflects the perfused microvessel area, permeability, and extravascular extracellular leakage space.[57,58] Only the latter technique is discussed because this is by far the most common method used. Low-molecular-weight extravascular and extracellular contrast agents (gadolinium chelates) shorten the T1 relaxation of water and results in an increase in signal intensity on T1-weighted MR images. One essential aspect of DCE MR imaging includes the dynamic MR imaging, referring to the temporal component, with complete coverage of the prostate with a fast T1-weighted sequence, which is required before, during, and after the bolus injection of a low-molecular-weight contrast agent (see **Table 1**, DCE MR imaging protocol). DCE MR imaging findings are related to differences in microvascular characteristics observed between normal and malignant prostatic tissues.[51] The obtained T1-weighted DCE MR imaging data can be assessed in two ways.

The first is a semiquantitative approach describing signal intensity changes by using a number of parameters, such as (1) the onset time of the signal intensity curve (t_0 = time from appearance in an artery to the arrival of contrast agent in the tissue of interest); (2) the slope and height of the enhancement curve (time-to-peak); (3) maximum signal intensity (peak enhancement); and (4) wash-in-washout gradient or plateau phase.[59] These parameters are limited by the fact that they may not accurately reflect contrast agent concentration in tissues and can be influenced by the MR imaging scanner settings (including gain and scaling factors).

The second is a quantitative approach using pharmokinetic modeling, which is usually applied to changes in the contrast agent concentrations in tissue. Concentration-time curves are mathematically fitted by using one of many described pharmokinetic models, and quantitative kinetic parameters are derived. These include (1) transfer constant of the contrast agent (K^{trans}); (2) rate constant (K_{ep}); and (3) interstitial extravascular extracellular space (V_e).[60] Uncertainties exist with regard to the reliability of kinetic parameters estimates derived from the application of kinetic models to T1-weighted DCE MR imaging datasets. The vascular input function used in the calculations also affects the reliability of the data obtained. Robust methods for measuring the arterial input function are essential. Currently, these methods are emerging but are still not widely available.[61]

Currently, there are no FDA-approved DCE MR imaging postprocessing software packages available. Every institution is using its own developed software for analyzing these large datasets. Some companies are developing these packages for data evaluation; however, too little data are available for discussion. Furthermore, quantitative evaluation of the kinetic parameters has not been performed. There are no thresholds available, like in MR spectroscopy, for differentiation between benign and malignant tissue. This is probably caused by the interpatient variability (variable vascular anatomy, atherosclerosis, cardiac output). Almost all imaging data in literature are evaluated based on qualitative assessment rather than quantitative thresholds.

Functional dynamic imaging parameters are estimated as follows: each MR imaging signal enhancement–time curve is first fitted to a general exponential signal intensity model. Consequently, the curve is reduced to a model with five parameters (t_0, time-to-peak, peak enhancement, and washin-washout gradient or plateau). The reduced signal enhancement–time curve is converted to a reduced tracer concentration–time curve (with the tracer concentration in millimoles per milliliter) such that peak enhancement is effectively converted to gadolinium concentration. In the authors' institution, the reduced plasma concentration–time curve is estimated by using a reference tissue method. Deconvolution of the plasma profile and estimation of the pharmacokinetic parameters conformed to the theoretic derivations but are implemented in the reduced signal space as $K^{trans} = V_e \cdot k_{ep}$, where V_e is an estimate of the extracellular volume (expressed as a percentage); K^{trans} is the volume transfer constant (1 per minute); and k_{ep} is the rate constant (1 per minute) between the extracellular extravascular space and the plasma space.

Clinical Application of Dynamic Contrast-Enhanced MR Imaging for Prostate Carcinoma

A fair number of studies have been performed to assess the value of DCE MR imaging in prostate cancer. Hara and colleagues[62] showed that DCE MR imaging was able to detect clinically important prostate cancer in 93% of the cases, with transrectal ultrasound–guided biopsy as the gold standard. In patients with at least two negative transrectal ultrasound–guided biopsy sessions and rising prostate-specific antigen level, MR imaging plays an important role.[63]

DCE MR imaging is of importance in localization and staging of prostate carcinoma, (**Fig. 2**); several studies have found that DCE MR imaging is superior to T2-weighted MR imaging for prostate cancer localization. The authors' group showed in a recent study that the area under the receiver operating curve for localizing prostate cancer increased significantly from 0.68 with T2-weighted imaging to 0.91 when adding DCE MR imaging.[26] DCE MR imaging is less accurate in the localization of tumor within the central gland, whereas peripheral zone localization is markedly improved. Although the literature is sparse on the additional value of DCE MR imaging in local staging, such imaging does seem to improve local staging performance. With the use of DCE MR imaging the staging performance of the less experienced showed a significant improvement of the area under the receiver-operating curve compared with T2-weighted imaging alone (0.66 and 0.82, respectively; $P = .01$).[48]

The application of DCE MR imaging for detection of local recurrence after radical prostatectomy or radiation therapy is increasingly being used. Haider and colleagues[64] found that DCE MR imaging performs better than T2-weighted imaging for the detection and localization of prostate cancer in the peripheral zone after external beam radiotherapy. DCE MR imaging had significantly better sensitivity (72% versus 38%), positive predictive value (46% versus 24%), and negative predictive value (95% versus 88%) compared with T2-weighted imaging. Sciarra and colleagues[65] reported the use of DCE MR imaging and MR spectroscopic imaging for the detection of local recurrence in patients postprostatectomy, and they concluded that the combination of these techniques is accurate for identification of local prostate cancer recurrence with biochemical failure (87% sensitivity and 94% specificity). This information could be helpful in the planning of salvage therapy.

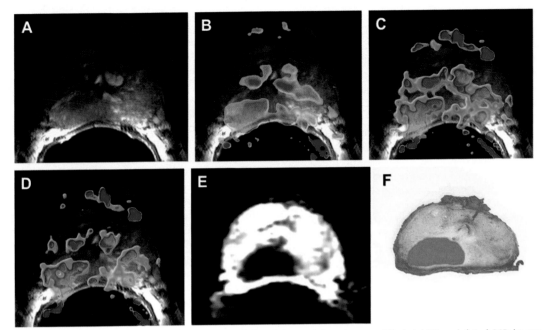

Fig. 2. A 68-year-old man with prostate cancer of the right peripheral zone. (*A*) Axial T2-weighted MR image shows a low signal intensity area in the right peripheral zone. Color parametric maps were calculated (*B*) and demonstrated increased washout in the right peripheral zone, (*C* and *D*) increased Ktrans and kep. (*E*) ADC map at the same level as in image A shows reduced ADC compared with the normal peripheral zone. (*F*) Histopathology confirmed these findings and showed a tumor with Gleason Score of 4+3 = 7.

CURRENT RESEARCH AND FOCUSES FOR THE FUTURE IN DIFFUSION-WEIGHTED MR IMAGING AND DYNAMIC CONTRAST-ENHANCED MR IMAGING OF THE PROSTATE

The technical feasibility of DWI and DCE MR imaging techniques for prostate imaging is now well established. Current and future research should focus on the additive values of DWI and DCE MR imaging to conventional and other MR imaging techniques of the prostate.

The performance of prostate DWI and DCE MR imaging is likely to gain from computer-assisted diagnosis.[66] The combination of the quantitative functional data makes these techniques very suitable for computer analysis and prospective malignancy likelihood calculations. It was recently shown in 18 patients imaged at 3 T, that computer-assisted diagnosis software had a good diagnostic accuracy of discriminating normal from malignant prostate tissue with an area (Az) under the receiver-operating curve of 0.77 for DWI alone. For differentiation between prostate cancer and normal peripheral zone the Az reached 0.89, whereas for differentiation from normal central gland the Az was limited to 0.64. This is in concordance with other reports.[13,14,30,32] Computer-assisted diagnosis seems to perform at least at a comparable level as conventional ADC mapping.

The strength of DWI and DCE MR imaging might be in its potential to characterize tumors and possibly predict tumor behavior, making it a valuable tool in selecting patients for different therapies or active surveillance.

SUMMARY

DWI is an advanced MR imaging technique that still needs to be clinically validated in addition to the more commonly used anatomic MR imaging sequences, such as high-resolution T2-weighted imaging. With the increasing availability of 3-T systems, and with the concomitant use of an endorectal coil, the quality of prostate DWI will further improve and this will likely increase its clinical usefulness.

DCE MR imaging of the prostate is increasingly recognized as a potential tool for imaging of prostate cancer, helping prostate cancer localization, and improving local staging performance for less experienced readers. This technique should always be used in conjunction with T2-weighted imaging. Differentiation of prostatitis and BPH from prostate cancer is inadequate with current anatomic MR imaging techniques. The combination of T2-weighted imaging, DWI, and DCE MR imaging (multimodality MR imaging) may overcome these limitations and may be able accurately to detect, localize, stage, and grade prostate carcinoma. In addition to these techniques MR spectroscopic imaging also is important to mention, and is discussed elsewhere in this issue.

ACKNOWLEDGMENTS

The authors thank Christina Hulsbergen–van der Kaa, MD, PhD, for sharing her experience on histopathologic assessment of the prostate.

REFERENCES

1. Crank J. The mathematics of diffusion. New York: Oxford University Press; 1956.
2. Stejskal EO, Tanner JE. Spin diffusion measurements: spin echoes in the presence of a time-dependent field–gradient. J Chem Phys 1965;42:288–92.
3. Basser PJ, Mattiello J, LeBihan D. Estimation of the effective self-diffusion tensor from the NMR spin echo. J Magn Reson 1994;103:247–54.
4. Bammer R, Skare S, Newbould R, et al. Foundations of advanced magnetic resonance imaging. NeuroRx 2005;2:167–95.
5. Basser PJ. Inferring microstructural features and the physiological state of tissues from diffusion-weighted images. NMR Biomed 1995;8:333–44.
6. Westin CF, Maier SE, Mamata H, et al. Processing and visualization for diffusion tensor MRI. Med Image Anal 2002;6:93–108.
7. Bammer R. Basic principles of diffusion-weighted imaging. Eur J Radiol 2003;45:169–84.
8. Schaefer PW, Copen WA, Lev MH, et al. Diffusion-weighted imaging in acute stroke. Magn Reson Imaging Clin N Am 2006;14:141–68.
9. Moseley ME, Butts K, Yenari MA, et al. Clinical aspects of DWI. NMR Biomed 1995;8:387–96.
10. Moseley ME, Kucharczyk J, Mintorovitch J, et al. Diffusion-weighted MR imaging of acute stroke: correlation with T2-weighted imaging and magnetic susceptibility-enhanced MR imaging in cats. AJNR Am J Neuroradiol 1990;11:423–9.
11. Lansberg MG, Norbash AM, Marks MP, et al. Advantages of adding diffusion-weighted magnetic resonance imaging to conventional magnetic resonance imaging for evaluating acute stroke. Arch Neurol 2000;57:1311–6.
12. Anderson AW, Xie J, Pizzonia J, et al. Effects of cell volume fraction changes on apparent diffusion in human cells. Magn Reson Imaging 2000;18:689–95.
13. Kumar V, Jagannathan NR, Kumar R, et al. Apparent diffusion coefficient of the prostate in men prior to biopsy: determination of a cut-off value to predict malignancy of the peripheral zone. NMR Biomed 2007;20:505–11.
14. Kim CK, Park BK, Lee HM, et al. Value of diffusion-weighted imaging for the prediction of prostate cancer location at 3T using a phased-array coil: preliminary results. Invest Radiol 2007;42:842–7.
15. Tamada T, Sone T, Toshimutsu S, et al. Age-related and zonal anatomical changes of apparent diffusion coefficient values in normal human prostatic tissues. J Magn Reson Imaging 2008;27:552–6.
16. Hricak H, Dooms GC, McNeal JE, et al. MR imaging of the prostate gland: normal anatomy. AJR Am J Roentgenol 1987;148:51–8.
17. Allen KS, Kressel HY, Arger PH, et al. Age-related changes of the prostate: evaluation by MR imaging. AJR Am J Roentgenol 1989;152:77–81.
18. Ren J, Huan Y, Wang H, et al. Diffusion-weighted imaging in normal prostate and differential diagnosis of prostate diseases. Abdom Imaging 2008 [Epub ahead of print].
19. Song SK, Qu Z, Garabedian EM, et al. Improved magnetic resonance imaging detection of prostate cancer in a transgenic mouse model. Cancer Res 2002;62:1555–8.
20. Manenti G, Carlani M, Mancino S, et al. Diffusion tensor magnetic resonance imaging of prostate cancer. Invest Radiol 2007;42:412–9.
21. Gibbs P, Pickles MD, Turnbull LW. Diffusion imaging of the prostate at 3.0 Tesla. Invest Radiol 2006;41:185–8.
22. White S, Hricak H, Forstner R, et al. Prostate cancer: effect of postbiopsy hemorrhage on interpretation of MR images. Radiology 1995;195:385–90.
23. Rajesh A, Coakley FV. MR imaging and MR spectroscopic imaging of prostate cancer. Magn Reson Imaging Clin N Am 2004;12:557–79.
24. Fütterer JJ, Heijmink SW, Spermon JR. Imaging the male reproductive tract: current trends and future directions. Radiol Clin North Am 2008;46:133–47.
25. Haider MA, van der Kwast TH, Tanguay J, et al. Combined T2-weighted and diffusion-weighted MRI for localization of prostate cancer. AJR Am J Roentgenol 2007;189:323–8.
26. Fütterer JJ, Heijmink SW, Scheenen TW, et al. Prostate cancer localization with dynamic contrast-enhanced MR imaging and proton MR spectroscopic imaging. Radiology 2006;241:449–58.
27. Hricak H. MR imaging and MR spectroscopic imaging in the pre-treatment evaluation of prostate cancer. Br J Radiol 2005;78:103–11.
28. Hosseinzadeh K, Schwarz SD. Endorectal diffusion-weighted imaging in prostate cancer to differentiate malignant and benign peripheral zone tissue. J Magn Reson Imaging 2004;20:654–61.
29. Shimofusa R, Fujimoto H, Akamata H, et al. Diffusion-weighted imaging of prostate cancer. J Comput Assist Tomogr 2005;29:149–53.
30. Miao H, Fukatsu H, Ishigaki T. Prostate cancer detection with 3-T MRI: comparison of diffusion-weighted and T2–weighted imaging. Eur J Radiol 2007;61:297–302.

31. Morgan VA, Kyriazi S, Ashley SE, et al. Evaluation of the potential of diffusion-weighted imaging in prostate cancer detection. Acta Radiol 2007;48:695–703.

32. Tanimoto A, Nakashima J, Kohno H, et al. Prostate cancer screening: the clinical value of diffusion-weighted imaging and dynamic MR imaging in combination with T2-weighted imaging. Magn Reson Imaging 2007;25:146–52.

33. Albertsen PC, Hanley JA, Gleason DF, et al. Competing risk analysis of men aged 55 to 74 years at diagnosis managed conservatively for clinically localized prostate cancer. JAMA 1998;280:975–80.

34. Desireddi NV, Roehl KA, Loeb S, et al. Improved stage and grade-specific progression-free survival rates after radical prostatectomy in the PSA era. Urology 2007;70:950–5.

35. Han M, Partin AW, Pound CR, et al. Long–term biochemical disease-free and cancer-specific survival following anatomic radical retropubic prostatectomy. The 15-year Johns Hopkins experience. Urol Clin North Am 2001;28:555–65.

36. Roach M III, Weinberg V, Sandler H, et al. Staging for prostate cancer: time to incorporate pretreatment prostate-specific antigen and Gleason score? Cancer 2007;109:213–20.

37. de Vries SH, Postma R, Raaijmakers R, et al. Overall and disease-specific survival of patients with screen-detected prostate cancer in the European randomized study of screening for prostate cancer, section Rotterdam. Eur Urol 2007;51:366–74.

38. Ruijter ET, Van de Kaa CA, Schalken JA, et al. Histological heterogeneity in multifocal prostate cancer: biological and clinical implications. J Pathol 1996;180:295–9.

39. Noguchi M, Stamey TA, McNeal JE, et al. Relationship between systematic biopsies and histological features of 222 radical prostatectomy specimens: lack of prediction of tumor significance for men with nonpalpable prostate cancer. J Urol 2001;166:104–9.

40. Grossklaus DJ, Coffey CS, Shappel SB, et al. Prediction of tumour volume and pathological stage in radical prostatectomy specimens is not improved by taking more prostate needle-biopsy cores. BJU Int 2001;88:722–6.

41. Wang L, Masaheri Y, Zhang J, et al. Assessment of biological aggressiveness of prostate cancer: correlation of MR signal intensity with Gleason grade after radical prostatectomy. Radiology 2008;246:168–76.

42. Nakanishi K, Kobayashi M, Nakaguchi K, et al. Whole-body MRI for detecting metastatic bone tumor: diagnostic value of diffusion-weighted images. Magn Reson Med Sci 2007;6(3):147–55.

43. Nemeth AJ, Henson JW, Mullins ME, et al. Improved detection of skull metastasis with diffusion-weighted MR imaging. AJNR Am J Neuroradiol 2007;28(6):1088–92.

44. Cornfeld DM, Weinreb JC. MR imaging of the prostate: 1.5T versus 3T. Magn Reson Imaging Clin N Am 2007;15:433–48.

45. Matsuoka A, Minato M, Harada M, et al. Comparison of 3.0- and 1.5-Tesla diffusion-weighted imaging in the visibility of breast cancer. Radiat Med 2008;26:15–20.

46. Heijmink SW, Fütterer JJ, Hambrock T, et al. Prostate cancer: body-array versus endorectal coil MR imaging at 3 T-comparison of image quality, localization, and staging performance. Radiology 2007;244:184–95.

47. Futterer JJ, Engelbrecht MR, Jager GJ, et al. Prostate cancer: comparison of local staging accuracy of pelvic phased-array coil alone versus integrated endorectal-pelvic phased-array coils: local staging accuracy of prostate cancer using endorectal coil MR imaging. Eur Radiol 2007;17:1055–65.

48. Fütterer JJ, Engelbrecht MR, Huisman HJ, et al. Staging prostate cancer with dynamic contrast-enhanced endorectal MR imaging prior to radical prostatectomy: experienced versus less experienced readers. Radiology 2005;237:541–9.

49. Padhani AR, Harvey CJ, Cosgrove DO. Angiogenesis imaging in the management of prostate cancer. Nat Clin Pract Urol 2005;2:596–607.

50. Folkman J. New perspectives in clinical oncology from angiogenesis research. Eur J Cancer 1996;32A:2534–9.

51. Alonzi R, Padhani A, Allen C. Dynamic contrast enhanced MRI in prostate cancer. Eur J Radiol 2007;63:335–50.

52. Carmeliet P, Jain RK. Angiogenesis in cancer and other diseases. Nature 2000;407:249–57.

53. Jackson MW, Bentel JM, Tilley WD. Vascular endothelial growth factor (VEGF) expression in prostate cancer and benign prostatic hyperplasia. J Urol 1997;157:2323–8.

54. Jain RK, Safabakhsh N, Sckell A, et al. Endothelial cell death, angiogenesis, and microvascular function after castration in an androgen-dependent tumor: role of vascular endothelial growth factor. Proc Natl Acad Sci U S A 1998;95:10820–5.

55. Collins DJ, Padhani AR. Dynamic magnetic resonance imaging of tumor perfusion. IEEE Eng Med Biol Mag 2004;23:65–83.

56. d'Arcy JA, Collins DJ, Padhani AR, et al. Informatics in radiology (infoRAD): magnetic resonance imaging workbench: analysis and visualization of dynamic contrast-enhanced MR imaging data. Radiographics 2006;26:621–32.

57. Sorensen AG, Tievsky AL, Ostergaard L, et al. Contrast agents in functional MR imaging. J Magn Reson Imaging 1997;7:47–55.

58. Barbier EL, Lamalle L, Decorps M. Methodology of brain perfusion imaging. J Magn Reson Imaging 2001;13:496–520.

59. Huisman HJ, Engelbrecht MR, Barentsz JO. Accurate estimation of pharmacokinetic contrast-enhanced dynamic MRI parameters of the prostate. J Magn Reson Imaging 2001;13:607–14.

60. Tofts PS, Brix G, Buckley DL, et al. Estimating kinetic parameters from dynamic contrast-enhanced T(1)-weighted MRI of a diffusable tracer: standardized quantities and symbols. J Magn Reson Imaging 1999;10:223–32.

61. Rijpkema M, Kaanders JH, Joosten FB, et al. Method for quantitative mapping of dynamic MRI contrast agent uptake in human tumors. J Magn Reson Imaging 2001;14:457–63.

62. Hara N, Okuizumi M, Koike H, et al. Dynamic contrast-enhanced MR imaging (DCE–MRI) is a useful modality for the precise detection and staging of early prostate cancer. Prostate 2005;62:140–7.

63. Beyersdorff D, Taupitz M, Winkelmann B, et al. Patients with a history of elevated prostate-specific antigen levels and negative transrectal US-guided quadrant or sextant biopsy results: value of MR imaging. Radiology 2002;224:701–6.

64. Haider MA, Chung P, Sweet J, et al. Dynamic contrast-enhanced magnetic resonance imaging for localization of recurrent prostate cancer after external beam radiotherapy. Int J Radiat Oncol Biol Phys 2008;70:425–30.

65. Sciarra A, Panebianco V, Di Silverio F, et al. Role of dynamic contrast-enhanced magnetic resonance (MR) imaging and proton MR spectroscopic imaging in the detection of local recurrence after radical prostatectomy for prostate cancer. Eur Urol 2008; 54(3):485–8.

66. Puech P, Betrouni N, Viard R, et al. Prostate cancer computer-assisted diagnosis software using dynamic contrast-enhanced MRI. Conf Proc IEEE Eng Med Biol Soc 2007;2007:5567–70.

Advances in MR Spectroscopy of the Prostate

John Kurhanewicz, PhD[a],*, Daniel B. Vigneron, PhD[b]

KEYWORDS

- Prostate cancer
- [1]H Magnetic resonance spectroscopic imaging (MRSI)
- Hyperpolarized ^{13}C MRSI • Citrate • Choline • Polyamines

Whereas MR imaging traces anatomy, ^{1}H magnetic resonance spectroscopic imaging (MRSI) is used to spatially detect deviations from normal biochemistry that occur in tumor tissue. Specifically, MR anatomic images, especially high spatial resolution combined endorectal coil pelvic phased array MR images, provide an excellent depiction of prostatic anatomy with regions of healthy prostate tissue demonstrating higher signal intensity than prostate cancer on T2-weighted images.[1] MRSI provides a noninvasive method of detecting small molecular biomarkers (choline-containing metabolites, polyamines and citrate) within the cytosol and extracellular spaces of the prostate and is performed in conjunction with high-resolution anatomic imaging (MR imaging) (**Fig. 1**).[2]

The robust acquisition of prostate MRSI requires very accurate volume selection and efficient outer volume suppression.[3–5] The resonances for citrate, choline, creatine, and polyamines occur at distinct frequencies or positions in the spectrum, although the peaks for choline, creatine, and polyamines overlap at 1.5 T (see **Fig. 1**C, D). The areas under these signals are related to the concentration of the respective metabolites, and changes in these concentrations can be used to identify cancer with good specificity.[6,7] Specifically, in spectra taken from regions of prostate cancer (see **Fig. 1**D), citrate and polyamines are significantly reduced or absent, while choline is elevated relative to spectra taken from surrounding healthy peripheral zone tissue (see **Fig. 1**C).

Commercial combined 1.5-T MR imaging/MRSI exams are currently available and a growing amount of published data has demonstrated that the metabolic biomarkers, choline, citrate, and polyamines, provided by three-dimensional (3-D) ^{1}H MRSI combined with the anatomic information provided by MR imaging can significantly improve the detection and characterization of prostate cancer in individual patients (see **Fig. 1**).[8,9] Recent patient studies have also demonstrated that the detection and characterization of prostate cancer can be improved through the addition of more sensitive spectroscopic imaging techniques (hyperpolarized ^{13}C MRSI),[10] diffusion-weighted imaging (DWI), dynamic contrast enhanced (DCE) imaging, and by performing the multiparametric imaging examination at 3 T.[9] In this article, the current status and recent advances in MR imaging/MRSI of prostate cancer will be described.

UNIQUE METABOLISM OF THE PROSTATE

The metabolic changes observed by ^{1}H MRSI take advantage of the well-documented unique metabolism of healthy prostate epithelial cells that have the specialized function of synthesizing and

Grant sponsors: National Institutes of Health: R01 CA102751; R01 CA111291, R01 EB007588, R01CA059897, R21 EB005363, and R01 CA079980; University of California Discovery Grant: ITL-BIO04-10148.

[a] University of California, San Francisco, Byers Hall, Room 102, 1700 4th Street, Box 2520, San Francisco, CA 94158, USA

[b] University of California, San Francisco, Byers Hall, Room 203E, 1700 4th Street, Box 2520, San Francisco, CA 94158, USA

* Corresponding author.

E-mail address: john.kurhanewicz@radiology.ucsf.edu (J. Kurhanewicz).

Magn Reson Imaging Clin N Am 16 (2008) 697–710

doi:10.1016/j.mric.2008.07.005

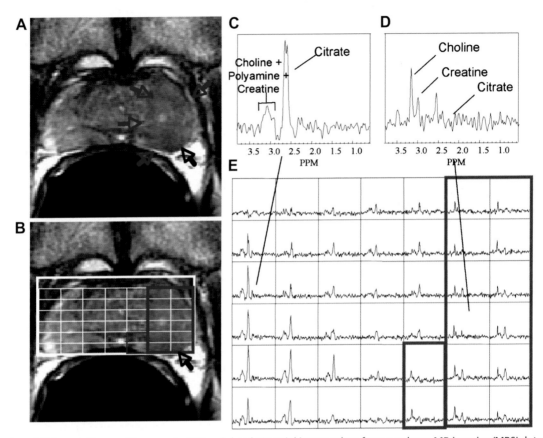

Fig. 1. (*A*) A reception-profile–corrected T2-weighted FSE axial image taken from a volume MR imaging/MRSI data set demonstrating a large region of hypointensity in the left midgland (*red arrows*) with suspected extracapsular extension (*black arrow*). The selected volume for spectroscopy (*bold white box*) and a portion of the 16 × 8 × 8 spectral phase encode grid overlaid (*fine white line*) on the T2-weighted image (*B*) with the corresponding 0.3 cm³ proton spectral array (*E*). Spectra in regions of cancer (*D*, and *red box* in *E*) demonstrate dramatically elevated choline and an absence of citrate and polyamines relative to regions of healthy peripheral zone tissue (*C*). In this fashion, metabolic abnormalities can be correlated with anatomic abnormalities from throughout the prostate. The strength of the combined MR imaging/MRSI examination has been found to be when changes in all three metabolic markers (choline, polyamines, and citrate) and imaging findings are concordant for cancer.

secreting large amounts of citrate, which is dramatically reduced or lost in prostate cancer.[11–14] The decrease in citrate with prostate cancer is because of changes in cellular function[15] and changes in the organization of the tissue, resulting in a loss of its characteristic ductal morphology.[16,17] The loss of citrate in prostate cancer is intimately linked with changes in zinc levels that are extraordinarily high in healthy prostate epithelial cells.[13,18] In healthy prostatic epithelial cells, the presence of high levels of zinc inhibit the enzyme aconitase, thereby preventing the oxidation of citrate in the Krebs cycle.[13,18] Costello and Franklin[13,14] have shown that these elevated levels of zinc are primarily because of increased expression of ZIP-type plasma membrane Zn uptake transporters (primarily Human ZIP-1). Human ZIP-1 is reduced and zinc levels are dramatically

reduced in prostate cancer and the malignant epithelial cells; there exists evidence that the loss of the capability to retain high levels of zinc is an important factor in the development and progression of prostate cancer.[13,18] It is also believed that the transformation of prostate epithelial cells to citrate-oxidizing cells, which increases energy production capability, is essential to the process of malignancy and metastasis.[12]

The elevation of choline-containing metabolites (phosphocholine [PC], glycerophosphocholine [GPC], free choline [Cho]) and the over and under-expression of key enzymes in phospholipid membrane synthesis and degradation, specifically choline kinase and a number of the phospholipases, has been associated with the presence, progression, and therapeutic response of a variety of human cancers including prostate.[8,19–21]

Specifically, high-resolution magic angle spinning (HR-MAS) spectroscopic studies of ex vivo surgical prostate tissues demonstrated elevated levels of ethanolamine- and choline-containing compounds and that elevated PC was the most robust predictor of prostate cancer.[22] In ^{1}H MRSI studies of prostate cancer patients, the elevation of the in vivo "choline" resonance has also been the most specific biomarker of prostate cancer presence,[8] and both in vivo and ex vivo spectroscopic studies have shown that the degree of elevation of choline roughly correlates with Gleason score.[8]

Healthy prostate epithelial cells also contain very high concentrations of polyamines, particularly spermine.[8,23,24] Similar to citrate, polyamines are dramatically reduced in prostate cancer and this reduction is associated with significant changes in the levels of expression of polyamine metabolism regulatory genes.[8,23] Ornithine decarboxylase catalyzes the first step of spermine synthesis, and has been found to be overexpressed in prostate cancer.[23] The polyamines spermidine and spermine have been implicated or involved in a wide variety of physiologic processes, most of which are closely related to cell proliferation.[25] The polyamines also exert diverse effects on protein synthesis and act as inhibitors of numerous enzymes including several kinases.[25] However, similar to citrate, high levels of spermine are found in the prostatic ducts and the observed changes in spermine may also be a result of the loss of ductal morphology or a reduction in the secretion of polyamines in cancer.[26]

CLINICAL APPLICATIONS OF 1.5-T MR IMAGING/MR SPECTROSCOPIC IMAGING
Detection and Localization of Cancer Within the Prostate

In clinical practice, reliable detection and localization of often small regions of prostate cancer is of increasing therapeutic importance owing to the emergence of "active surveillance" and focal ablative therapy.[27] In addition, tumor localization has been related to the risk of postprostatectomy tumor recurrence, with a higher risk when surgical margins are positive at the base than at the apex.[6] It has been demonstrated in multiple studies that MRSI can be used to improve the ability of MR imaging to identify the location and extent of cancer within the prostate (see **Fig. 1**).[6,7,28–31] A study of 53 biopsy-proven prostate cancer patients before radical prostatectomy and step-section pathologic examination demonstrated a significant improvement in cancer localization to a sextant biopsy of the prostate (left and right—base, midgland, and apex) of the prostate using combined MR imaging/MRSI versus MR imaging alone. A combined positive result from both MR imaging and MRSI indicated the presence of tumor with high specificity (91%) while high sensitivity (95%) was attained when either test alone indicated the presence of cancer.[7] In another study it was found that the addition of a positive sextant biopsy finding to concordant MR imaging/MRSI findings further increased the specificity (98%) of cancer localization to a prostatic sextant, whereas high sensitivity (94%) was again obtained when any of the tests alone were positive for cancer.[6] However, more recent studies in early-stage prostate cancer patients have indicated that combined 1.5 MR imaging/MRSI does poorly at detecting and localizing small low-grade tumors.[28,31,32] One recent study demonstrated that overall sensitivity of MR spectroscopic imaging was 56% for tumor detection, increasing from 44% in lesions with Gleason score of 3 + 3 to 89% in lesions with Gleason score greater than or equal to 4 + 4.[32] The inability to detect small low-grade tumors by 1.5-T MRSI is primarily because of averaging of surrounding benign tissue in spectroscopic volumes containing cancer, owing to the spatial resolution of 1.5-T MRSI (0.34 mL, $\approx$ 7 mm on a side). In a recent multicenter trial of prostate MR imaging/MRSI (ACRIN 6659), the clinical downstaging (smaller lower grade disease) of prostate cancer in patients going on for surgery had a significant impact on the sensitivity and specificity of tumor detection. Complete data were available for 110 patients. MR imaging alone and combined MR imaging/MRSI were of similar poor accuracy in peripheral zone tumor localization (area under the curve [AUC] of 0.60 versus 0.58, respectively, $P > .05$).[33] At 3 T, spatial resolution of MRSI can be increased approximately twofold (0.16 mL, $\approx$ 5 mm on a side) in the same acquisition time (**Fig. 2**), and this will be clearly needed for the imaging of men with early-stage, small-volume (< 0.5 mL) prostate cancer. Another study demonstrated that DCE MR imaging can detect and determine the volume of smaller foci of prostate cancer with greater overall accuracy than MR imaging/MRSI. Sensitivity, specificity, and positive and negative predictive values for cancer detection by DCE MR imaging were 77%, 91%, 86%, and 85% for foci greater than 0.2 mL, and 90%, 88%, 77%, and 95% for foci greater than 0.5 mL, respectively.[34]

Tumor Volume Estimation

The pathologic finding that larger tumors are more likely to be of an advanced stage suggests measurement of tumor volume may provide important

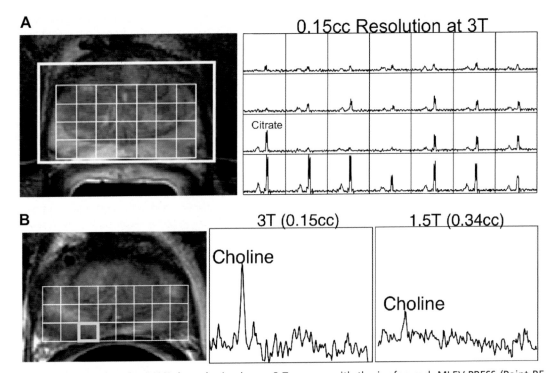

Fig. 2. Prostate MR imaging/MRSI data obtained on a 3-T scanner with the j-refocused, MLEV-PRESS (Point RE-Solved Spectroscopy) MRSI sequence (101). (*A*) T2-weighted MR imaging and a 3D MR spectral array are shown for a pretherapy patient. The 3D MRSI data were acquired in 17 minutes with a spatial resolution of 0.15 cm³ using the specialized acquisition sequence to obtain upright citrate resonances at an echo time of 85 ms on a 3-T MR scanner. (*B*) 3-T MR imaging and MRSI data are shown for the same prostate cancer patient with biopsy proven cancer in the right midgland. The higher resolution obtainable at 3-T MRSI (*middle*) depicted more clearly the elevated choline levels as compared with the corresponding 1.5-T data (*right*) acquired on the same day.

information on prognosis that is independent of direct morphologic assessment of extracapsular extension.[35] This has important implications for the potential prognostic role of imaging in prostate cancer, since: "it is beyond the capability of any current imaging study to detect microscopic local tumor extension."[36] Two recent studies suggest that MR imaging/MRSI and DCE MR imaging may noninvasively provide estimates of cancer volume at diagnosis. One study investigated the estimation of prostate cancer tumor volume by endorectal MR imaging and MRSI in 37 patients who were scanned before radical prostatec-tomy.[31] This study demonstrated that for nodules greater than 0.5 cm³, tumor volume measurements by MR imaging, MRSI, and combined MR imaging and MRSI were all positively correlated with histopathologic volume (Pearson's correlation coefficients of 0.49, 0.59, and 0.55, respectively), but only measurements by MRSI and combined MR imaging/MRSI reached statistical significance ($P < .05$). The findings also suggested that the addition of MRSI to MR imaging increased the overall accuracy of prostate cancer tumor volume

measurement, although measurement variability still limited consistent quantitative tumor volume estimation, particularly for small tumors (under 0.5 cm³).

Detection of High-grade Prostate Cancer

The histology of prostate cancer is variable, ranging from well (Gleason score $\leq 3 + 4$) to poorly differentiated (Gleason score 4/3, 8, 9, 10).[37] The evaluation of the dominant histologic pattern is important, because poorly differentiated tumors are more aggressive, and are predictive of cancer stage. Specifically, in a study of 113 patients undergoing radical prostatectomy,[38] 63% of patients with a Gleason score of 6 or less had organ-confined disease, compared with 33% of patients with a Gleason score of 7% and 0% of patients with a Gleason score of 8. Limitations of the Gleason score are clustering of assigned values to 6 and 7, and high interobserver variability.[39] MRSI may be able to provide an noninvasive assessment of cancer grade for all of the cancer foci within the prostate, potentially with reduced interobserver variability and grade clustering. Early biochemical studies have indicated that citrate levels in prostatic adenocarcinomas are grade dependent, with citrate levels being low in well-differentiated, low-grade prostatic cancer and effectively absent in poorly differentiated high-grade prostatic cancer.[40,41] More recent proton HR-MAS spectroscopy studies of intact human prostate tissues have demonstrated a significant, grade-dependent elevation of choline and ethanolamine containing phospholipid membrane metabolites in prostate cancer.[19,20] In an MR imaging/MRSI study of 32 patients before surgery, there was a statistically significant relationship between the choline and creatine to citrate ratio and Gleason score.[42] However, these results were obtained for lesions that were identified on pathology and that also had a concordant MR imaging finding of low T2 signal intensity. In a study of 123 patients, where this approach was not taken, there was only a trend in the choline + creatine/citrate ratio with Gleason score. In clinical practice, the pathologic location of the lesion is not known and MRSI voxels contain a complex mixture of malignant and benign tissue types that reduce its ability to determine cancer grade.[32] This can be improved with the improved spectral resolution obtainable on 3-T MRSI.

Predicting Organ-confined (No Extracapsular Extension or Seminal Vesicle Invasion) Prostate Cancer

A more accurate prediction of organ-confined prostate cancer at the time of diagnosis would allow the determination of whether "focal therapy" is appropriate for a given patient. The use of T2-weighted fast spin echo imaging and a pelvic phased-array incorporating an endorectal coil can markedly improved the evaluation of extracapsular extension (ECE; accuracy = 81%, sensitivity = 84%, and specificity = 80%) and seminal vesicle invasion (SVI; accuracy = 96%, sensitivity = 83%, and specificity = 98%), thereby improving the staging of prostatic cancer.[43] However, the detection of ECE and SVI by MR imaging is becoming more difficult because men are being diagnosed at earlier stages of disease, and because the microscopic spread of cancer through the prostatic capsule or into the seminal vesicles cannot be directly seen on MR imaging. Two studies have suggested that the addition of MRSI to MR imaging data can improve prostate cancer staging. In one study of 53 patients with early-stage prostate cancer, tumor volume estimates based on MRSI findings were combined with MR imaging criteria[44] to assess the ability of combined MR imaging/MRSI to predict extracapsular cancer spread. It was found that tumor volume per lobe estimated by MRSI was significantly ($P < .01$) higher in patients with ECE than in patients without ECE. Moreover, the addition of an MRSI estimate of tumor volume to MR imaging findings for ECE[43] improved the diagnostic accuracy and decreased the interobserver variability of MR imaging in the diagnosis of extracapsular extension of prostate cancer.[44]

Adding MR Imaging/MR Spectroscopic Imaging to Clinical Nomograms

An important advance in the staging of prostate cancer has been the development of multivariable risk prediction instruments such as the Partin tables[45] and nomograms, which combine clinical stage, serum prostate specific antigen (PSA) levels, and grade of biopsy results to predict at the time of diagnosis the pathologic stage of the cancer and indolent disease, respectively.[46,47] Recent studies have demonstrated that addition of 1.5-T MR imaging/MRSI findings can to significantly improve the predictive ability of these nomograms. In a study of 24 prostate cancer patients before radical prostatectomy, the addition of endorectal MR imaging results contributed significant incremental value to the biopsy-based nomograms for predicting SVI.[48] It was found that the nomogram plus endorectal MR imaging (0.87) had a significantly larger ($P < .05$) AUC than either endorectal MR imaging alone (0.76) or the nomogram alone (0.80).[48] In another study of 383 prostate cancer patients before radical prostatectomy, 1.5-T MR imaging/MRSI data were added to a biopsy-based staging nomogram for predicting organ-confined prostate cancer (OCPC, no ECE or SVI) to assess its incremental value. The increase in predictive accuracy provided by the addition of 1.5-T MR/MRSI findings were significant in all patient risk groups but were greatest in the intermediate- and high-risk groups ($P < .01$ for both).[49]

Predicting Indolent Disease

Because of increased screening using serum PSA and extended-template transrectal ultrasound (TRUS)-guided biopsies, thousands of patients with prostate cancer are being identified at an earlier and potentially more treatable stage.[50] However, the risk of overdetection, detecting a cancer that would not become clinically significant during that patient's lifetime if left untreated, has been estimated to vary between 15% and 84%.[51–53] Therefore, there is an increased interest in "active surveillance," but clinical parameters alone are not sufficient to predict a benign disease course. A recent study suggests that the addition of MR imaging/MRSI data to clinical parameters can improve this prediction. In a study of 220 patients before surgery, the addition of MR imaging (AUC 0.803) and 1.5-T MR imaging/MRSI (AUC 0.854) to biopsy-based nomograms (basic AUC 0.57, comprehensive 0.73) was found to significantly improve the prediction of indolent prostate cancer using a surgical definition of indolent disease (no SVI, ECE and <0.5 cm³ of cancer with no pattern 4 or 5 cancer) as the standard of reference.

Cancer Detection in Men with Prior Negative Biopsies

Another important group of patients being referred for an MR imaging/MRSI examination before therapy is composed of men who have elevated or rising PSA levels but negative TRUS-guided biopsies. These patients tend to have very enlarged central glands as a result of benign prostatic hyperplasia (BPH), which present sampling problems for TRUS-guided biopsies, or they have cancers in difficult locations to biopsy such as the apex or in the lateral or anterior locations within the prostate.[54] A recent publication has demonstrated that MR imaging/MRSI can improve the identification of regions of cancer for targeting of TRUS-guided biopsies in patients with prior negative TRUS biopsy.[55,56]

Therapeutic Selection and Planning

Several possible roles for MR imaging and MRSI have been suggested in radiation treatment planning. Staging by MR imaging/MRSI at diagnosis has been found to be of incremental prognostic significance in patients with moderate and high-risk tumors going on for radiation therapy.[57] Specifically, the finding of more than 5 mm of extracapsular extension before radiation seems to be of particular negative prognostic significance, and the latter group may be candidates for more aggressive supplemental therapy.[57] For the patient in **Fig. 3**, the MR imaging/MRSI findings were concordant, indicating a large volume of T2 hypointensity (see **Fig. 1A**, *red arrows*) and associated abnormal spectroscopic voxels (significantly elevated choline and reduced polyamine and citrate (**Fig. 3A**, *red arrows*)) bilaterally at the midgland and apex of the prostate. Additionally, there was a mild bulge of the prostate and irregularity of the prostatic capsule in the left midgland, indicative of extracapsular extension. However, there was no evidence of seminal vesicle invasion or pelvic lymphadenopathy within the pelvis.

Based on these findings, it was clear that aggressive therapy would be necessary. The patient subsequently underwent high-dose rate brachytherapy combined with 22 sessions of external beam radiation therapy, and neoadjuvant androgen-deprivation therapy.

Using fiducial markers and image fusion software, it has been shown that CT overestimates the clinical target volume by 34% when compared with MR imaging,[58] and that dose-volume planning with MR imaging would decrease radiation dose to the bladder, rectum, and femoral heads. This result is hardly unexpected, given the limited soft tissue contrast of CT in the prostate and perineum, particularly when CT is performed without intravenous contrast enhancement, as is the usual protocol for radiation planning CT scans. Several recent research studies have directly integrated MR imaging/MRSI data into the radiation treatment plan to optimize radiation dose selectively to regions of prostate cancer using either intensity modulated radiotherapy (IMRT)[59–61] or brachytherapy[62–65]; however, this is not being done in routine clinical practice.

MR Imaging and MRSI in Posttreatment Follow-up

A growing number of patients receiving a MR imaging/MRSI are referred for suspected local cancer recurrence after various therapies (hormonal deprivation therapy, radiation therapy, cryosurgery, and radical prostatectomy). Recurrent cancer is typically suspected in these patients because of a detectable or rising PSA. However, the use of PSA testing to monitor therapeutic efficacy is not ideal since PSA is not specific for prostate cancer, and it can take 2 years or more for PSA levels to reach a nadir following radiation therapy (both external beam and brachytherapy).[66,67] Further, the interpretation of PSA data is more complicated for patients undergoing therapies such as hormone deprivation therapy that have a direct effect on the production of PSA. Conventional imaging methods, including TRUS, CT, and MR imaging, often cannot distinguish healthy from malignant tissue following therapy because of therapy-induced changes in tissue structure.[68,69] The only definitive way to determine if residual or recurrent tissue is malignant is the histologic analysis of random biopsies, which are subject to sampling errors and are more difficult to pathologically interpret after therapy.

The spectroscopic criteria used to identify residual/recurrent prostate cancer needs to be adjusted because of a time-dependent loss of prostate metabolites following therapy. For

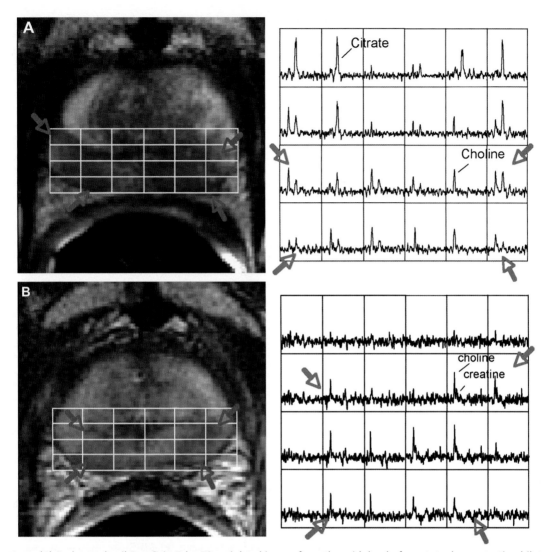

Fig. 3. (*A*) Endorectal coil Fast Spin Echo T2-weighted image from the midgland of prostate demonstrating bilateral low signal intensity (*red arrows*) in the regions of biopsy-proven prostate cancer. The overlying white grid shows the locations where the MRSI spectra are taken from (*right*). Regions of prostate cancer (*red arrow*) demonstrate elevated choline and reduced citrate relative to regions of healthy tissue. (*B*) A T2-weighted image and corresponding spectral array taken from the same location as in (*A*) 4 years after combined radiation and androgen deprivation therapy. There are a number of voxels demonstrating metabolic atrophy consistent with effective treatment; however, there remain bilateral regions of elevated choline that were confirmed to be recurrent prostate cancer at biopsy.

example, prostatic citrate production and secretion have been shown to be regulated by hormones,[15] and an early dramatic reduction of citrate and polyamines after initiation of complete hormonal blockade has been observed by MRSI.[70] There was slower loss of choline and creatine with increasing duration of hormone deprivation therapy.[70] This loss of prostatic metabolites correlates with the presence of tissue atrophy and is considered to be an indicator of effective therapy.[70] Similar time-dependent

reductions in prostate metabolites also occurred after radiation therapy.[71,72]

Studies have also demonstrated the ability of MR imaging/MRSI to discriminate residual or recurrent prostate cancer from residual benign tissue and atrophic/necrotic tissue after cryosurgery,[73–75] hormone deprivation therapy,[70,76] and radiation therapy.[71,77] These studies have relied on elevated choline to creatine as a metabolic marker for prostate cancer because polyamines and citrate tend to disappear early after therapy in both residual healthy and malignant tissues. **Fig. 3**B shows the same patient as in 3A, 4 years after therapy. Consistent with effective radiation therapy, there were a number of spectroscopic voxels that demonstrated a complete loss of all prostate metabolites (metabolic atrophy). However, residual metabolic abnormalities (choline to creatine $\geq$ 1.5) persisted bilaterally in the midgland toward the apex and this region was later confirmed as residual cancer by TRUS-guided biopsy. A recent MR imaging/MRSI study of 21 prostate cancer patients with biochemical failure after external-beam radiation therapy demonstrated that the presence of three or more voxels having a choline/creatine of 1.5 or greater in a hemiprostate showed a sensitivity and specificity of 87% and 72%, respectively, for the diagnosis of local cancer recurrence. The detection of residual cancer at an early stage following treatment and the ability to monitor the time course of therapeutic response would allow earlier intervention with additional therapy and provide a more quantitative assessment of therapeutic efficacy.

LIMITATIONS OF MR IMAGING/MRSI

Combined 1.5-T MR imaging/MRSI has recognized limitations, including the potential for false positive and false negative results. The limitations include postbiopsy changes, confounding benign pathologies (prostatitis, BPH), mixing of cancer and healthy tissue with small-volume (<0.5 mL) early-stage cancer, and an insufficient understanding of the histologic and biological basis of false positives and false negatives. Postbiopsy hemorrhage results in both over- and underestimation of tumor extent at MR imaging and MRSI.[78–80] The timing of MR imaging and MRSI of the prostate following transrectal biopsy is therefore important. Early studies have recommended an interval of 3 weeks between transrectal biopsy and MR imaging.[78–80] However, there has been a trend toward increased prostate sampling during transrectal biopsy; and currently more than six core biopsies are frequently obtained.[81] The increase in prostate sampling has raised new questions about the optimal timing of MR imaging and MRSI following transrectal biopsy, and the impact of postbiopsy hemorrhage on interpretation of MR imaging and MRSI. In a recent study of 43 patients with biopsy-proven prostate cancer undergoing endorectal MR imaging and MRSI before radical prostatectomy confirming organ-confined disease, the outcome variables of capsular irregularity and spectral degradation were correlated with the predictor variables of time from biopsy and degree of postbiopsy

hemorrhage.[82] The authors found capsular irregularity was unrelated to time from biopsy or to degree of hemorrhage. Spectral degradation was inversely related to time from biopsy (P < .01); the mean percentage of degraded peripheral zone voxels was 18.5% within 8 weeks of biopsy compared with 7% after 8 weeks. Spectral degradation was unrelated to the degree of hemorrhage. The authors concluded that in organ-confined prostate cancer, capsular irregularity can be seen at any time after biopsy irrespective of the degree of hemorrhage, whereas spectral degradation is seen predominantly in the first 8 weeks. MR staging criteria and guidelines for scheduling studies after biopsy may require appropriate modification.

Only a few studies have investigated the MR imaging and MRSI appearances of acute and chronic prostatitis, but these initial reports suggest that in at least some cases prostatitis may mimic cancer. Engelhard and colleagues[83] found that biopsy-proven prostatitis correlated with areas of low T2 signal intensity at MR imaging. Theoretically, the inflammatory process of prostatitis might be expected to reduce the level of citrate seen at MRSI, although Van Dorsten and colleagues[84] failed to find any difference between healthy peripheral zone spectra and peripheral zone spectra from 12 patients thought to have prostatitis. Further studies with better pathologic correlation are required to elucidate the true spectroscopic findings in prostatitis. Cancers within the central gland (transition zone and central zone) also have proven to be particularly difficult to discriminate on MR imaging/MRSI. There is significant overlap of low signal intensity on T2-weighted images and metabolism on MRSI in regions of central gland tumor with predominately stromal BPH.[85] Regions of predominately glandular BPH have very elevated levels of citrate and polyamines since they are secretory products of healthy and hyperplastic glandular tissues. While in predominately stromal tissues, such as predominately stromal BPH, citrate and polyamine levels are very low similar to what is observed in cancer. Like cancer, there can also be somewhat elevated choline, since there is increased cellular proliferation in BPH as in cancer.

While prostatitis and stromal BPH are the most common benign confounding factors in overcalling prostate cancer by MR imaging/MRSI, prostate cancer can also be undercalled as a result of signals arising from surrounding benign tissues masking the metabolic fingerprint of cancer, particularly for small infiltrative disease. Specifically, benign glandular tissues have very high signal intensity on T2-weighted MR imaging as well as very high levels of polyamines and citrate, and these signals will dominate the prostate spectrum. Predominately mucinogenic prostate cancer is also very difficult to detect on MR imaging/MRSI. On T2-weighted MR imaging they have high signal intensity because of the presence of the pockets of mucin. On MRSI, the spectral signal intensity is often very low because of the low density of prostate cancer cells.

FUTURE DIRECTIONS—HYPERPOLARIZED ^{13}C METABOLIC IMAGING OF THE PROSTATE

Whereas the current commercially available clinical MR imaging/^{1}H MRSI prostate examination relies on changes in choline, citrate, and polyamine metabolism, lactate and alanine have largely been ignored because of the difficulty of suppressing the large signals from periprostatic lipids that overlap lactate and alanine.[86] Significantly higher concentrations of lactate and alanine have been found in prostate cancer biopsies compared with healthy biopsy tissue. High levels of lactate in cancer is consistent with prior studies and has been associated with increased glycolysis and cell membrane biosynthesis.[87,88] ^{18}F-2-deoxy-2-fluoro-D-glucose (FDG) positron emission tomography (PET) studies have shown high rates of glucose uptake in several human cancers and that the glucose uptake correlates directly with the aggressiveness of the disease and inversely with the patient's prognosis.[89,90] The high glucose uptake leads to increased lactate production in most tumors even though some of

them have sufficient oxygen, a condition know as the Warburg Effect[91] or aerobic glycolysis.[87] The increased glycolysis provides the parasitic cancer cells with an energy source that is independent of its oxygen supply, a carbon source for the biosynthesis of cell membranes that begins with lipogenesis,[88] and an acid source that likely enables the cells to invade neighboring tissue.[87] New hyperpolarized ^{13}C spectroscopic imaging techniques[10,92,93] and advances in lipid suppression and spectral edited ^{1}H spectroscopic imaging[5,94] provide the opportunity to observe changes in lactate and alanine in clinical MR imaging/MRSI exams.

^{13}C labeled substrates have recently been polarized using dynamic nuclear polarization (DNP) techniques to obtain tens of thousand-fold enhancement of the ^{13}C nuclear magnetic resonance (NMR) signals from the substrate as well as its metabolic products.[92,95,96] Preliminary DNP studies in rats, rat xenograft tumors, and a transgenic mouse model of prostate cancer (**Fig. 4**) have demonstrated greater than 50,000-fold enhancements in the polarization of [1-^{13}C] pyruvate and its metabolic products, lactate and alanine, providing sufficient MR signal for high spatial and temporal resolution spectroscopic imaging of the metabolites.[10,93,97] Pyruvate is ideal for these studies because the signal from C-1 carbon relaxes very slowly as a result of its long T1 and it is at the entry point to several important energy and biosynthesis pathways. In particular, it is converted to lactate in glycolysis, to alanine for protein synthesis and/or lipogenesis, and to acetyl-CoA

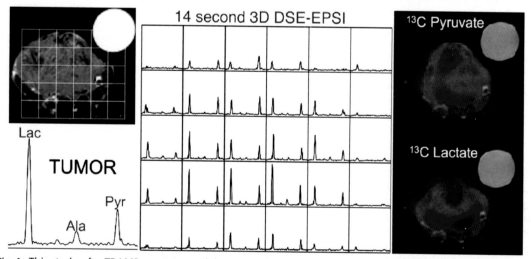

Fig. 4. This study of a TRAMP prostate model tumor using the HyperSense system for pre-polarization demonstrated not only high ^{13}C lactate in the tumor but also differences in metabolite distributions in the tumor. The data were acquired in 14 seconds and show high uptake of hyperpolarized pyruvate throughout much of the tumor, except for a presumably necrotic region at the center. The lactate image demonstrated a focus of high metabolic activity in the posterior aspect of the tumor, which is indicative of biologically aggressive cancer.

and oxaloacetate to support the citric acid cycle and biosynthesis of membrane lipids. Several studies involving preclinical murine models of human prostate cancer have suggested that that hyperpolarized [^{13}C-1] lactate levels measured after the injection of hyperpolarized [^{13}C-1] pyruvate provide a noninvasive way to detect primary and metastatic disease and characterize the aggressiveness (histologic stage) of prostate cancer (see **Fig. 4**).[10,98]

SUMMARY

Commercial MR imaging/MRSI packages for staging prostate cancer on 1.5-T MR scanners are now available and the technology is becoming mature enough to begin assessing its clinical utility in large patient cohort studies using surgical pathology or clinical outcomes as the standard of reference. Before therapy, prostate cancer can be discriminated from benign tissues based on a combination of reduced signal intensity on T2 MR imaging, increased choline and reduced citrate and polyamines on MRSI. After therapy, the loss of all metabolites (metabolic atrophy) has been associated with effective therapy, while residual prostate cancer has been identified based on the presence of three or more voxels having choline/creatine greater than 1.5 with an accuracy of 80%. Recent studies have demonstrated that 1.5-T MR imaging/MRSI has the potential to significantly improve the local evaluation of prostate cancer presence and volume and has been shown to have a significant incremental benefit in the prediction of pathologic stage when added to nomograms incorporating nonimaging preoperative risk factors. Combined 1.5-T MR imaging/MRSI also has recognized limitations, including the potential for false positive and false negative results, particularly for small-volume (< 0.5 mL) early-stage cancer. Recent studies have shown that accuracy can be improved by performing MR imaging/MRSI at higher magnetic field strengths (3 T),[26,99] and through the addition of other functional MR techniques, namely DWI and DCE imaging.[9] There are currently no commercially available 3-T MR imaging/MRSI/DWI/DCE staging examinations but the ability to accomplish this examination on clinical 3-T scanners in a clinical reasonable time has been demonstrated and commercial products should be available within the next couple of years.[9] Hyperpolarized ^{13}C labeled metabolic substrates have shown potential to revolutionize the way we use MR imaging in the risk assessment of prostate cancer patients.[98,100,101] While preclinical hyperpolarized ^{13}C studies have been very encouraging, future studies are necessary to determine the feasibility of adding hyperpolarized ^{13}C spectroscopic imaging to a clinical multiparametric MR staging examination of prostate cancer patients and for determining how all of the metabolic biomarkers can be best combined to provide the most accurate assessment of prostate cancer.

REFERENCES

1. Hricak H, White S, Vigneron D, et al. Carcinoma of the prostate gland: MR imaging with pelvic phased-array coils versus integrated endorectal–pelvic phased-array coils. Radiology 1994;193: 703–9.
2. Kurhanewicz J, Vigneron DB, Hricak H, et al. Three-dimensional H-1 MR spectroscopic imaging of the in situ human prostate with high (0.24–0.7-cm3) spatial resolution. Radiology 1996;198:795–805.
3. Tran TK, VIgneron DB, Sailasuta N, et al. Very selective supression pulses for clinical MRSI studies of brain and prostate cancer. Magn Reson Med 2000;43:23–33.
4. Schricker AA, Pauly JM, Kurhanewicz J, et al. Dual-band spectral-spatial RF pulses for prostate MR spectroscopic imaging. Magn Reson Med 2001; 46:1079–87.
5. Cunningham CH, Vigneron DB, Chen AP, et al. Design of symmetric-sweep spectral-spatial RF pulses for spectral editing. Magn Reson Med 2004;52:147–53.
6. Wefer AE, Hricak H, Vigneron DB, et al. Sextant localization of prostate cancer: comparison of sextant biopsy, magnetic resonance imaging and magnetic resonance spectroscopic imaging with step section histology. J Urol 2000;164:400–4.
7. Scheidler J, Hricak H, Vigneron DB, et al. Prostate cancer: localization with three-dimensional proton MR spectroscopic imaging–clinicopathologic study. Radiology 1999;213:473–80.
8. Kurhanewicz J, Swanson MG, Nelson SJ, et al. Combined magnetic resonance imaging and spectroscopic imaging approach to molecular imaging of prostate cancer. J Magn Reson Imaging 2002; 16:451–63.
9. Kurhanewicz J, Vigneron D, Carroll P, et al. Multiparametric magnetic resonance imaging in prostate cancer: present and future. Curr Opin Urol 2008;18:71–7.
10. Chen AP, Albers MJ, Cunningham CH, et al. Hyperpolarized C-13 spectroscopic imaging of the TRAMP mouse at 3T—initial experience. Magn Reson Med 2007;58:1099–106.
11. Costello LC, Franklin RB. Concepts of citrate production and secretion by prostate. 1. Metabolic relationships. Prostate 1991;18:25–46.
12. Costello LC, Franklin RB. Bioenergetic theory of prostate malignancy. Prostate 1994;25:162–6.

13. Costello LC, Franklin RB. Novel role of zinc in the regulation of prostate citrate metabolism and its implications in prostate cancer. Prostate 1998;35: 285–96.

14. Franklin RB, Ma J, Zou J, et al. Human ZIP1 is a major zinc uptake transporter for the accumulation of zinc in prostate cells. J Inorg Biochem 2003;96: 435–42.

15. Costello LC, Franklin RB. Concepts of citrate production and secretion by prostate: 2. Hormonal relationships in normal and neoplastic prostate. Prostate 1991;19:181–205.

16. Kahn T, Beurrig K, Schmitz-Dreager B, et al. Prostatic carcinoma and benign prostatic hyperplasia: MR imaging with histopathologic correlation. Radiology 1989;173:847–51.

17. Schiebler ML, Tomaszewski JE, Bezzi M, et al. Prostatic carcinoma and benign prostatic hyperplasia: correlation of high-resolution MR and histopathologic findings. Radiology 1989;172:131–7.

18. Liang JY, Liu YY, Zou J, et al. Inhibitory effect of zinc on human prostatic carcinoma cell growth. Prostate 1999;40:200–7.

19. Swanson MG, Vigneron DB, Tabatabai ZL, et al. Proton HR-MAS spectroscopy and quantitative pathologic analysis of MRI/3D-MRSI-targeted postsurgical prostate tissues. Magn Reson Med 2003; 50:944–54.

20. Swanson MG, Zektzer AS, Tabatabai ZL, et al. Quantitative analysis of prostate metabolites using (1)H HR-MAS spectroscopy. Magn Reson Med 2006;55:1257–64.

21. Ackerstaff E, Pflug BR, Nelson JB, et al. Detection of increased choline compounds with proton nuclear magnetic resonance spectroscopy subsequent to malignant transformation of human prostatic epithelial cells. Cancer Res 2001;61: 3599–603.

22. Keshari K, Swanson M, Simko J, et al. "Quantification of choline and ethanolamine containing phospholipids in healthy and malignant prostate tissue". Presented at the Proceedings of the International Society of Magnetic Resonance in Medicine. Berlin, May 19–25, 2007.

23. Saverio B, Pierpaola D, Serenella A, et al. Tumor progression is accompanied by significant changes in the levels of expression of polyamine metabolism regulatory genes and clusterin (sulfated glycoprotein 2) in human prostate cancer specimens. Cancer Res 2000;60:28–34.

24. Swanson MG, Vigneron DB, Tran TK, et al. Single-voxel oversampled J-resolved spectroscopy of in vivo human prostate tissue. Magn Reson Med 2001;45:973–80.

25. Heby O. Role of polyamines in the control of cell proliferation and differentiation. Differentiation 1981;19:1–20.

26. Chen AP, Cunningham CH, Kurhanewicz J, et al. High-resolution 3D MR spectroscopic imaging of the prostate at 3 T with the MLEV-PRESS sequence. Magn Reson Imaging 2006;24:825–32.

27. Carroll PR, Presti JJ, Small E, et al. Focal therapy for prostate cancer 1996: maximizing outcome. Urology 1997;84–94.

28. Dhingsa R, Qayyum A, Coakley FV, et al. Prostate cancer localization with endorectal MR imaging and MR spectroscopic imaging: effect of clinical data on reader accuracy. Radiology 2004;230: 215–20.

29. Hasumi M, Suzuki K, Taketomi A, et al. The combination of multi-voxel MR spectroscopy with MR imaging improve the diagnostic accuracy for localization of prostate cancer. Anticancer Res 2003;23:4223–7.

30. Hasumi M, Suzuki K, Oya N, et al. MR spectroscopy as a reliable diagnostic tool for localization of prostate cancer. Anticancer Res 2002;22: 1205–8.

31. Coakley FV, Kurhanewicz J, Lu Y, et al. Prostate cancer tumor volume: measurement with endorectal MR and MR spectroscopic imaging. Radiology 2002;223:91–7.

32. Zakian KL, Sircar K, Hricak H, et al. Correlation of proton MR spectroscopic imaging with gleason score based on step-section pathologic analysis after radical prostatectomy. Radiology 2005;234: 804–14.

33. Weinreb J, Blume J, Coakley F, et al. Endorectal MR and MR spectroscopic imaging for sextant localization of prostate cancer prior to radical prostatectomy: results of the ACRIN 6659 prospective multi-institutional clinicopathological study. Radiology, Submitted.

34. Villers A, Puech P, Mouton D, et al. Dynamic contrast enhanced, pelvic phased array magnetic resonance imaging of localized prostate cancer for predicting tumor volume: correlation with radical prostatectomy findings. J Urol 2006;176:2432–7.

35. D'Amico AV, Chang H, Holupka E, et al. Calculated prostate cancer volume: the optimal predictor of actual cancer volume and pathologic stage. Urology 1997;49:385–91.

36. Smith JA Jr, Scardino PT, Resnick MI, et al. Transrectal ultrasound versus digital rectal examination for the staging of carcinoma of the prostate: results of a prospective, multi-institutional trial. J Urol 1997; 157:902–6.

37. Gleason D. Histologic grading of prostate cancer: a perspective. Hum Pathol 1992;23:273–9.

38. Wills ML, Sauvageot J, Partin AW, et al. Ability of sextant biopsies to predict radical prostatectomy stage. Urology 1998;51:759–64.

39. McLean M, Srigley J, Banerjee D, et al. Interobserver variation in prostate cancer Gleason

scoring: are there implications for the design of clinical trials and treatment strategies? Clin Oncol (R Coll Radiol) 1997;9:222–5.

40. Cooper JF, Farid I. The role of citric acid in the physiology of the prostate. 3. Lactate/citrate ratios in benign and malignant prostatic homogenates as an index of prostatic malignancy. J Urol 1964;92:533–6.

41. Kurhanewicz J, Dahiya R, Macdonald JM, et al. Citrate alterations in primary and metastatic human prostatic adenocarcinomas: 1H magnetic resonance spectroscopy and biochemical study. Magn Reson Med 1993;29:149–57.

42. Kurhanewicz J, Vigneron DB, Nelson SJ. Three-dimensional magnetic resonance spectroscopic imaging of brain and prostate cancer. Neoplasia 2000;2:166–89.

43. Yu KK, Hricak H, Alagappan R, et al. Detection of extracapsular extension of prostate carcinoma with endorectal and phased-array coil MR imaging: multivariate feature analysis. Radiology 1997;202:697–702.

44. Yu KK, Scheidler J, Hricak H, et al. Prostate cancer: prediction of extracapsular extension with endorectal MR imaging and three-dimensional proton MR spectroscopic imaging. Radiology 1999;213:481–8.

45. Partin AW, Yoo J, Carter HB, et al. The use of prostate specific antigen, clinical stage and Gleason score to predict pathological stage in men with localized prostate cancer. J Urol 1993;150:110–4.

46. Graefen M, Augustin H, Karakiewicz PI, et al. Can predictive models for prostate cancer patients derived in the United States of America be utilized in European patients? A validation study of the Partin tables. Eur Urol 2003;43:6–10 [discussion: 11].

47. Steyerberg EW, Roobol MJ, Kattan MW, et al. Prediction of indolent prostate cancer: validation and updating of a prognostic nomogram. J Urol 2007;177:107–12 [discussion: 112].

48. Wang L, Hricak H, Kattan MW, et al. Prediction of seminal vesicle invasion in prostate cancer: incremental value of adding endorectal MR imaging to the Kattan nomogram. Radiology 2007;242:182–8.

49. Wang L, Hricak H, Kattan MW, et al. Prediction of organ-confined prostate cancer: incremental value of MR imaging and MR spectroscopic imaging to staging nomograms. Radiology 2006;238:597–603.

50. Han M, Partin AW, Piantadosi S, et al. Era specific biochemical recurrence-free survival following radical prostatectomy for clinically localized prostate cancer. J Urol 2001;166:416–9.

51. Draisma G, Boer R, Otto SJ, et al. Lead times and overdetection due to prostate-specific antigen screening: estimates from the European Randomized Study of Screening for Prostate Cancer. J Natl Cancer Inst 2003;95:868–78.

52. Etzioni R, Penson DF, Legler JM, et al. Overdiagnosis due to prostate-specific antigen screening: lessons from US prostate cancer incidence trends. J Natl Cancer Inst 2002;94:981–90.

53. Carroll PR. Early stage prostate cancer—do we have a problem with over-detection, overtreatment or both? J Urol 2005;173:1061–2.

54. Coakley FV, Hricak H. Radiologic anatomy of the prostate gland: a clinical approach. Radiol Clin North Am 2000;38:15–30.

55. Prando A, Kurhanewicz J, Borges AP, et al. Prostatic biopsy directed with endorectal MR spectroscopic imaging findings in patients with elevated prostate specific antigen levels and prior negative biopsy findings: early experience. Radiology 2005;236:903–10.

56. Yuen JS, Thng CH, Tan PH, et al. Endorectal magnetic resonance imaging and spectroscopy for the detection of tumor foci in men with prior negative transrectal ultrasound prostate biopsy. J Urol 2004;171:1482–6.

57. Westphalen AC, McKenna DA, Kurhanewicz J, et al. Role of magnetic resonance imaging and magnetic resonance spectroscopic imaging before and after radiotherapy for prostate cancer. J Endourol 2008;22:789–94.

58. Sannazzari GL, Ragona R, Ruo Redda MG, et al. CT-MRI image fusion for delineation of volumes in three-dimensional conformal radiation therapy in the treatment of localized prostate cancer. Br J Radiol 2002;75:603–7.

59. Pickett B, Vigneault E, Kurhanewicz J, et al. Static field intensity modulation to treat a dominant intraprostatic lesion to 90 Gy compared to seven field 3-dimensional radiotherapy. Int J Radiat Oncol Biol Phys 1999;44:921–9.

60. van Lin EN, Futterer JJ, Heijmink SW, et al. IMRT boost dose planning on dominant intraprostatic lesions: gold marker-based three-dimensional fusion of CT with dynamic contrast-enhanced and 1H-spectroscopic MRI. Int J Radiat Oncol Biol Phys 2006;65:291–303.

61. Xia P, Pickett B, Vigneault E, et al. Forward or inversely planned segmental multileaf collimator IMRT and sequential tomotherapy to treat multiple dominant intraprostatic lesions of prostate cancer to 90 Gy. Int J Radiat Oncol Biol Phys 2001;51:244–54.

62. DiBiase SJ, Hosseinzadeh K, Gullapalli RP, et al. Magnetic resonance spectroscopic imaging-guided brachytherapy for localized prostate cancer. Int J Radiat Oncol Biol Phys 2002;52:429–38.

63. Pouliot J, Kim Y, Lessard E, et al. Inverse planning for HDR prostate brachytherapy used to boost dominant intraprostatic lesions defined by magnetic resonance spectroscopy imaging. Int J Radiat Oncol Biol Phys 2004;59:1196–207.

64. Zaider M, Zelefsky MJ, Lee EK, et al. Treatment planning for prostate implants using magnetic-resonance

spectroscopy imaging. Int J Radiat Oncol Biol Phys 2000;47:1085–96.

65. Kim Y, Hsu IC, Lessard E, et al. Class solution in inverse planned HDR prostate brachytherapy for dose escalation of DIL defined by combined MRI/MRSI. Radiother Oncol 2008;88:148–55.

66. Blasko JC, Wallner K, Grimm PD, et al. Prostate specific antigen based disease control following ultrasound guided 125iodine implantation for stage T1/T2 prostatic carcinoma. J Urol 1995;154:1096–9.

67. Zagars GK, Pollack A. External beam radiotherapy dose response of prostate cancer. Int J Radiat Oncol Biol Phys 1997;39:1011–8.

68. Coakley FV, Hricak H, Wefer AE, et al. Brachytherapy for prostate cancer: endorectal MR imaging of local treatment-related changes. Radiology 2001;219:817–21.

69. Chen M, Hricak H, Kalbhen CL, et al. Hormonal ablation of prostatic cancer: effects on prostate morphology, tumor detection, and staging by endorectal coil MR imaging. AJR Am J Roentgenol 1996;166:1157–63.

70. Mueller-Lisse UG, Swanson MG, Vigneron DB, et al. Time-dependent effects of hormone-deprivation therapy on prostate metabolism as detected by combined magnetic resonance imaging and 3D magnetic resonance spectroscopic imaging. Magn Reson Med 2001;46:49–57.

71. Roach M 3rd, Kurhanewicz J, Carroll P. Spectroscopy in prostate cancer: hope or hype? Oncology (Williston Park) 2001;15:1399–410 [discussion: 1415–396, 1418].

72. Pickett B, Ten Haken RK, Kurhanewicz J, et al. Time to metabolic atrophy after permanent prostate seed implantation based on magnetic resonance spectroscopic imaging. Int J Radiat Oncol Biol Phys 2004;59:665–73.

73. Kalbhen CL, Hricak H, Chen M, et al. Prostate carcinoma: MR imaging findings after cryosurgery. Radiology 1996;198:807–11.

74. Parivar F, Hricak H, Shinohara K, et al. Detection of locally recurrent prostate cancer after cryosurgery: evaluation by transrectal ultrasound, magnetic resonance imaging, and three-dimensional proton magnetic resonance spectroscopy. Urology 1996; 48:594–9.

75. Parivar F, Kurhanewicz J. Detection of recurrent prostate cancer after cryosurgery. Curr Opin Urol 1998;8:83–6.

76. Mueller-Lisse UG, Vigneron DB, Hricak H, et al. Localized prostate cancer: effect of hormone deprivation therapy measured by using combined three-dimensional H-1 MR spectroscopy and MR imaging: clinicopathologic case-controlled study. Radiology 2001;221:380–90.

77. Pickett B, Kurhanewicz J, Coakley F, et al. Use of MRI and spectroscopy in evaluation of external beam radiotherapy for prostate cancer. Int J Radiat Oncol Biol Phys 2004;60:1047–55.

78. Chelsky MJ, Schnall MD, Seidmon EJ, et al. Use of endorectal surface coil magnetic resonance imaging for local staging of prostate cancer. J Urol 1993; 150(2 Pt 1):391–5.

79. Schnall MD, Imai Y, Tomaszewski J, et al. Prostate cancer: local staging with endorectal surface coil MR imaging. Radiology 1991;178:797–802.

80. White S, Hricak H, Forstner R, et al. Prostate cancer: effect of postbiopsy hemorrhage on interpretation of MR images. Radiology 1995;195:385–90.

81. Bauer JJ, Zeng J, Zhang W, et al. Lateral biopsies added to the traditional sextant prostate biopsy pattern increases the detection rate of prostate cancer. Prostate Cancer Prostatic Dis 2000;3:43–6.

82. Qayyum A, Coakley FV, Lu Y, et al. Organ-confined prostate cancer: effect of prior transrectal biopsy on endorectal MRI and MR spectroscopic imaging. AJR Am J Roentgenol 2004;183:1079–83.

83. Engelhard K, Hollenbach HP, Deimling M, et al. Combination of signal intensity measurements of lesions in the peripheral zone of prostate with MRI and serum PSA level for differentiating benign disease from prostate cancer. Eur Radiol 2000;10: 1947–53.

84. van Dorsten FA, van der Graaf M, Engelbrecht MR, et al. Combined quantitative dynamic contrast-enhanced MR imaging and (1)H MR spectroscopic imaging of human prostate cancer. J Magn Reson Imaging 2004;20:279–87.

85. Zakian KL, Eberhardt S, Hricak H, et al. Transition zone prostate cancer: metabolic characteristics at 1H MR spectroscopic imaging—initial results. Radiology 2003;229:241–7.

86. Nelson SJ, Vigneron DB, Star-Lack J, et al. High spatial resolution and speed in MRSI. NMR Biomed 1997;10:411–22.

87. Gatenby RA, Gillies RJ. Why do cancers have high aerobic glycolysis? Nat Rev Cancer 2004;4:891–9.

88. Costello LC, Franklin RB. 'Why do tumour cells glycolyse?': from glycolysis through citrate to lipogenesis. Mol Cell Biochem 2005;280:1–8.

89. Mochiki E, Kuwano H, Katoh H, et al. Evaluation of 18F-2-deoxy-2-fluoro-D-glucose positron emission tomography for gastric cancer. World J Surg 2004;28:247–53.

90. Kunkel M, Reichert TE, Benz P, et al. Overexpression of Glut-1 and increased glucose metabolism in tumors are associated with a poor prognosis in patients with oral squamous cell carcinoma. Cancer 2003;97:1015–24.

91. Warburg O, Wind F, Negelein E. Uber den Stoffwechsel von Tumouren im Korper. Klin Wochenschr 1926;5:829–32.

92. Ardenkjaer-Larsen JH, Fridlund B, Gram A, et al. Increase in signal-to-noise ratio of >10,000 times

in liquid-state NMR. Proc Natl Acad Sci USA 2003; 100:10158–63.

93. Kohler SJ, Yen Y, Wolber J, et al. In vivo (13)carbon metabolic imaging at 3T with hyperpolarized (13)C-1-pyruvate. Magn Reson Med 2007;58:65–9.

94. Star-Lack J, Spielman D, Adalsteinsson E, et al. In vivo lactate editing with simultaneous detection of choline, creatine, NAA, and lipid singlets at 1.5 T using PRESS excitation with applications to the study of brain and head and neck tumors. J Magn Reson 1998;133:243–54.

95. Golman K, Olsson LE, Axelsson O, et al. Molecular imaging using hyperpolarized 13C. Br J Radiol 2003;76(Spec No 2):S118–27.

96. Mansson S, Johansson E, Magnusson P, et al. 13C imaging-a new diagnostic platform. Eur Radiol 2006;16:57–67.

97. Golman K, Zandt RI, Lerche M, et al. Metabolic imaging by hyperpolarized 13C magnetic resonance imaging for in vivo tumor diagnosis. Cancer Res 2006;66:10855–60.

98. Albers MJ, Chen AP, Bok R, et al. Monitoring prostate cancer progression in a transgenic murine model using 3T hyperpolarized 13C MRS. Presented at the ISMRM Fifteenth Scientific Meeting. Berlin, May 19–15, 2007.

99. Cunningham CH, Vigneron DB, Marjanska M, et al. Sequence design for magnetic resonance spectroscopic imaging of prostate cancer at 3 T. Magn Reson Med 2005;53:1033–9.

100. Golman K, Ardenaer-Larsen JH, Petersson JS, et al. Molecular imaging with endogenous substances. Proc Natl Acad Sci U S A 2003;100: 10435–9.

101. Cunningham CH, Chen AP, Albers MJ, et al. Double spin-echo sequence for rapid spectroscopic imaging of hyperpolarized (13)C. J Magn Reson 2007;187:357–62.

Index

Note: Page numbers of article titles are in **boldface** type.

Magn Reson Imaging Clin N Am 16 (2008) 711–715
doi:10.1016/S1064-9689(08)00112-8

Moving?

Make sure your subscription moves with you!

To notify us of your new address, find your **Clinics Account Number** (located on your mailing label above your name), and contact customer service at:

E-mail: elspcs@elsevier.com

800-654-2452 (subscribers in the U.S. & Canada)
1-407-563-6020 (subscribers outside of the U.S. & Canada)

Fax number: 407-363-9661

Elsevier Periodicals Customer Service
6277 Sea Harbor Drive
Orlando, FL 32887-4800

*To ensure uninterrupted delivery of your subscription, please notify us at least 4 weeks in advance of move.

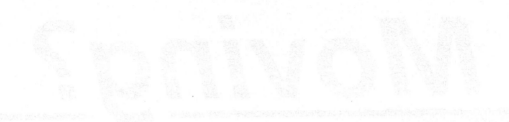

United States Postal Service

Statement of Ownership, Management, and Circulation
(All Periodicals Publications Except Requestor Publications)

1. Publication Title	2. Publication Number	3. Filing Date
Magnetic Resonance Imaging Clinics of North America	0 1 1 - 9 0 0 9	9/15/08

4. Issue Frequency	5. Number of Issues Published Annually	6. Annual Subscription Price
Feb, May, Aug, Nov	4	$253.00

7. Complete Mailing Address of Known Office of Publication (Not printer) (Street, city, county, state, and ZIP+4)

Elsevier Inc.
360 Park Avenue South
New York, NY 10010-1710

Contact Person
Stephen Bushing

Telephone (Include area code)
215-239-3688

8. Complete Mailing Address of Headquarters or General Business Office of Publisher (Not printer)

Elsevier Inc., 360 Park Avenue South, New York, NY 10010-1710

9. Full Names and Complete Mailing Addresses of Publisher, Editor, and Managing Editor (Do not leave blank)

Publisher (Name and complete mailing address)

John Schrefer , Elsevier, Inc. , 1600 John F. Kennedy Blvd. Suite 1800, Philadelphia, PA 19103-2899

Editor (Name and complete mailing address)

Lisa Richman, Elsevier, Inc. , 1600 John F. Kennedy Blvd. Suite 1800, Philadelphia, PA 19103-2899

Managing Editor (Name and complete mailing address)

Catherine Bewick, Elsevier, Inc. , 1600 John F. Kennedy Blvd. Suite 1800, Philadelphia, PA 19103-2899

10. Owner (Do not leave blank. If the publication is owned by a corporation, give the name and address of the corporation immediately followed by the names and addresses of all stockholders owning or holding 1 percent or more of the total amount of stock. If not owned by a corporation, give the names and addresses of the individual owners. If owned by a partnership or other unincorporated firm, give its name and address as well as those of each individual owner. If the publication is published by a nonprofit organization, give its name and address.)

Full Name	Complete Mailing Address
Wholly owned subsidiary of	4520 East-West Highway
Reed/Elsevier, US holdings	Bethesda, MD 20814

11. Known Bondholders, Mortgagees, and Other Security Holders Owning or Holding 1 Percent or More of Total Amount of Bonds, Mortgages, or Other Securities. If none, check box ☐ None

Full Name	Complete Mailing Address
N/A	

12. Tax Status (For completion by nonprofit organizations authorized to mail at nonprofit rates) (Check one)
The purpose, function, and nonprofit status of this organization and the exempt status for federal income tax purposes:
☐ Has Not Changed During Preceding 12 Months
☐ Has Changed During Preceding 12 Months (Publisher must submit explanation of change with this statement)

PS Form 3526, September 2006 (Page 1 of 3 (Instructions Page 3)) PSN 7530-01-000-9931 PRIVACY NOTICE: See our Privacy policy in www.usps.com

---

13. Publication Title	14. Issue Date for Circulation Data Below
Magnetic Resonance Imaging Clinics of North America	August 2008

15. Extent and Nature of Circulation		Average No. Copies Each Issue During Preceding 12 Months	No. Copies of Single Issue Published Nearest to Filing Date
a. Total Number of Copies (Net press run)		3675	3400
b. Paid Circulation (By Mail and Outside the Mail)	(1) Mailed Outside-County Paid Subscriptions Stated on PS Form 3541. (Include paid distribution above nominal rate, advertiser's proof copies, and exchange copies)	2215	2046
	(2) Mailed In-County Paid Subscriptions Stated on PS Form 3541 (Include paid distribution above nominal rate, advertiser's proof copies, and exchange copies)		
	(3) Paid Distribution Outside the Mails Including Sales Through Dealers and Carriers, Street Vendors, Counter Sales, and Other Paid Distribution Outside USPS®	780	752
	(4) Paid Distribution by Other Classes Mailed Through the USPS (e.g. First-Class Mail®)		
c. Total Paid Distribution (Sum of 15b (1), (2), (3), and (4))	▲	2995	2798
d. Free or Nominal Rate Distribution (By Mail and Outside the Mail)	(1) Free or Nominal Rate Outside-County Copies Included on PS Form 3541	60	32
	(2) Free or Nominal Rate In-County Copies Included on PS Form 3541		
	(3) Free or Nominal Rate Copies Mailed at Other Classes Mailed Through the USPS (e.g. First-Class Mail)		
	(4) Free or Nominal Rate Distribution Outside the Mail (Carriers or other means)		
e. Total Free or Nominal Rate Distribution (Sum of 15d (1), (2), (3) and (4))	▲	60	32
f. Total Distribution (Sum of 15c and 15e)	▲	3055	2830
g. Copies not Distributed (See instructions to publishers #4 (page #3))		620	570
h. Total (Sum of 15f and g)	▲	3675	3400
i. Percent Paid (15c divided by 15f times 100)		98.04%	98.87%

16. Publication of Statement of Ownership

☐ If the publication is a general publication, publication of this statement is required. Will be printed in the **November 2008** issue of this publication. ☐ Publication not required

17. Signature and Title of Editor, Publisher, Business Manager, or Owner

[signature] — Executive Director of Subscription Services | Date September 15, 2008

Stephen Bushing - Executive Director of Subscription Services

I certify that all information furnished on this form is true and complete. I understand that anyone who furnishes false or misleading information on this form or who omits material or information requested on the form may be subject to criminal sanctions (including fines and imprisonment) and/or civil sanctions (including civil penalties).

PS Form 3526, September 2006 (Page 2 of 3)